STUDENT WORKBOOK FOR

Understanding Human Structure and Function

STUDENT WORKBOOK FOR

Understanding Human Structure and Function

Valerie C. Scanlon, PhD
College of Mount Saint Vincent
Riverdale, New York

Tina Sanders
Medical Illustrator
Castle Creek, New York
Formerly
Head Graphic Artist
Tompkins Courtland Community College
Dryden, New York

 F. A. DAVIS COMPANY • Philadelphia

F. A. Davis Company
1915 Arch Street
Philadelphia, PA 19103

Printed in the United States of America

Last digit indicates print number: 10 9 8 7

Publisher, Nursing: Robert G. Martone
Nursing Editor: Alan Sorkowitz
Production Editor: Jessica Howie Martin
Cover Designer: Louis J. Forgione

As new scientific information becomes available through basic and clinical research, recommended treatments and drug therapies undergo changes. The author and publisher have done everything possible to make this book accurate, up to date, and in accord with accepted standards at the time of publication. The author, editors, and publisher are not responsible for errors or omissions or for consequences from application of the book, and make no warranty, expressed or implied, in regard to the contents of the book. Any practice described in this book should be applied by the reader in accordance with professional standards of care used in regard to the unique circumstances that may apply in each situation. The reader is advised always to check product information (package inserts) for changes and new information regarding dose and contraindications before administering any drug. Caution is especially urged when using new or infrequently ordered drugs.

To the Student

The purpose of this student workbook is to help you learn the material in the basic anatomy and physiology course you are about to take. How much you learn and how well you learn it is up to you, so it is important to remember that real learning depends on many factors.

1. Time. Try to give yourself enough study time to learn effectively. This may not always be easy, but it is worth striving for. Cramming the night before an exam may work once in a while, but setting aside some time for study every day is usually a much more successful strategy.

2. Self-discipline. Don't be discouraged by the amount of material you have to learn. Keep at it, and you will find that the more you learn, the easier it becomes to learn.

3. Know when to memorize and when to understand. Some material simply must be memorized, but other material requires true comprehension. For example, each bone in the body has a name, and you will have to memorize the name of each bone and its location in the body. Will this memorization serve a purpose? Indeed it will, for when you learn the actions of muscles, you will have to know the bones to which each muscle is attached. Memorization is often the foundation for comprehension.

4. Ask questions—of your teacher, your fellow students, and yourself. When you don't understand something, ask your teacher or a classmate, and you'll probably get an answer. But what kind of questions can you ask yourself? Very simple yet very important ones. If you are studying a part of the body, ask yourself: What is its name? Where is it? What is it made of? What does it do? For such things as cells, tissues, or organs, we can summarize these questions as name, location, structure, and function. For a process that takes place within the body, the questions will be a little different, but still simple. Ask yourself: What is happening? What is the purpose for this? If you can answer these questions, you truly comprehend and understand the process.

When I give study questions to my own students, I pay attention to their comments and suggestions. Were my questions helpful? If not, why not? Their answers are very important to me and help me to better help them learn. Even though you are not in my class, your comments and suggestions are more than welcome. After all, this book was written for you, to help you learn, continue your education, and become a successful member of the profession you have chosen. I would be pleased to hear from you. Please send your comments to me in care of F. A. Davis Company, 1915 Arch Street, Philadelphia, PA 19103.

Valerie C. Scanlon
Dobbs Ferry, New York

How to Use This Workbook

Each chapter in this workbook corresponds to the same chapter in the textbook. The workbook chapters are organized into sections that correspond to the major sections of the textbook's chapters, so that you may proceed from topic to topic before completing the entire chapter in the textbook.

Types of Exercises

The types of exercises within each section include completion (fill-in) questions, matching columns, and diagrams with labeling and coloring exercises.

Completion Questions. For these questions, you are asked to supply the missing word or words in a statement. For example:

All the bones of the body are collectively called the _____ .
On the line provided, you would write *skeleton*.

Matching Columns. In these exercises, you are asked to match the terms in one column with the descriptive phrases in another column. For example:

Match each holiday with its proper custom. Use each letter once.

1) Valentine's Day _____   A. Fireworks

2) Halloween _____   B. Costumes and pumpkins

3) July 4th _____   C. Turkey dinner

4) Thanksgiving _____   D. Flowers and candy

In this matching column, there is only one letter per answer line: 1) D   2) B   3) A   4) C

For some matching columns, there will be more than one letter on some answer lines. When the directions say "Use each letter once," they mean that *every* letter belongs on one or another of the answer lines. There will *never* be any extra answers. For example:

Match each part of a week with the proper days. Use each letter once. One answer line will have two correct letters, and the other will have three.

1) Weekend _____   A. Sunday

2) Weekdays _____   B. Tuesday

C. Thursday

D. Saturday

E. Wednesday

To answer this question completely, your answers should be: 1) A, D   2) B, C, E

Occasionally, a letter or letters may be used more than once in a matching column. When this happens, the directions will clearly state this. Remember to read the directions carefully, and remember also that there will never be any unused answers.

Diagram Exercises.   Many diagrams have been included in this workbook to give you opportunities for the visual application of your knowledge. In *labeling exercises,* you will provide names for the parts indicated by the numbered leader lines on the diagram.

Some of the diagrams include a color key for *coloring* certain parts. Colors help add emphasis to a diagram and may help you retain a mental picture of that part of the body. Use the color key below the illustration to indicate the colors you have used for each part. In most cases, the choice of colors is up to you, but there are some traditional colors. Arteries, for example, are always red in anatomic illustrations. Veins are blue, lymphatic structures are green, and nerves are yellow. These colors may be used for other structures, of course, but they should always be used for the structures mentioned above.

Clinical Applications

The situations and questions in this section of each chapter have been taken from the text material that briefly refers to diseases and disorders. These are simple applications and are meant to make the text material more relevant and meaningful for you.

Checking Your Answers

When you have completed a chapter section, check your answers against the Answer Key included at the end of this workbook. If you have answered a question incorrectly, reread the appropriate section in the textbook as a review. Try to figure out *why* you made the mistake. Was it simply not knowing the answer? Not reading the question carefully? Confusing two terms that sound alike? Whatever the reason, if you can determine why you made the mistake, you probably won't make it again (when it counts!). Remember also that, once you have completed a section and made any necessary corrections, that section becomes a concise summary of the essential information on that topic and may be used for a quick review or more intensive studying.

End-of-Chapter Tests

When you complete each chapter, you will find two comprehensive chapter exams. Both of these exams are in a multiple-choice format. Answers to them can be found in the Answer Key at the back of the workbook.

Multiple-Choice Test #1.   This test consists of traditional multiple-choice questions for which you are asked to select the correct answer from four choices. For example:

Which of these is a plant?

a) earthworm   b) fern   c) frog   d) dog

Circle or underline the correct answer, which is *b*.

This type of question tests your knowledge and your ability to recognize the correct answer. When you take this test, answer all the questions. If you are not sure, take a guess and make a note for yourself about why you have made this particular choice. Then, when you check your answers, you can pay special attention to these to see if your thinking was correct. As always, if you do make a mistake, try to determine why, so that you will not make the same mistake again.

Multiple-Choice Test #2.   The questions on this test evaluate your level of knowledge, reading ability, and thinking ability. Each question asks you to select the statement that is NOT true about a particular topic, and then to correct the false statement to make it true. For example:

Which statement is NOT true of dogs?

a) Dogs have four legs and two ears.

b) Many dogs can be taught to do simple tricks.

c) Many dogs are friendly and loyal.

d) Very young dogs are called kittens.

Reword your choice to make it a correct statement.

_____

In this example, choice *d* is not true and is therefore the correct answer. You may want to underline the part of the answer choice that is not true (in this case, *kittens*) to help you focus your thinking. Then, rewrite the statement (or just the incorrect part) to make it true: *Very young dogs are called puppies.*

Will you have to read carefully and think clearly when you take a test like this? Surely you will, but if you do well on a self-test such as this, you can be confident that you know and understand the material.

Contents

Chapter 1

Organization and General Plan of the Body

This chapter describes how the body is organized, from simple to more complex levels. Also in this chapter, the terminology used to describe the body is presented.

LEVELS OF ORGANIZATION

Complete each statement, and give appropriate examples.

1. a) The simplest level of organization is the _____ level.

    b) Give three examples of organic chemicals. _____ , _____ ,

    _____

    c) Give three examples of inorganic chemicals. _____ , _____ ,

    _____

2. a) The most complex level of organization is the _____ level.

    b) Give three examples of this level. _____ , _____ ,

    _____

3. a) The simplest *living* level of organization is the _____ level.

    b) When cells with similar structure and function are grouped and work together, they form a

    _____ .

    c) A group of tissues that is arranged in a particular way to accomplish specific functions is called an

    _____ .

4. Match each group of tissues with its function (a letter) and its example in the body (a number).

    Each letter and number is used once.

    1) Epithelial tissue _____

    2) Connective tissue _____

    Functions
    A. Supports, transports, or stores materials
    B. Contracts and brings about movement

3) Muscle tissue _____

4) Nerve tissue _____

C. Transmits impulses that regulate body functions

D. Covers or lines surfaces

Examples

1. The lining of the stomach and the epidermis of the skin
2. The heart and skeletal muscles
3. Bone, blood
4. Spinal cord, brain

5. a) The structure of a tissue, cell, or organ is called its _____ . The function of the tissue, cell, or organ is called its _____ .

b) Describe one way the physiology of a bone (an organ) is related to its anatomy.

_____

HOMEOSTASIS

Complete each statement.

1. A person who is in a state of homeostasis may also be said to be in a state of good _____ .

2. Homeostasis means that despite constant changes, the body remains relatively _____ .

3. Changes that affect the body may take place where? _____ or _____

4. For each of these changes, describe in simple terms what will happen to maintain homeostasis. (Note: Some responses may include conscious decisions.)

1) Eating lunch _____

2) Inhaling _____

3) Experiencing a headache _____

4) Cutting your finger _____

5) Going outside on a cold day _____

TERMS OF LOCATION

Define each term given, and provide the term with the opposite meaning.

1. Inferior: _____

    Opposite: _____

2. Proximal: _____

    Opposite: _____

3. Lateral: _____

    Opposite: _____

4. Peripheral: _____

    Opposite: _____

5. Superficial: _____

    Opposite: _____

6. Anterior: _____

    Opposite: _____

7. Dorsal: _____

    Opposite: _____

8. Internal: _____

    Opposite: _____

BODY PARTS AND AREAS

1. Below are anterior and posterior views of the body in anatomical position.

   Label the following areas:

frontal	brachial	inguinal	popliteal	femoral	volar
temporal	buccal	iliac	cervical	deltoid	plantar
nasal	orbital	gluteal	mammary	occipital	patellar
pectoral	parietal	lumbar	cranial	sacral	perineal
axillary	umbilical				

A   B

2. Complete the following by choosing the correct directional term from the pair given and by defining each term for a body area.

   1) a) The deltoid area is _____ (medial or lateral) to the cervical area.

      b) Deltoid refers to the _____ .

      c) Cervical refers to the _____ .

   2) a) The femoral area is _____ (proximal or distal) to the patellar area.

      b) Femoral refers to the _____ .

      c) Patellar refers to the _____ .

   3) a) The occipital and lumbar areas are on the _____ (anterior or posterior) side of the body.

      b) Occipital refers to the _____ .

      c) Lumbar refers to the _____ .

   4) a) The pectoral and umbilical areas are on the _____ (dorsal or ventral) side of the body.

      b) Pectoral refers to the _____ .

      c) Umbilical refers to the _____ .

   5) a) The volar area is _____ (superior or inferior) to the plantar area.

      b) Volar refers to the _____ .

      c) Plantar refers to the _____ .

   6) a) The cutaneous area is _____ (superficial or deep) to the muscles.

      b) Cutaneous refers to the _____ .

   7) a) The ribs are _____ (internal or external) to the pulmonary area.

      b) Pulmonary refers to the _____ .

   8) The nerves in the hand are part of the _____ (central or peripheral) nervous system, and the brain is part of the _____ (central or peripheral) nervous system.

BODY CAVITIES

1. Match each statement with the body cavity(ies) it pertains to.

   Some answer lines will have more than one correct letter. Use each letter once; one letter is used twice.

   1) Cranial cavity _____
   2) Thoracic cavity _____
   3) Spinal cavity _____

   A. Lined with the parietal pleura
   B. Contains the spinal cord
   C. Lined with meninges
   D. Contains the heart and lungs
   E. Lined with the peritoneum

4) Pelvic cavity _____

5) Abdominal cavity _____

F. Contains the internal reproductive organs and urinary bladder

G. Contains the brain

H. The inferior boundary is the diaphragm

I. The superior boundary is the diaphragm

J. Contains the liver and pancreas

2. Below is a diagram of the major body cavities.

Label each numbered cavity and the brackets: dorsal or ventral cavity.

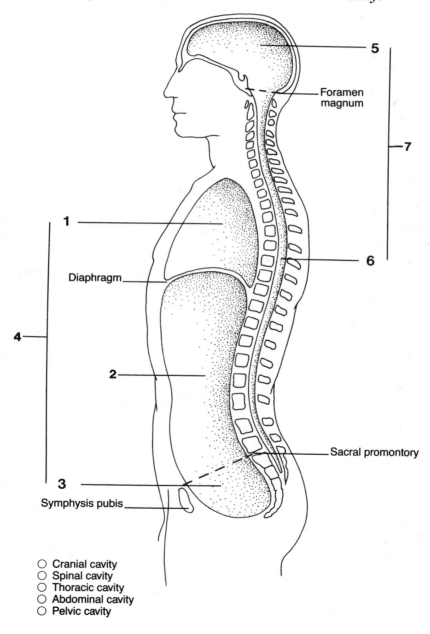

Foramen magnum

Diaphragm

Sacral promontory

Symphysis pubis

○ Cranial cavity
○ Spinal cavity
○ Thoracic cavity
○ Abdominal cavity
○ Pelvic cavity

BODY SECTIONS

1. Match the following sections with the correct descriptions.

    Use each letter once.

    1) Sagittal section _____

    2) Cross section _____

    3) Frontal section _____

    4) Transverse section _____

    5) Longitudinal section _____

    A. A plane along the long axis of an organ
    B. A plane that divides the body into right and left portions
    C. A plane that divides the body into upper and lower portions
    D. A plane perpendicular to the long axis of an organ
    E. A plane that divides the body into front and back portions

2. On the diagrams below, label each plane or section.

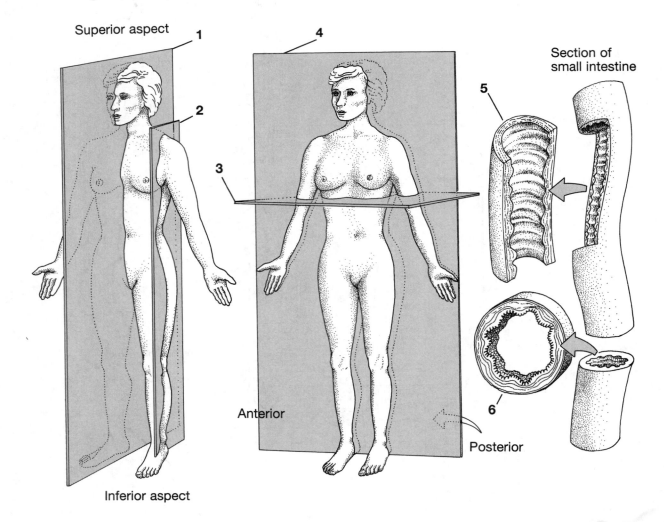

Superior aspect

Inferior aspect

Anterior

Posterior

Section of small intestine

ORGAN SYSTEMS

Integumentary
Nervous
Lymphatic
Urinary

Skeletal
Endocrine
Respiratory
Reproductive

Muscular
Circulatory
Digestive

1. Take your answers from the list above, and name the organ system described by each statement.

1) _____ Moves the skeleton and produces heat.

2) _____ Transports oxygen and nutrients to tissues.

3) _____ Produces egg or sperm to continue the human species.

4) _____ Supports the body and protects internal organs.

5) _____ Removes waste products from the blood.

6) _____ Exchanges oxygen and carbon dioxide between the blood and air.

7) _____ Regulates body functions by means of impulses.

8) _____ Regulates body functions by means of hormones.

9) _____ Destroys pathogens that enter the body.

10) _____ Changes food to simpler chemicals to be absorbed.

11) _____ Is a barrier to pathogens and to chemicals.

2. Name the organ system to which each of the following organs belongs (take your answers from the list above).

1) _____ Heart

2) _____ Kidneys

3) _____ Spinal cord

4) _____ Skin

5) _____ Trachea

6) _____ Muscles

7) _____ Ribs

8) _____ Ovaries

9) _____ Pancreas

10) _____ Spleen

11) _____ Thyroid gland

12) _____ Testes

13) _____ Lungs

14) _____ Esophagus

15) _____ Tendons

16) _____ Eyes

17) _____ Pituitary gland

18) _____ Arteries

19) _____ Sweat glands

20) _____ Stomach

CLINICAL APPLICATIONS

1. Surgery involving the intestines requires an incision through the abdominal wall. Name the layers that must be cut to enter the abdominal cavity.

1) _____ (part of the integumentary system)

2) _____ (provides for movement of the trunk)

3) _____ (the lining of the abdominal cavity)

2. Meningitis is a serious disease caused by certain bacteria. Name the membranes affected and the organs they cover.

Membranes: _____   Organs: _____

_____

3. Briefly explain each of the following, and include the common name for each anatomical term.

1) Renal failure: _____

2) Cardiac arrest: _____

3) Pulmonary vein: _____

4) Hepatic coma: _____

5) Gastric ulcer: _____

4. Look at the digestive organs depicted in the diagram below, and name the abdominal quadrant(s) in which each of these organs is found (some may be in more than one).

1) Stomach _____   3) Small intestine _____

2) Liver _____   4) Large intestine _____

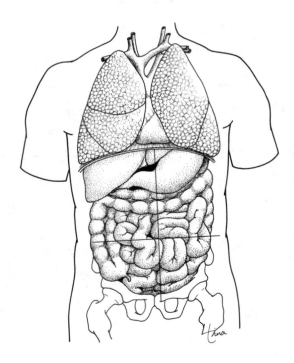

MULTIPLE CHOICE TEST # 1

Choose the correct answer for each question.

1. A synonym is a word that has the same meaning as another word. A synonym for ventral is:
   a) anterior   b) dorsal   c) posterior   d) lateral

2. An antonym is a word that has the opposite meaning of another word. An antonym for medial is:
   a) distal   b) dorsal   c) peripheral   d) lateral

3. The most superior body cavity is the:
   a) abdominal cavity   b) spinal cavity   c) thoracic cavity   d) cranial cavity

4. The diaphragm separates the:
   a) thoracic and abdominal cavities   c) cranial and spinal cavities
   b) abdominal and pelvic cavities   d) thoracic and pelvic cavities

5. The body is cut in a mid-transverse section, and is now separated into two parts that may be called:
   a) anterior-posterior   b) superior-inferior   c) dorsal-ventral   d) medial-lateral

6. A cross section of an artery would look like a:
   a) rectangle   b) hollow circle   c) cylinder   d) hollow cube

7. The most inferior body cavity is the:
   a) thoracic cavity   b) abdominal cavity   c) pelvic cavity   d) cranial cavity

8. The most superior body system is the:
   a) nervous system   c) muscular system
   b) skeletal system   d) integumentary system

9. A tissue found on the surface of an organ must be a(an):
   a) epithelial tissue   b) connective tissue   c) muscle tissue   d) nerve tissue

10. A tissue that causes contractions of the stomach to mix food with gastric juice must be a type of:
    a) epithelial tissue   b) connective tissue   c) muscle tissue   d) nerve tissue

11. The tissue that enables you to think and answer all these questions is:
    a) epithelial tissue   b) connective tissue   c) muscle tissue   d) nerve tissue

12. A tissue that supports body parts or transports materials within the body is a type of:
    a) epithelial tissue   b) connective tissue   c) muscle tissue   d) nerve tissue

13. Homeostasis means that the internal environment of the body is:
    a) exactly the same at all times
    b) relatively stable in spite of constant changes
    c) constantly changing drastically
    d) not changing at all

14. The two organ systems that regulate body functions by means of impulses and hormones are the:
    a) skeletal and muscular   c) digestive and respiratory
    b) nervous and endocrine   d) urinary and circulatory

15. The two organ systems that are *most* responsible for protecting the body against pathogens are the:
    a) integumentary and lymphatic   c) digestive and urinary
    b) skeletal and circulatory   d) muscular and endocrine

16. Which of the following is NOT an aspect of the anatomy of an organ?
    a) size   b) type of cells present   c) shape   d) function

17. In order to describe abdominal locations more precisely, the abdomen may be divided into (the division most often used clinically):
    a) two halves   b) four quadrants   c) eight sections   d) 12 sections

MULTIPLE CHOICE TEST # 2

Read each question and the four answer choices carefully. When you have made a choice, follow the instructions to complete your answer.

1. The chemical level of organization of the body includes all of the the following *except:*
   a) water   b) oxygen   c) protein   d) muscles

   *For your choice, name the level of organization to which it **does** belong.*

   _____

2. The organ level of organization includes all of the following *except* the:
   a) arteries   b) liver   c) blood   d) kidneys

   *For your choice, name the level of organization to which it **does** belong.*

   _____

3. Which sequence lists the levels of organization in the proper order of increasing complexity?
   a) chemicals, cells, tissues, organs, organ systems
   b) chemicals, tissues, organs, cells, organ systems
   c) cells, chemicals, organs, tissues, organ systems
   d) cells, chemicals, tissues, organs, organ systems

4. Which type of tissue is NOT paired with its correct general function?
   a) muscle—specialized to contract
   b) connective—specialized to support, transport, or store materials
   c) nerve—specialized to protect body parts
   d) epithelial—specialized to cover or line body surfaces

   For your choice, state its correct general function.

   _____

5. Which statement is NOT true of homeostasis?
   a) it is a state of good health
   b) external changes bring about specific responses by the body
   c) internal changes have no effect on homeostasis
   d) the proper functioning of all the organ systems contributes to homeostasis

   Reword your choice to make it a correct statement.

   _____

6. Which membrane is NOT paired with its proper location?
   a) peritoneum—lines abdominal organs
   b) meninges—lines the cranial cavity
   c) visceral pleura—covers the lungs
   d) parietal pleura—lines the thoracic cavity

   For your choice, state its proper location.

   _____

7. A mid-sagittal section of the head would cut through all of the following *except* these two:
   a) nose   b) eyes   c) mouth   d) brain   e) ears

   For your choices, explain why they would not be cut by this section.

   _____

8. A mid-frontal section of the body would NOT separate the:
   a) inguinal area from the gluteal area
   b) frontal area from the occipital area
   c) pectoral area from the lumbar area
   d) cervical area from the femoral area

   For your choice, name the type of section that would separate these two areas.

   _____

9. Which statement is NOT true of cells?
   a) the human body contains many different types of cells
   b) cells are made of inorganic and organic chemicals
   c) cells are the smallest living subunits of structure and function
   d) a group of cells with similar structure and function is called an organ

   Reword your choice to make it a correct statement.

   _____

10. Which statement is NOT true of body cavities.
    a) the diaphragm separates the thoracic and pelvic cavities
    b) the dorsal cavity consists of the cranial and spinal cavities
    c) the ventral cavity consists of the thoracic, abdominal, and pelvic cavities
    d) the pleural membranes are the serous membranes of the thoracic cavity

    Reword your choice to make it a correct statement.

    _____

Chapter 2

Some Basic Chemistry

This chapter presents the simple chemistry necessary to an understanding of anatomy and physiology. The functions of the important inorganic and organic chemicals are described as they relate to the working of the human body.

ELEMENTS, ATOMS, AND BONDS

1. A substance made of only one type of atom is called an _____ .

2. Name the element represented by each chemical symbol.

   Fe _____   Na _____   Cl _____

   Ca _____   I _____   Cu _____

   O _____   P _____   Zn _____

   C _____   Mg _____   Co _____

   H _____   N _____   Mn _____

   K _____   S _____   F _____

3. The subunits of atoms are _____ , _____ , and

   _____ .

4. a) The atomic subunit that has a negative charge is the _____ , and the subunit that

   has a positive charge is the _____ .

   b) The subunit that has no charge is the _____ .

   c) Which of these subunits are found in the atomic nucleus? _____ and

   _____

   d) Which of these subunits are present in equal numbers in an atom? _____ and

   _____

   e) Which of these subunits gives an atom its bonding capabilities? _____

5. An atom that has lost or gained electrons and now has a positive or negative charge is called an

_____ .

6. The bonding of two or more atoms results in the formation of a _____ .

7. The bond formed when one atom loses electrons that are gained by other atoms is called an

_____ bond.

8. The bond formed when two or more atoms share electrons is called a _____ bond.

9. a) Name a molecule that exists naturally as a gas. _____

   b) Name a molecule that exists naturally as a liquid. _____

   c) Name a molecule that exists naturally as a solid. _____

10. The type of bond that may be weakened in an aqueous (water) solution is the

_____ bond.

11. The atoms of organic molecules such as carbohydrates and proteins are bonded by

_____ bonds.

12. The diagram below depicts the formation of a molecule of sodium chloride.

   Label the following: the protons in each atom, the electron orbitals in each atom, and the transfer of an electron.

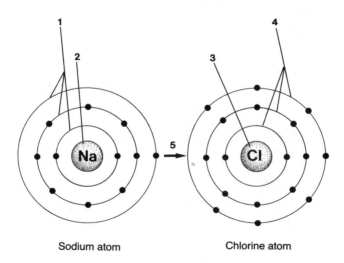

Sodium atom   Chlorine atom

13. The weak bonds that maintain the three-dimensional shape of proteins and nucleic acids are called

_____ bonds.

14. a) A reaction in which smaller molecules bond to form a new, larger molecule is called a

_____ reaction.

b) A reaction in which bonds are broken and a large molecule is changed to smaller ones is called a

_____ reaction.

INORGANIC COMPOUNDS

Complete the following:

1. The most abundant compound in the human body is _____ .

2. a) Water is a solvent, which means that many substances will _____ in water.

   b) State a specific way that water as a solvent is important to the body.

   _____

3. a) Water is a lubricant, which means that it prevents _____ between surfaces.

   b) State a specific way that water as a lubricant is important to the body.

   _____

4. Water absorbs a great deal of heat as it evaporates. State why this is important to the body.

   _____

5. a) Water found in blood vessels is called (NOT blood) _____ .

   b) Water found within cells is called _____ .

   c) Water found in lymph vessels is called _____ .

   d) Water found between cells is called _____ .

Below is a diagram of the water compartments. Name each of the specific forms of water within each compartment.

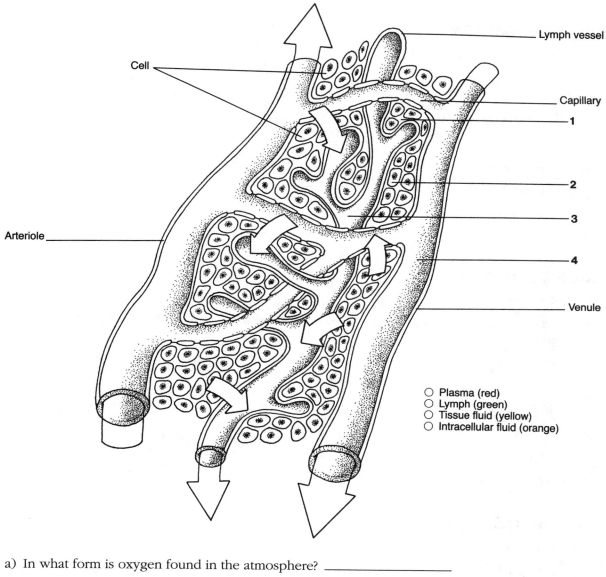

Lymph vessel

Cell

Capillary

1

2

3

Arteriole

4

Venule

○ Plasma (red)
○ Lymph (green)
○ Tissue fluid (yellow)
○ Intracellular fluid (orange)

6. a) In what form is oxygen found in the atmosphere? _____

   b) State the chemical formula of oxygen. _____

   c) Within the body, oxygen is essential for the process called _____ , which produces _____ for cellular processes that require energy.

7. a) Carbon dioxide is produced in the body as a waste product of the process of _____ .

b) State the chemical formula of carbon dioxide. _____

c) If excess CO_2 is present in body fluids, these fluids will become too _____ .

CELL RESPIRATION

1. Complete the summary reaction of cell respiration by naming the four products of the reaction:

$C_6H_{12}O_6$ + O_2 → _____ + _____ + _____ + _____
(glucose)

2. State what happens to each of the two molecular products.

_____

_____

3. State the purpose of each of the two energy forms produced. _____

_____

_____

TRACE ELEMENTS

1. Match these elements with their proper functions in the body.

   Each letter is used at least once, and two letters are used twice. Some answer lines will have more than one correct letter.

   1) Iron _____
   2) Sulfur _____
   3) Calcium _____
   4) Iodine _____
   5) Phosphorus _____
   6) Sodium and potassium _____

   A. Part of some proteins such as insulin
   B. Provides strength in bones and teeth
   C. Part of hemoglobin in red blood cells
   D. Part of the hormone thyroxine
   E. Necessary for muscle contraction
   F. Part of DNA and RNA
   G. Necessary for blood clotting
   H. Necessary for nerve impulse transmission

ACIDS, BASES, AND pH

1. a) State the range of the pH scale: _____ to _____ .

   b) In this scale, the number that indicates a neutral pH is _____ .

   c) Neutral means that there are as many _____ ions as there are _____ ions in the solution.

   d) The portion of the pH scale from 0 to 6.99 represents solutions that are _____ .

   e) The portion of the pH scale from 7.01 to 14 represents solutions that are _____ .

2. a) State the normal pH range of blood: _____

   b) This pH range means that blood is slightly _____ (acidic or alkaline).

3. Chemicals in body fluids that help prevent drastic pH changes are called _____ .

4. A buffer system changes strong acids or bases to substances that _____ .

ORGANIC COMPOUNDS

1. Structure—Match each structural description with its proper organic compound.

   ### *Use each letter once.*

   1) Glucose _____

   2) Pentose sugar _____

   3) Sucrose _____

   4) Starch _____

   5) Glycogen _____

   6) Cellulose _____

   7) True fat _____

   8) Phospholipid _____

   9) Cholesterol _____

   10) Amino acids _____

   11) Proteins _____

   A. A polysaccharide made by plants for energy storage
   B. Made of one glycerol and one, two, or three fatty acids
   C. A six-carbon monosaccharide or hexose sugar
   D. A steroid
   E. Made of many amino acids
   F. A polysaccharide for energy storage in animal cells
   G. The molecular subunits of proteins
   H. A five-carbon monosaccharide
   I. A diglyceride that includes a phosphate group
   J. A polysaccharide that is part of plant cell walls
   K. A disaccharide

2. Functions—Match each description of function with its proper organic compound.

   ### *Use each letter once. Three lines will have two correct letters each.*

   1) Glucose _____

   2) Pentose sugars _____

   3) Sucrose _____

   4) Starch _____

   5) Glycogen _____

   6) Cellulose _____

   7) True fats _____

   8) Phospholipid _____

   9) Cholesterol _____

   10) Amino acids _____

   11) Proteins _____

   A. Changed to vitamin D in the skin on exposure to sunlight
   B. A polysaccharide that is digested to glucose and used for energy production
   C. An energy storage molecule in subcutaneous tissue
   D. The primary energy source for cells
   E. Bonded by peptide bonds to form proteins
   F. A diglyceride that is part of cell membranes
   G. Part of DNA and RNA
   H. These include enzymes and antibodies
   I. A sugar that is digested to monosaccharides to produce energy
   J. The storage form for glucose in the liver and muscles
   K. A polysaccharide that promotes peristalsis in the colon
   L. Used to synthesize the steroid hormones
   M. These include hemoglobin and insulin
   N. Also called fiber

CHEMICAL STRUCTURE—REVIEW

1. Below is the diagram of a chemical molecule. Name the elements in this molecule.

_____ , _____ , _____ , and _____

2. a) Name this molecule. _____

   b) Name the type of bond that holds its elements together. _____

3. a) Name the larger molecules that are made of many of this type of smaller molecule.

   _____

   b) State three functions of these larger molecules in the body.

   1) _____

   2) _____

   3) _____

4. Below is another important chemical molecule. Name the elements in this molecule.

_____ , _____ , and _____

5. State the chemical formula of this molecule. _____ (If you do not recognize it, simply
   count the number of each type of atom.)

6. a) Name this molecule. _____

   b) State its function in the body. _____

   c) Name three larger molecules that are made of many of this smaller molecule, and state a function of each.

   1) _____

   2) _____

   3) _____

ENZYMES

1. Enzymes are proteins that increase the rate of reactions without the need for additional energy.

   Another way to say this is that enzymes are _____ in the body.

2. The diagram below shows a synthesis reaction catalyzed by an enzyme.

   Label the enzyme-substrate complex, the active site of the enzyme, the product of the reaction, and the enzyme after the reaction.

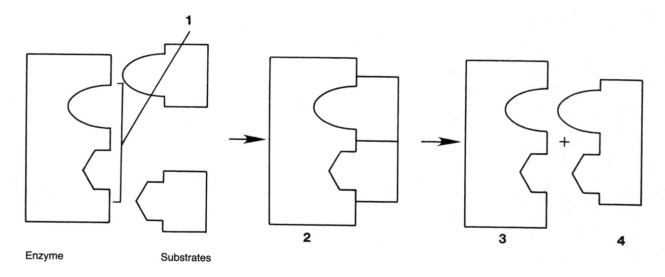

Enzyme   Substrates

○ Active site
○ Substrates
○ Product

3. An increase in body temperature, such as a fever, may inactivate enzymes because the higher

   temperature changes the _____ of the enzymes.

4. A state of acidosis may inactivate enzymes because excess _____ ions block the

   _____ of these enzymes.

DNA, RNA, AND ATP

1. Both DNA and RNA are made of subunits called nucleotides. A nucleotide consists of

   three smaller molecules: _____ , _____ , and _____ .

2. Structure—Match each statement with the proper nucleic acid molecule.

   Use each letter once. Each answer line will have two correct letters.

   1) DNA _____

   2) RNA _____

   3) ATP _____

   A. A single strand of nucleotides
   B. A double strand of nucleotides
   C. A single nucleotide with three phosphate
      groups
   D. Contains the nitrogenous bases A,T,C, and G
   E. Is an energy transfer molecule
   F. Contains the nitrogenous bases A,U,C, and G

3. Below is a diagram of the DNA double helix.

Complete the DNA nucleotides according to the complementary base pairing found in DNA.

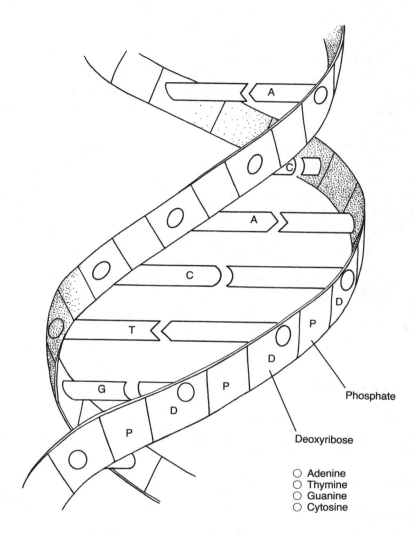

Phosphate

Deoxyribose

○ Adenine
○ Thymine
○ Guanine
○ Cytosine

4. Functions—Match each statement with the proper nucleic acid molecule.

Use each letter once. Two answer lines will have two correct letters.

1) DNA _____

2) RNA _____

3) ATP _____

A. Directly involved in protein synthesis
B. Formed when energy is released in cell respiration
C. Makes up the chromosomes in the nucleus of a cell
D. Provides energy for cellular reactions
E. The genetic code for hereditary characteristics

CLINICAL APPLICATIONS

1. a) Mr. B. has severe emphysema and cannot exhale efficiently. As CO_2 accumulates, the pH of his body fluids will _____ (increase or decrease), and he will be in the state called

   _____ .

   b) In this state, Mr. B.'s blood pH might be:
      a) 7.32   b) 7.38   c) 7.40   d) 7.42   e) 7.50

2. Mrs. T. is 72 years old and has osteoporosis, a condition in which the bones have become fragile and tend to fracture more easily. Which mineral is NOT present in sufficient amounts in Mrs. T.'s bones?
   a) iron   b) sodium   c) iodine   d) calcium   e) potassium

3. Following a car accident, Mr. M. is hospitalized and is receiving an intravenous solution of dextrose (glucose) in water. The direct purpose of this solution is to: (choose one answer)
   a) replace the RBCs lost in hemorrhage
   b) provide an energy source for cell respiration
   c) provide the molecules needed for protein synthesis
   d) provide the molecules to repair tissues

4. Ms. C. is 16 years old, and her doctor has advised her to eat foods rich in iron. The most probable reason for this recommendation is to: (choose one answer)
   a) provide for adequate hemoglobin synthesis to prevent anemia
   b) promote the growth of bones
   c) provide for the synthesis of thyroxine by the thyroid gland
   d) provide a primary energy source

MULTIPLE CHOICE TEST # 1

Choose the correct answer for each question.

1. The direct source of energy for cells is usually:
   a) protein   b) glucose   c) DNA   d) fats

2. An atom that has a charge after losing or gaining electrons is called:
   a) a molecule   b) an ion   c) a compound   d) a substance

3. The smallest part of an element is:
   a) an atom   b) a molecule   c) an ion   d) a compound

4. The normal pH range of blood is:
   a) 7.05–7.25   b) 7.40–7.50   c) 7.15–7.35   d) 7.35–7.45

5. Which formulas depict *ions* of sodium and chlorine?
   a) Na^+, Cl^- b) Na, Cl   c) Na, Cl^+ d) Na^{+2}, Cl^{-2}

6. Which formula shows a molecule with covalent bonds?
   a) $CaCl_2$ b) H_2O c) NaCl   d) Ca^{+2}

7. Which two compounds are important for energy storage in the body?
   a) proteins and phospholipids
   b) glucose and cholesterol
   c) glycogen and true fats
   d) DNA and cellulose

8. Intracellular fluid is the name for water found in:
   a) tissue spaces   b) arteries and veins   c) cells   d) lymph vessels

9. Enzymes are molecules that catalyze reactions and are all:
   a) carbohydrates   b) steroids   c) fats   d) proteins

10. The trace element most essential for oxygen transport in the blood is:
    a) calcium   b) iron   c) iodine   d) sodium

11. Which of the following pH values are correct?
    a) acid 5, neutral 7, alkaline 9
    b) acid 1, neutral 3, alkaline 5
    c) acid 7, neutral 8, alkaline 9
    d) acid 6, neutral 8, alkaline 10

12. Which of the following organic molecules is NOT paired with its correct subunits?
    a) glycogen—glucose
    b) proteins—monosaccharides
    c) DNA and RNA—nucleotides
    d) true fats—fatty acids and glycerol

13. An enzyme may become inactive when:
    a) body temperature rises excessively
    b) the pH of body fluids becomes too acidic
    c) homeostasis is maintained
    d) all of the above
    e) a and b only
    f) b and c only

14. Which of the following is the genetic code in our cells?
    a) glucose in cell respiration
    b) proteins in enzymes
    c) RNA in chromosomes
    d) DNA in chromosomes

15. The energy transfer molecule formed in cell respiration is:
    a) DNA   b) protein   c) glucose   d) ATP

16. The waste product of cell respiration is:
    a) water   b) heat   c) carbon dioxide   d) ATP

17. The two elements that provide strength in bones and teeth are:
    a) Fe and Na   b) I and Cl   c) Na and K   d) Ca and P

18. A carbohydrate is made of the elements:
    a) oxygen, calcium, nitrogen
    b) carbon, nitrogen, chlorine
    c) hydrogen, nitrogen, oxygen
    d) carbon, hydrogen, oxygen

19. The polysaccharide that is NOT an energy source is:
    a) glycogen   b) cellulose   c) starch   d) sucrose

20. The molecule used to synthesize the hormones estrogen and testosterone is:
    a) cholesterol   b) DNA   c) proteins   d) phospholipids

MULTIPLE CHOICE TEST #2

Read each question and the four answer choices carefully. When you have made a choice, follow the instructions to complete your answer.

1. Which of the following is NOT an element?
   a) carbon   b) water   c) oxygen   d) iron

   Explain why your choice is not an element.

   _____

2. Which statement is NOT true of chemical bonds?
   a) covalent bonds involve the sharing of electrons between atoms
   b) covalent bonds are often weakened when in a water solution
   c) ionic bonds involve the loss of electron(s) by one atom and the gain of these electron(s) by another atom
   d) inorganic molecules such as salts are formed by ionic bonds

   Reword your choice to make it a correct statement.

   _____

3. Which statement is NOT true of water compartments?
   a) tissue fluid is water found surrounding cells
   b) plasma is water found in blood vessels
   c) lymph is water found in lymph vessels
   d) intracellular fluid is water found between cells

   Reword your choice to make it a correct statement.

   _____

4. Which statement is NOT true of cell respiration?
   a) oxygen is required for the complete breakdown of a glucose molecule
   b) the oxygen required comes from breathing
   c) glucose is a fat molecule obtained from food
   d) the purpose of cell respiration is to produce ATP to provide energy for cellular processes

   Reword your choice to make it a correct statement.

   _____

5. Which statement is NOT true of the products of cell respiration?
   a) the heat energy produced has no purpose in the body
   b) the CO_2 formed is exhaled
   c) the water formed becomes part of intracellular fluid
   d) the ATP produced is used for cellular functions that require energy

   Reword your choice to make it a correct statement.

   _____

6. Which trace element is paired with its proper function?
   a) iron is part of bones and teeth
   b) sulfur is part of some proteins such as insulin
   c) calcium is part of the hormone thyroxine
   d) iodine is part of hemoglobin

   Rearrange the three incorrect pairings to make them correct.

   _____

7. Which statement is NOT true of pH and buffer systems?
   a) a buffer system prevents drastic changes in the pH of body fluids
   b) the normal pH range of blood is 7.0–8.0

c) the neutral point on the pH scale is 7.0
d) an acidic solution contains more H^+ ions than OH^- ions

Reword your choice to make it a correct statement.

_____

8. Which statement is NOT true of the functions of water in the body?
   a) the sense of taste depends on the solvent ability of water
   b) in sweating, excess body heat evaporates water on the skin surface
   c) water is a lubricant and prevents friction as food moves through the digestive tract
   d) the excretion of waste products in urine depends on the lubricant action of water

Reword your choice to make it a correct statement.

_____

9. Which organic compound is paired with its proper function?
   a) glycogen—a form of energy storage in adipose tissue
   b) true fats—part of DNA and RNA
   c) cholesterol—used to synthesize the steroid hormones
   d) pentose sugars—a form of energy storage in the liver

Rearrange the three incorrect pairings to make them correct.

_____

10. Which of the following is NOT a function of proteins?
    a) hemoglobin transports nutrients in RBCs
    b) muscle structure and contraction
    c) part of the structure of skin and tendons
    d) enzymes to catalyze reactions

Reword your choice to make it a correct function.

_____

11. Which statement is NOT true of enzymes and their functioning?
    a) all enzymes are carbohydrates
    b) the theory of enzyme functioning is called the Active Site Theory
    c) the shape of an enzyme is related to the type of reaction it will catalyze
    d) changes in body temperature or pH may affect the functioning of enzymes

Reword your choice to make it a correct statement.

_____

12. Which statement is NOT true of the nucleic acids?
    a) DNA makes up the chromosomes of cells
    b) RNA is a single strand of nucleotides
    c) RNA is the genetic code for our hereditary characteristics
    d) RNA functions in the process of protein synthesis

Reword your choice to make it a correct statement.

_____

13. Which statement is NOT true of ATP?
    a) it is a specialized nucleotide
    b) it is a product of cell respiration
    c) it is needed for energy-requiring cellular reactions
    d) it contains three potassium groups

    Reword your choice to make it a correct statement.

    _____

14. Which statement is NOT true of chemical reactions?
    a) synthesis reactions involve the breaking of bonds
    b) synthesis reactions usually require energy
    c) decomposition reactions involve the breaking of bonds
    d) decomposition reactions change large molecules to smaller ones

    Reword your choice to make it a correct statement.

    _____

Chapter 3

Cells

Cells are the smallest living units of the structure and function of the body. This chapter describes cellular structure and some of the general activities that cells carry out within the body.

CELL STRUCTURE

1. Match the following major parts of a cell with their proper descriptions.

   Use each letter once. Each answer line will have two or more correct letters.

   1) Cell membrane _____
   2) Cytoplasm _____
   3) Nucleus _____

   A. Contains the chromosomes of a cell
   B. Made of phospholipids, protein, and cholesterol
   C. Is the control center of a cell because of the genes it contains
   D. A watery solution of minerals, organic molecules, and gases
   E. Forms the outermost boundary of a cell
   F. Contains the nucleolus
   G. Permits certain substances to enter or leave the cell
   H. Found between the cell membrane and the nucleus
   I. Is selectively permeable
   J. Mature red blood cells lack this structure

2. Name the three organic molecules that make up cell membranes: _____ , _____ , and _____ .

   Use your answers above to complete the following:

   1) Provides stability for the cell membrane _____
   2) Forms pores in the cell membrane _____
   3) Are antigens, in combination with oligosaccharides _____

4) Permit the diffusion of lipid-soluble substances into or out of the cell _____

5) Are receptor sites for hormones _____

3. The diagram below depicts a typical cell. Label all the cellular structures indicated.

4. Match each cell organelle with its proper structure (a letter statement) and its proper function (a number statement).

   Use each letter or number only once.

   1) Endoplasmic reticulum _____

   2) Ribosomes _____

   3) Golgi apparatus _____

   Structure
   A. Made of protein and ribosomal RNA
   B. Double-membrane structures; the inner membrane has folds called cristae

4) Mitochondria _____

5) Lysosomes _____

6) Centrioles _____

7) Cilia _____

8) Flagella _____

C. Two rod-shaped structures perpendicular to one another

D. A single, long, thread-like projection

E. An extensive series of membranous tubules that extend from the nuclear membrane to the cell membrane; may be rough or smooth

F. Short thread-like projections through the cell membrane

G. Single-membrane structures that contain tissue-digesting enzymes

H. A series of flat, membranous sacs

Function

1. The site of protein synthesis
2. The site of ATP production
3. Digest worn out cell parts or ingested bacteria
4. Provides motility for a sperm cell
5. Sweep materials across the cell surface
6. Passageway for transport of materials within the cell
7. Organize the spindle fibers during cell division
8. Synthesize carbohydrates and secrete materials from the cell

CELLULAR TRANSPORT MECHANISMS

1. Match each cellular transport process with its proper definition (a letter statement) and the proper example of the process in the body (a number statement).

   Use each letter or number only once.

   1) Diffusion _____

   2) Osmosis _____

   3) Facilitated diffusion _____

   4) Active transport _____

   5) Filtration _____

   6) Phagocytosis _____

   7) Pinocytosis _____

   Definition

   A. Diffusion of molecules, requiring carrier enzymes

   B. The engulfing of something by a stationary cell

   C. The movement of molecules from an area of greater concentration to an area of lesser concentration

   D. The engulfing of something by a moving cell

   E. The use of energy to move molecules from an area of lesser concentration to an area of greater concentration

   F. The diffusion of water through a semi-permeable membrane

   G. Water and dissolved materials move through a membrane from an area of higher pressure to an area of lower pressure

Example
1. The absorption of water by the small intestine or kidneys
2. The movement of oxygen from the blood to the cells of the body
3. Blood pressure in capillaries forces plasma out to become tissue fluid
4. The engulfing of bacteria by white blood cells
5. The intake of glucose by cells of the body
6. The reabsorption of small proteins by cells of the kidney tubules
7. The absorption of amino acids or glucose by the cells of the small intestine

2. The diagram below represents one alveolus (air sac) in the lung; the alveolus is surrounded by a pulmonary capillary. Indicate the relative concentrations of oxygen and carbon dioxide based on your knowledge of diffusion.

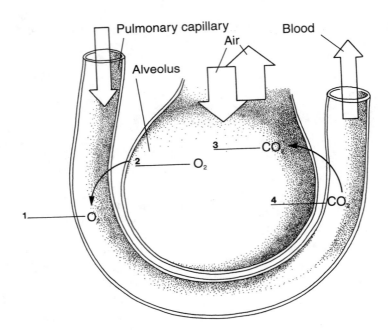

3. The diagram at the top of the next page represents a small section of the lining of the small intestine, with certain food molecules within the cavity of the intestine. For each nutrient, name the mechanism by which it is absorbed.

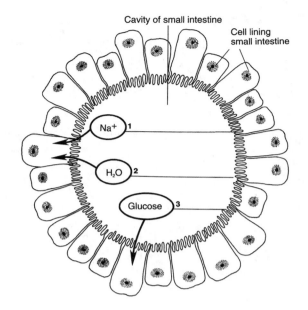

Cavity of small intestine

Cell lining
small intestine

Na^+ 1

H_2O 2

Glucose   3

4. Using human cells as a reference point, complete each statement by using the phrases: "a higher," "a lower," or "the same."

   1) An isotonic solution has _____ concentration of dissolved material as does a cell.

   2) A hypertonic solution has _____ concentration of dissolved material than does a cell.

   3) A hypotonic solution has _____ concentration of dissolved materials than does a cell.

5. The diagrams below depict human red blood cells in three different solutions. Notice what, if anything, has happened to the cells.

   Based on your knowledge of osmosis, indicate which solution is hypertonic, which is hypotonic, and which is isotonic to the cells.

1) _____   2) _____   3) _____

DNA AND THE GENETIC CODE

1. a) DNA makes up the _____ of a cell, which are found in the nucleus.

   b) Human cells contain how many of these DNA structures? _____

2. A DNA molecule is made of _____ (one, two, three, or four) strands of nucleotides twisted into a spiral called a _____ .

3. The complementary base-pairing of DNA means that adenine is always paired with

   _____ , and cytosine is always paired with _____ .

4. A gene is a segment of DNA that is the genetic code for one _____ .

5. A protein is made of the smaller molecules called _____ .

6. a) The DNA code for one amino acid consists of how many bases? _____

   b) Therefore, the name for this code may also be the _____ code.

   c) The other name for a triplet is a _____ .

RNA AND PROTEIN SYNTHESIS

1. An RNA molecule consists of how many strands of nucleotides? _____

2. One type of RNA copies the genetic code of a DNA gene; this type is called _____ RNA, which may be abbreviated _____ .

3. The bases found in mRNA are adenine, guanine, cytosine, and _____ .

4. An mRNA molecule is synthesized from the DNA in the _____ (part) of a cell, but then moves to the cytoplasm and becomes attached to which type of cell organelle?

   _____

5. A second type of RNA picks up amino acids in the cytoplasm of a cell; this type is called

   _____ RNA, which may be abbreviated _____ .

6. A tRNA has a triplet of bases called an anticodon, which matches the _____ on the mRNA, and ensures that the amino acid is positioned in its proper place in the protein.

7. Enzymes to form _____ bonds between amino acids are contained in the

   _____ to which the mRNA is attached.

8. The expression of the genetic code that gives us our hereditary characteristics is summarized in the sequence below. Fill in the missing parts of the sequence.

   DNA → 1._____ → Proteins → 2._____ ――――――――→ Hereditary
                                                                      characteristics

                              3._____ → Catalyze _____↑
                                                    reactions

9. The diagram below depicts the process of protein synthesis taking place in a cell.

   Label each of the following: nucleus, DNA, mRNA, tRNA, ribosome, amino acids, and peptide bond.

MITOSIS AND MEIOSIS

1. With respect to the processes of cell division, match the following statements.

   Use each letter once. Each answer line will have four correct letters.

   1) Mitosis _____

   2) Meiosis _____

   A. Two identical cells are produced
   B. One cell with the diploid number of chromosomes divides once
   C. Four cells are produced

D. One cell with the diploid number of chromosomes divides twice
E. Each cell produced has the haploid number of chromosomes
F. The cells produced are egg or sperm cells
G. The cells produced are needed for the growth and repair of tissues
H. Each cell produced has the diploid number of chromosomes

2. Before mitosis or meiosis takes place, a cell is said to be in a stage called interphase. During this time, DNA replication takes place. Explain what happens in DNA replication.

_____

3. Match the stages of mitosis with the events that take place during each.

   Use each letter once. Each answer line will have more than one correct letter.

   1) Prophase _____
   2) Metaphase _____
   3) Anaphase _____
   4) Telophase _____

   A. The pairs of chromatids line up on the equator of the cell
   B. The centrioles organize the formation of the spindle fibers
   C. The spindle fibers pull each set of chromosomes toward opposite poles of the cell
   D. The chromosomes coil up and become visible as short rods; each is a pair of chromatids connected at the centromere
   E. Each chromatid is now considered a separate chromosome
   F. The centromeres divide
   G. The nuclear membrane disappears
   H. Each set of chromosomes uncoils, and nuclear membranes are reformed
   I. Cytokinesis, the division of the cytoplasm, follows

4. State two sites in the human body where mitosis takes place constantly, and explain why this rapid mitosis is necessary.

   1) Site _____ Reason _____
   2) Site _____ Reason _____

5. Name one type of adult human cell that cannot reproduce itself by mitosis, and explain the significance of this.

   a) Type of cell _____
   b) Significance _____

   _____

6. The diagrams below depict the stages of mitosis in a cell with a diploid number of four.

   Label each cell as one of the following: interphase, prophase, metaphase, anaphase, telophase, cytokinesis. Then arrange the letters in the proper sequence.

a _____   b _____   c _____

d _____   e _____   f _____

Sequence: _____, _____, _____, _____, _____, _____.

CLINICAL APPLICATIONS

1. Mr. D. is receiving chemotherapy for cancer. This medication inhibits the process of mitosis, which slows the production of malignant cells. Also affected, however, are other cells that undergo rapid mitosis. Mr. D. may develop anemia if the _____ is affected this way.

2. a) Intravenous solutions are often isotonic, which means that their concentrations of water and dissolved materials are _____ as the concentrations found in the blood plasma.

   b) If distilled water were mistakenly administered intravenously, the red blood cells at the site would _____ (gain or lose) water by the process of _____ (filtration or osmosis) and would eventually _____ (swell or shrivel).

3. a) Certain antibiotics that are used to treat bacterial infections inhibit the synthesis of the nucleic acids DNA and RNA. While this may slow the growth of bacteria, the same processes in human cells may also be inhibited. Without DNA synthesis, what cellular process could not take place?

   _____

   b) Without RNA synthesis, what cellular process would not take place? _____

MULTIPLE CHOICE TEST # 1

Choose the correct answer for each question.

1. The cell organelles most directly associated with cell division are the:
   a) Golgi apparatus   b) centrioles   c) ribosomes   d) lysosomes

2. The hereditary material of cells is _____ that is found in the _____ of the cell.
   a) protein/ribosomes   c) glucose/nucleus
   b) DNA/chromosomes   d) RNA/ribosomes

3. The major structural parts of a cell are the:
   a) cell membrane, nucleus, cytoplasm   c) cytoplasm, nucleolus, endoplasmic reticulum
   b) nucleus, nucleolus, mitochondria   d) ribosomes, cell membrane, Golgi apparatus

4. The cell organelle most directly associated with the production of cellular proteins is:
   a) mitochondria   b) lysosomes   c) Golgi apparatus   d) ribosomes

5. The cellular transport mechanism that depends on carrier enzymes in the cell membrane is:
   a) filtration   b) osmosis   c) diffusion   d) facilitated diffusion

6. The cellular transport mechanism that depends on blood pressure is:
   a) diffusion   b) filtration   c) phagocytosis   d) active transport

7. A water-salt solution with the same salt concentration as in cells is called:
   a) isotonic   b) hypertonic   c) hypotonic   d) lemon-lime tonic

8. Mitosis produces cells that have:
   a) only one chromosome each
   b) the diploid number of chromosomes, 46 for people
   c) the haploid number of chromosomes, 23 for people
   d) double the number of chromosomes, 46 for people

9. Meiosis produces cells that have:
   a) the diploid number of chromosomes, 23 for people
   b) the haploid number of chromosomes, 46 for people
   c) the haploid number of chromosomes, 23 for people
   d) double the number of chromosomes, 92 for people

10. The organic molecules in the cell membrane that form pores and receptor sites for hormones are:
    a) cholesterol   b) phospholipids   c) proteins   d) carbohydrates

11. Meiosis is necessary to produce:
    a) skin cells   b) bone cells   c) muscle cells   d) egg or sperm cells

12. Mitosis is necessary for:
    a) production of new nerve cells
    b) continuation of the human species by reproduction
    c) growth and repair of tissues
    d) production of egg and sperm cells

13. The function of cilia is to:
    a) sweep materials across a surface
    b) provide locomotion (movement) for human cells

    c) move the chromosomes during mitosis

    d) support cells and keep them stable

14. The nucleus of a cell:
    a) forms the outer boundary of a cell and protects the cell
    b) contains most of the cell organelles
    c) regulates the activities of a cell by means of the genetic material it contains
    d) regulates what enters or leaves the cell to protect the cell from pathogens

15. The function of the Golgi apparatus of a cell is to synthesize:
    a) proteins   b) lipids   c) new genes   d) carbohydrates

16. Diffusion is defined as the movement of molecules:
    a) from an area of lesser concentration to an area of greater concentration
    b) from an area of greater pressure to an area of lower pressure
    c) from an area of lower energy to an area of higher energy
    d) from an area of greater concentration to an area of lesser concentration

17. A gene is the genetic code for one:
    a) cell   b) protein   c) organ   d) chromosome

18. The complementary base-pairing of DNA is:
    a) A–T and G–C   b) A–C and G–T   c) A–G and C–T   d) A–U and C–G

19. The complementary base-pairing of DNA with mRNA is:
    a) A–C and G–U   b) A–U and G–C   c) A–G and C–U   d) A–T and U–C

20. Human cells that cannot undergo mitosis in an adult include:
    a) stomach lining cells and muscle cells   c) bone marrow cells and skin cells
    b) nerve cells and muscle cells   d) skin cells and nerve cells

MULTIPLE CHOICE TEST # 2

Read each question and the four answer choices carefully. When you have made a choice, follow the instructions to complete your answer.

1. Which cellular transport mechanism is NOT paired with its correct definition?
    a) osmosis—the diffusion of water through a membrane
    b) filtration—the movement of water and dissolved materials through a membrane from an area of higher pressure to an area of lower pressure
    c) active transport—the movement of molecules from an area of greater concentration to an area of lesser concentration
    d) phagocytosis—the engulfing of something by a moving cell

For your choice, state the correct definition.

_____

2. Which cell organelle is NOT paired with its proper function?
    a) mitochondria—the site of cell respiration and ATP production
    b) lysosomes—contain enzymes to digest worn out cell parts
    c) endoplasmic reticulum—membranous tubules that are passageways within the cell
    d) ribosomes—the site of carbohydrate synthesis

For your choice, state its correct function.

_____

3. Which statement is NOT true of DNA?
   a) DNA makes up the chromosomes of cells
   b) DNA exists as a single strand of nucleotides called a double helix
   c) DNA is the genetic code for hereditary characteristics
   d) a gene is the genetic code for one protein

   Reword your choice to make it a correct statement.

   _____

4. Which statement is NOT true of the process of protein synthesis?
   a) the site of protein synthesis is the ribosomes in the cytoplasm
   b) tRNA molecules pick up amino acids and bring them to the proper mRNA triplet
   c) amino acids are bonded to one another by ionic bonds
   d) mRNA is formed in the nucleus as a copy of a DNA gene

   Reword your choice to make it a correct statement.

   _____

5. Which stage of mitosis is NOT paired with a correct event of that stage?
   a) telophase—a nuclear membrane reforms around each new set of chromosomes
   b) metaphase—the pairs of chromatids line up on the equator of the cell
   c) prophase—the chromosomes become visible and spindle fibers form
   d) anaphase—each pair of chromatids becomes attached to a spindle fiber

   *For your choice, state what **does** happen during this stage.*

   _____

6. Which statement is NOT true of the cell membrane?
   a) the phospholipids permit diffusion of lipid-soluble substances
   b) it forms the outer boundary of the cell
   c) it is impermeable, meaning that only certain substances may pass through
   d) some of the proteins form pores to permit the entry or exit of molecules

   Reword your choice to make it a correct statement.

   _____

7. Which statement is NOT true of mitosis in an adult?
   a) nerve cells only reproduce when there is damage to the brain
   b) skin cells reproduce to replace those worn off the skin surface
   c) red blood cells are continuously replaced by the red bone marrow
   d) muscle cells are unable to reproduce themselves

   Reword your choice to make it a correct statement.

   _____

8. Which cellular transport mechanism is NOT paired with its proper function in the body?
   a) pinocytosis—the reabsorption of small proteins by the kidney tubules
   b) diffusion—the exchange of gases between the air in the lungs and the blood

c) osmosis—the absorption of salts by the small intestine

d) filtration—the formation of tissue fluid as plasma is forced out of capillaries

For your choice, state a correct function of the mechanism.

_____

9. Which statement is NOT true of solutions?

a) human cells in a hypertonic solution would remain undamaged

b) a hypotonic solution has a lower concentration of dissolved materials than do human cells

c) blood plasma is isotonic to red blood cells

d) human cells in a hypotonic solution would swell

Reword your choice to make it a correct statement.

_____

Chapter 4

Tissues and Membranes

This chapter describes the tissues, which are groups of cells with similar structure and functions. The four major groups of tissues are: epithelial tissue, connective tissue, muscle tissue, and nerve tissue. Each of these groups has very specific characteristics and actions.

EPITHELIAL TISSUE

1. The diagrams below depict some of the types of epithelial tissue.

   Label each type with its complete name.

1) _____

2) _____

3) _____

4) _____

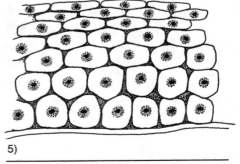

5) _____

2. Match each epithelial tissue with its proper structure (a letter statement) and functions in the body (one or more number statements).

Use each letter and number once. Each answer line will have one correct letter and may have more than one correct number.

1) Simple squamous epithelium _____

2) Stratified squamous epithelium _____

3) Transitional epithelium _____

4) Cuboidal epithelium _____

5) Columnar epithelium _____

6) Ciliated epithelium _____

Structure

A. Many layers of cells; surface cells are flat
B. Columnar cells with cilia on their free surfaces
C. One layer of cells that are taller than they are wide
D. One layer of cube-shaped cells
E. One layer of flat cells
F. Many layers of cells; surface cells are alternately rounded or flat

Function

1. Forms the alveoli of the lungs and permits diffusion of gases
2. Secretes the hormones of the thyroid gland
3. Forms the epidermis of the skin
4. Forms the stomach lining and secretes gastric juice
5. Forms capillaries to permit exchanges of materials
6. Secretes the saliva of salivary glands
7. Permits stretching of the urinary bladder as it fills
8. Lines arteries and veins and is smooth to prevent abnormal blood clotting
9. Forms the lining of the mouth and the esophagus
10. Lines the trachea, and sweeps mucus and bacteria toward the pharynx
11. Forms the lining of the small intestine and absorbs nutrients
12. Lines the fallopian tubes to sweep an ovum toward the uterus
13. May have microvilli to increase the surface area for absorption

3. Glands are made of epithelial tissue, and there are several different categories. Match each type of gland with its proper structure (one or two letter statements) and an example in the body (a number statement).

Use each letter and number once. One answer line will have two correct letters.

1) Unicellular glands _____

2) Exocrine glands _____

3) Endocrine glands _____

Structure

A. Consist of only one cell
B. Have no ducts; their secretions enter capillaries

C. Have ducts to take their secretions to their site
   of action
D. Their secretions are called hormones

Example
1. The thyroid gland and pituitary gland
2. Goblet cells that secrete mucus
3. The salivary glands and sweat glands

CONNECTIVE TISSUE

1. Match each connective tissue with its proper structure (a letter statement) and functions in the body
   (one or more number statements).

   Use each letter and number once. Each answer line will have one correct letter and may
   have more than one correct number.

   1) Blood _____

   2) Areolar connective tissue _____

   3) Adipose tissue _____

   4) Fibrous connective tissue _____

   5) Elastic connective tissue _____

   6) Bone _____

   7) Cartilage _____

Structure
A. Made primarily of elastin fibers
B. Made of cells in the fluid matrix called plasma
C. Made of osteocytes in a matrix of calcium salts
   and collagen
D. Made of cells specialized to store fat
E. Made of fibroblasts in a matrix of tissue fluid,
   collagen, and elastin fibers
F. Made of chrondrocytes in a matrix that is
   smooth and flexible
G. Made primarily of collagen fibers

Function
1. Beneath the skin and the epithelium of
   mucous membranes; has white blood cells to
   destroy pathogens
2. Forms tendons that connect muscles to bones
3. Surrounds the alveoli of the lungs and
   contributes to normal exhalation
4. Transports oxygen and nutrients and contains
   cells to destroy pathogens
5. Supports the body
6. Provides a smooth surface to prevent friction
   on joint surfaces
7. Stores excess energy in subcutaneous tissue
8. The cells are produced in red bone marrow
   and lymphatic tissue
9. Forms ligaments that connect bone to bone
10. Forms rings to keep the trachea open
11. In the walls of the large arteries where it helps
    maintain blood pressure
12. Protects some internal organs from
    mechanical injury

2. The diagrams below depict some of the types of connective tissue.

Label each type with its complete name.

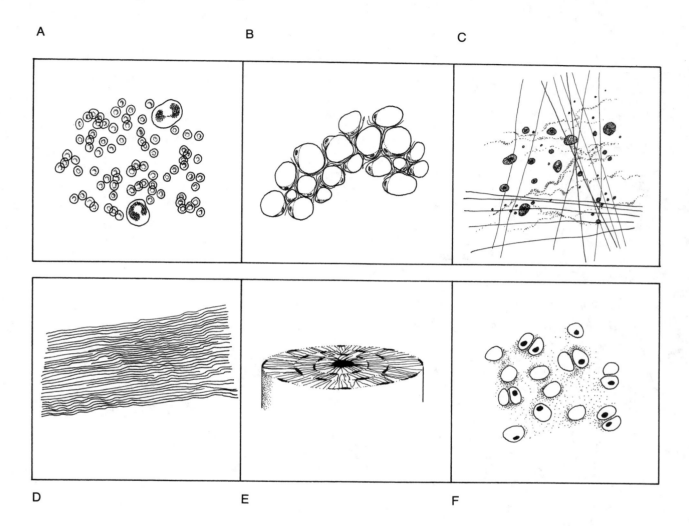

A   B   C

D   E   F

MUSCLE TISSUE

1. All three types of muscle tissue are specialized to contract and bring about movement of some kind.

   Each statement below is a structural or functional aspect of one of the three types of muscle tissue. Indicate the type to which the statement applies by writing SK for skeletal muscle, SM for smooth muscle, or C for cardiac muscle on the line before the statement.

   1) _____ The cells are tapered and have one nucleus each.

   2) _____ Attached to bones, moves the skeleton.

3) _____ Enables arteries to constrict or dilate to maintain blood pressure.

4) _____ The cells are branched and each has one nucleus.

5) _____ Also called striated muscle tissue, since the cylindrical cells appear to have striations.

6) _____ Produces a significant amount of body heat.

7) _____ Forms the walls of the chambers of the heart; its function is to pump blood.

8) _____ Also called visceral muscle, since it is found in many internal organs.

9) _____ Produces involuntary waves of contraction, called peristalsis, in the intestines.

10) _____ Each cell has several nuclei.

11) _____ The cells contract by themselves; nerve impulses regulate only the rate of contraction.

12) _____ Also called voluntary muscle, because nerve impulses are required for contraction.

13) _____ In the iris of the eye, it will constrict or dilate the pupil.

2. The diagrams below depict the three types of muscle tissue.

   Label each type with its complete name.

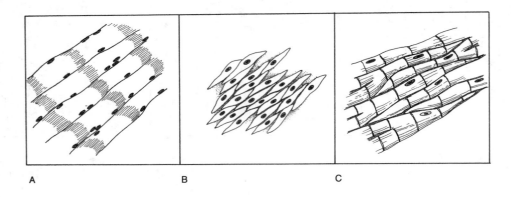

A   B   C

NERVE TISSUE

1. The name for nerve cells is _____ , and these cells are specialized to generate and

   transmit _____ .

2. Below is a diagram of a neuron.

   Label the following structures: cell body, nucleus, axon, dendrites.

3. a) The axon of a neuron carries impulses _____ (toward or away from) the cell
      body.

   b) The dendrites of a neuron carry impulses _____ (toward or away from) the cell
      body.

4. a) In the peripheral nervous system, the specialized cells that form the myelin sheath are called

      _____ .

   b) In the central nervous system, the specialized cells are called _____ .

5. a) The space between the axon of one neuron and the dendrites or cell body of the next neuron is

      called the _____ .

   b) Here, the transmission of nerve impulses depends on chemicals called _____ .

6. Name two organs made of nerve tissue. _____ and _____

7. State two general functions of nerve tissue in these organs or the nervous system as a whole.

   _____ and _____

MEMBRANES

1. Match each epithelial membrane with its proper locations and functions.

   Use each letter once. One answer line will have seven correct letters, and the other will have five correct letters.

   1) Serous membranes _____

   2) Mucous membranes _____

   A. Line the respiratory and digestive tracts
   B. Line closed body cavities
   C. Made of simple squamous epithelium
   D. Cover organs in closed body cavities
   E. Line the urinary and reproductive tracts
   F. Secrete serous fluid to prevent friction
   G. Secrete mucus to keep the living surface cells wet
   H. Include the pleural membranes
   I. Line body tracts that open to the environment
   J. Include the peritoneum and mesentery
   K. May contain goblet cells
   L. Include the pericardial membranes

2. a) The serous membranes that are found in closed body cavities are shown in the diagrams below.

   Label both membranes in each pair, and then complete the statements using proper terminology.

Abdominal Cavity

○ Parietal layer
○ Visceral layer

Thoracic Cavity

Cardiac Cavity

b) The _____ pleura lines the chest cavity, and the _____ pleura covers the lungs.

c) The _____ lines the abdominal cavity, and the _____ covers the abdominal organs.

d) The _____ pericardium lines the fibrous pericardium _____ , and the _____ pericardium covers the heart muscle.

3. Match each connective tissue membrane with the statement that describes its proper location and function.

   Use each letter once.

   1) Superficial fascia _____
   2) Deep fascia _____
   3) Synovial _____
   4) Fibrous pericardium _____
   5) Perichondrium _____
   6) Periosteum _____
   7) Meninges _____

   A. Lines joint cavities and secretes fluid to prevent friction when joints move
   B. Forms a sac around the heart
   C. Covers cartilage and contains capillaries
   D. Cover the brain and spinal cord and contain cerebrospinal fluid
   E. Covers bone and contains blood vessels that enter the bone
   F. Between the skin and the muscles; contains adipose tissue
   G. Covers each skeletal muscle and anchors tendons

CLINICAL APPLICATIONS

1. A 9-year-old boy has a simple fracture of the humerus, the bone of the upper arm. This fracture will heal relatively rapidly because bone has a good _____ to transport nutrients and oxygen to the site of repair.

2. A 26-year-old football player has torn cartilage in his knee joint. Such damage will be repaired slowly or not at all because cartilage itself has no _____ .

3. a) A victim of a diving accident has had his spinal cord severed in the lower cervical region, and no nerve impulses pass below this level. As a result, the _____ muscles below the neck are paralyzed because they no longer receive nerve impulses to initiate contraction.

   b) However, the _____ continues to contract because cardiac muscle cells are able to contract without the stimulus of nerve impulses.

4. A child with a ruptured appendix is receiving antibiotics to treat peritonitis. This serious infection involves the _____ , the membrane that lines the _____ cavity.

5. An elderly man has arthritis of the knees. The joint pain that accompanies arthritis may be due to inflammation of the _____ membrane that lines the joint cavities or damage to the _____ (type of tissue) that covers the joint surfaces of bones.

MULTIPLE CHOICE TEST # 1

Choose the correct answer for each question.

1. An endocrine gland has:
   a) a duct   b) no duct   c) no secretion   d) no blood supply

2. An example of an exocrine gland is the:
   a) salivary gland   b) thyroid gland   c) pituitary gland   d) adrenal gland

3. The type of epithelium in which the surface cells alternate from round to flat is:
   a) cuboidal   b) columnar   c) stratified squamous   d) transitional

4. The type of connective tissue with a liquid matrix called plasma is:
   a) cartilage   b) bone   c) adipose   d) blood

5. Axon, dendrite, and cell body are the three parts of:
   a) the brain   b) nerve tissue   c) a neuron   d) the central nervous system

6. The type of connective tissue with a solid matrix made of calcium salts is:
   a) areolar   b) bone   c) cartilage   d) fibrous

7. The type of muscle tissue also known as voluntary muscle is:
   a) smooth   b) cardiac   c) visceral   d) skeletal

8. The membrane that lines the digestive tract is a:
   a) serous membrane   b) synovial membrane   c) mucous membrane   d) fascia

9. The serous membrane that lines the thoracic cavity is the:
   a) visceral pleura   b) peritoneum   c) parietal pleura   d) mesentery

10. In the fallopian tube, an egg cell is moved toward the uterus by:
    a) ciliated epithelium   b) striated muscle   c) nerve tissue   d) cuboidal epithelium

11. To increase their surface area for absorption, columnar cells in the small intestine have:
    a) microvilli   b) cilia   c) goblet cells   d) ducts

12. The strong tissue that forms tendons and ligaments is:
    a) skeletal muscle   c) bone
    b) fibrous connective tissue   d) elastic connective tissue

13. The type of epithelium that makes up the outer layer of skin is:
    a) simple squamous   c) stratified squamous
    b) stratified columnar   d) simple columnar

14. The tissue that is thin enough to form capillaries and permit exchanges of materials is:
    a) smooth muscle   c) areolar connective tissue
    b) elastic connective tissue   d) simple squamous epithelium

15. The type of muscle tissue that produces a significant amount of body heat is:
    a) skeletal   b) smooth   c) cardiac   d) visceral

16. Cardiac muscle is found in:
    a) the heart and arteries   c) the heart only
    b) arteries only   d) arteries, veins, and the heart

17. The membranes that cover the brain and spinal cord are the:
    a) visceral cranial membranes   c) synovial membranes
    b) periosteum   d) meninges

18. The space between two neurons where a neurotransmitter carries the impulse is called a:
    a) cell body   b) matrix   c) Schwann cell   d) synapse

19. The unicellular glands that secrete mucus in the respiratory tract are:
    a) goblet cells   b) endocrine glands   c) microvilli   d) serous glands

20. The tissue that transports nutrients and oxygen throughout the body is:
    a) nerve tissue   b) blood   c) areolar connective tissue   d) serous tissue

21. The type of muscle tissue that provides peristalsis in the intestines is:
    a) skeletal   b) voluntary   c) striated   d) smooth

22. The type of connective tissue that stores excess energy in the form of fat is:
    a) fibrous   b) cartilage   c) elastic   d) adipose

MULTIPLE CHOICE TEST # 2

Read each question and the four answer choices carefully. When you have made a choice,
follow the instructions to complete your answer.

1. Which tissue does NOT contribute to the functioning of the trachea?
   a) ciliated epithelium sweeps mucus and pathogens to the pharynx
   b) cartilage rings keep the trachea open
   c) goblet cells produce mucus
   d) columnar epithelium absorbs nutrients

   For your choice, state the correct location of the tissue with this function.

   _____

2. Which tissue does NOT contribute to the functioning of an artery?
   a) simple squamous epithelium forms the lining and prevents abnormal clotting
   b) cardiac muscle pumps blood
   c) elastic connective tissue helps maintain normal blood pressure
   d) smooth muscle tissue helps maintain normal blood pressure

   For your choice, state the correct location of the tissue with this function.

   _____

3. Which epithelial membrane is NOT paired with its proper location?
   a) peritoneum—lines the thoracic cavity
   b) mucous membrane—lines the urinary tract
   c) mesentery—covers the abdominal organs
   d) visceral pleura—covers the lungs

   For your choice, state its correct location.

   _____

4. Which of the following does NOT contribute to the structure and function of bones?
   a) the periosteum is a membrane that covers the bone
   b) calcium salts in the bone matrix provide strength
   c) cartilage on joint surfaces is smooth to prevent friction
   d) bones are moved by smooth muscle

   Reword your choice to make it a correct statement.

   _____

5. Which statement is NOT true of glands?
   a) exocrine glands have ducts to transport their secretions to other sites
   b) the secretions of endocrine glands are called hormones
   c) endocrine glands have no ducts, and their secretions enter capillaries
   d) an example of an exocrine gland is the thyroid gland

   Reword your choice to make it a correct statement.

   _____

6. Which statement is NOT true of muscle tissue?
   a) skeletal muscle in the iris of the eye changes the size of the pupil
   b) cardiac muscle forms the heart and pumps blood
   c) smooth muscle provides peristalsis in the intestines
   d) skeletal muscle moves the skeleton

   For your choice, name the muscle tissue that does have this function.

   _____

7. Which statement is NOT true of nerve tissue?
   a) transmission of impulses at synapses depends on chemicals called neurotransmitters
   b) nerve tissue makes up the peripheral nerves, spinal cord, and brain
   c) Schwann cells produce the myelin sheath for peripheral neurons
   d) the axon of a neuron carries impulses toward the cell body

   Reword your choice to make it a correct statement.

   _____

8. Which statement is NOT true of blood?
   a) white blood cells destroy pathogens and provide immunity
   b) nutrients and waste products are transported by red blood cells
   c) red blood cells contain hemoglobin to carry oxygen
   d) platelets are important for clotting to prevent blood loss

   Reword your choice to make it a correct statement.

   _____

9. Which statement is NOT true of the connective tissues?
   a) adipose tissue stores protein as a potential energy source
   b) fibrous connective tissue makes up tendons that connect muscle to bone
   c) areolar connective tissue is found between the skin and the muscles
   d) elastic connective tissue around the alveoli contributes to normal exhalation

   Reword your choice to make it a correct statement.

   _____

10. Which statement is NOT true of the epithelial tissues?
    a) transitional epithelium permits expansion of the urinary bladder
    b) simple cuboidal epithelium in the salivary glands secretes saliva
    c) stratified squamous epithelium of the outer layer of skin has living cells on the surface
    d) simple squamous epithelium in the alveoli permits exchange of gases

    Reword your choice to make it a correct statement.

    _____

Chapter 5

The Integumentary System

This chapter describes the integumentary system, which consists of the skin and the subcutaneous tissue. Each part is made of specific tissues that have very specific functions.

GENERAL STRUCTURE AND FUNCTIONS

1. Match each major part of the integumentary system with its proper structure (a letter statement) and function (a number statement).

   Use each letter and number once.

   1) Epidermis _____

   2) Dermis _____

   3) Subcutaneous tissue _____

   Structure

   A. Made of areolar connective and adipose tissue
   B. The outer layer of the skin, made of stratified squamous epithelium
   C. The inner layer of the skin, made of modified fibrous connective tissue

   Function

   1. Contains the accessory structures of the skin, such as receptors and sweat glands
   2. Connects the dermis to the muscles and stores fat
   3. Mitosis constantly renews this layer that forms a barrier between the body and the external environment

EPIDERMIS

1. The epidermis is the outer layer of the skin and may be further subdivided into layers of its own.

   a) Name the epidermal layer in which mitosis takes place. _____

   b) Name the epidermal layer that is composed of dead cells. _____

2. a) In the stratum corneum, all that is left of the cells is the protein _____ .

   b) The stratum corneum is an effective barrier that prevents the loss of _____ from the body and also prevents the entry of _____ and _____ .

3. If the skin is subjected to constant pressure, a thicker area of epidermis will be formed. More cells are produced by the process of _____ in the _____ (layer).

4. If the skin is subjected to friction, layers of the epidermis may be separated, and _____ will collect in the area and form a _____ .

5. a) Melanocytes produce the protein _____ , which is a pigment.

   b) What is the stimulus for increased melanin production? _____

   c) Explain the function of melanin (NOT to give the skin color).

DERMIS

1. Match the following parts of the dermis with their proper descriptions.

   Use each letter once.

   1) Fibroblasts _____

   2) Collagen fibers _____

   3) Elastin fibers _____

   4) Papillary layer _____

   5) Hair follicles _____

   6) Nail follicles _____

   7) Sebaceous glands _____

   8) Eccrine sweat glands _____

   9) Apocrine sweat glands _____

   10) Ceruminous glands _____

   11) Receptors _____

   A. Contains capillaries to nourish the stratum germinativum of the epidermis
   B. Provide information about changes in the external environment
   C. The protein that gives the dermis its strength
   D. Produce a lipid substance called sebum
   E. The cells that produce collagen and elastin
   F. Mitosis at the root produces the hair shaft
   G. Produce their secretion in times of stress or strong emotions
   H. Produce their secretion during exercise or in a warm environment
   I. Mitosis at the root produces the nail
   J. The protein that gives the dermis elasticity
   K. Produce cerumen, or earwax

2. a) The free nerve endings in the dermis are the receptors for the cutaneous sense of _____ .

   b) The encapsulated nerve endings in the dermis are the receptors for the cutaneous senses of _____ , _____ , _____ , and _____ .

   c) Explain why the skin of the palm is more sensitive to touch than is the skin of the shoulder.

3. a) The ends of fingers and toes are protected from mechanical injury by _____ .

   b) Name the protein these structures are made of. _____

4. a) The secretion that prevents drying of the eardrum is _____ .

   b) The secretion that prevents drying of the skin and hair is _____ .

   c) The secretion that helps lower body temperature is _____ .

5. a) One function of human hair is to keep dust out of the _____ or

   _____ .

   b) Another function is to provide insulation from the cold for the _____ (part of the body).

   c) Name the protein hair is made of. _____

6. In stress situations, the _____ in the dermis will constrict to shunt blood to more vital organs.

7. a) The vitamin formed in the skin is vitamin _____ , which is made from

   _____ when the skin is exposed to _____ .

   b) The function of this vitamin is to promote the absorption of _____ and

   _____ in the small intestine.

8. The diagram below is a section through the skin and subcutaneous tissue.

   Label the parts indicated.

SUBCUTANEOUS TISSUE

1. The other name for subcutaneous tissue is the _____ .

2. a) The subcutaneous tissue is located between the _____ and the

   _____ .

   b) Name the two types of connective tissue in this layer. _____ and

   _____

3. The areolar connective tissue contains many white blood cells that destroy _____ that

   have entered _____ .

4. a) The adipose tissue contains cells that are specialized to store _____ as a source of

   potential _____ .

   b) State two other functions of subcutaneous fat. _____

   and _____

MAINTENANCE OF BODY TEMPERATURE

1. The role of the skin in the maintenance of body temperature depends on the _____ glands and the small arteries called _____ .

2. a) In a _____ environment, the eccrine glands secrete more sweat onto the skin surface.

   b) Excess body heat is then lost in the process of _____ of the sweat.

3. a) In a cold environment, the arterioles in the dermis will _____ (constrict or dilate).

   b) This will _____ (increase or decrease) blood flow through the dermis, and body heat will be _____ (lost or retained).

4. a) In a warm environment, the arterioles in the dermis will _____ (constrict or dilate).

   b) This will _____ (increase or decrease) blood flow through the dermis, and body heat will be _____ (lost or retained).

5. The tissue in the walls of the arterioles that permits vasoconstriction or vasodilation is

   _____ .

CLINICAL APPLICATIONS

1. a) A severe third-degree burn involves the loss of the stratum _____ .

   b) For a patient with extensive third-degree burns, two potentially serious problems are

   _____ and _____ .

2. Mrs. M. is 72 years old. Her doctor has advised her to be sure to use a fan in hot weather. This is

   important because the _____ glands of elderly people are not as active, and the body

   temperature might _____ sharply during hot weather.

MULTIPLE CHOICE TEST # 1

Choose the correct answer for each question.

1. The outer layer of the skin is the:
   a) papillary layer   b) dermis   c) subcutaneous tissue   d) epidermis

2. The mechanism of heat loss that depends upon evaporation is:
   a) fat storage   c) vasodilation in the dermis
   b) sweating   d) vasoconstriction in the dermis

3. The protein in epidermal cells that makes the skin relatively waterproof is:
   a) keratin   b) collagen   c) melanin   d) elastin

4. The tissue that stores fat in subcutaneous tissue is:
   a) adipose tissue   c) areolar connective tissue
   b) fibrous connective tissue   d) stratified squamous epithelium

5. The glands of the skin that are most concerned with the maintenance of body temperature are:
   a) apocrine   b) eccrine   c) sebaceous   d) ceruminous

6. In the dermis, the receptors for pain are:
   a) encapsulated nerve endings   c) free nerve endings
   b) axons   d) collagen fibers

7. Vitamin D is formed in the skin when the skin is exposed to:
   a) pressure   b) friction   c) stress   d) ultraviolet rays

8. The layer of the dermis that contains capillaries to nourish the stratum germinativum of the epidermis is the:
   a) follicle layer   b) papillary layer   c) collagen layer   d) subcutaneous layer

9. The part of a hair follicle that undergoes mitosis to form the hair is the:
   a) hair root   b) hair shaft   c) generative layer   d) keratin portion

10. The part of the epidermis that undergoes mitosis is the:
    a) stratum corneum   c) stratum germinativum
    b) papillary layer   d) stratum melanin

11. The protein that protects inner living skin from the damaging effects of ultraviolet rays is:
    a) keratin   b) collagen   c) elastin   d) melanin

12. The layer of skin that, if unbroken, prevents the entry of most pathogens is the:
    a) stratum germinativum   c) stratum corneum
    b) papillary layer   d) collagen layer

13. The proteins that make up most of the dermis are:
    a) keratin and collagen   c) elastin and melanin
    b) collagen and elastin   d) melanin and keratin

14. Cells that increase their secretion when stimulated by ultraviolet rays are:
    a) fibroblasts   b) adipocytes   c) keratin cells   d) melanocytes

15. The secretion that prevents drying of the eardrum is:
    a) cerumen   b) sebum   c) sweat   d) tissue fluid

16. At the ends of fingers and toes, nails are produced in structures called:
   a) fibroblasts   b) nail glands   c) follicles   d) mitosis

17. Many white blood cells, which destroy pathogens that enter breaks in the skin, are found in the:
   a) adipose cells
   b) areolar connective tissue
   c) stratum corneum
   d) keratinized layer

18. The dermis is strong because of the presence of:
   a) keratin   b) elastin fibers   c) collagen fibers   d) areolar connective tissue

19. For a person with extensive third-degree burns, serious potential problems are infection and:
   a) dehydration   b) loss of tissue fluid   c) both of these   d) neither of these

20. Some human hair functions to keeps dust out of the:
   a) nose and mouth   b) eyes and mouth   c) ears and mouth   d) eyes and nose

MULTIPLE CHOICE TEST # 2

Read each question and the four answer choices carefully. When you have made a choice, follow the instructions to complete your answer.

1. Which statement is NOT true of the subcutaneous tissue?
   a) white blood cells in the areolar connective tissue destroy pathogens that enter through breaks in the skin
   b) adipose tissue stores carbohydrates as a form of potential energy
   c) it is found between the dermis and the muscles
   d) adipose tissue cushions some bony prominences

   Reword your choice to make it a correct statement.

   _____

2. Which statement is NOT true of the tissues of the skin?
   a) the epidermis is made of simple squamous epithelium
   b) the dermis is made of a modified fibrous connective tissue
   c) fibroblasts in the dermis produce collagen fibers and elastin fibers
   d) in the epidermis, the surface layers of cells are dead

   Reword your choice to make it a correct statement.

   _____

3. Which statement is NOT true of the glands in the dermis?
   a) cerumen is produced by ceruminous glands in the ear canals
   b) apocrine sweat glands increase their secretions in response to emotions
   c) sebum from sebaceous glands prevents drying and cracking of the skin
   d) secretion of sweat by eccrine sweat glands is important to excrete excess body water

   Reword your choice to make it a correct statement.

   _____

4. Which statement is NOT true of the epidermis?
   a) the stratum corneum consists of keratinized dead cells that prevent the loss or entry of water
   b) mitosis takes place in the stratum germinativum, and new cells are pushed toward the skin surface
   c) melanocytes produce melanin that protects living skin layers from bacteria
   d) an unbroken stratum corneum prevents the entry of pathogens and many chemicals

   Reword your choice to make it a correct statement.

   _____

5. Which statement is NOT true of the role of the skin in the maintenance of body temperature?
   a) in a cold environment, vasoconstriction in the dermis conserves body heat
   b) in a warm environment, eccrine glands secrete more sweat onto the skin surface
   c) in a warm environment, vasodilation in the dermis promotes heat loss
   d) in sweating, excess body heat is lost in the process of osmosis of sweat

   Reword your choice to make it a correct statement.

   _____

6. Which statement is NOT true of the accessory skin structures?
   a) hair helps insulate the head from cold
   b) nails protect the ends of the fingers and toes from mechanical injury
   c) the receptors in the epidermis are for the cutaneous senses of touch, pressure, heat, cold, and pain
   d) eyelashes and eyebrows keep dust and perspiration out of the eyes

   Reword your choice to make it a correct statement.

   _____

7. Which statement is NOT true of the dermis?
   a) collagen fibers provide strength
   b) the papillary layer has capillaries to nourish the stratum germinativum
   c) elastin fibers permit the skin to be stretched and then returned to its original shape
   d) it is located between the stratum corneum and the subcutaneous tissue

   Reword your choice to make it a correct statement.

   _____

8. Which of the following does NOT happen when the sun's ultraviolet rays strike the skin?
   a) melanocytes increase their production of melanin
   b) cholestrol in the skin is converted to vitamin C
   c) the epidermal cells take in the melanin produced and become darker in color
   d) living cells in the stratum germinativum may be damaged

   Reword your choice to make it a correct statement.

   _____

9. Which statement is NOT true of the skin?
   a) the skin covers the body and is considered an organ
   b) the epidermis is the inner layer, and the dermis is the outer layer

c) functions include maintenance of body temperature and prevention of the entry of pathogens

d) functions include detection of changes in the external environment and production of vitamin D

Reword your choice to make it a correct statement.

_____

10. Which of the following is NOT made of the protein keratin?
    a) the fingernails and toenails
    b) the hair shafts
    c) the pigment of hair and skin
    d) the stratum corneum

For your choice, state what it is made of.

_____

Chapter 6

The Skeletal System

The skeletal system consists of the bones that make up the skeleton, the ligaments that connect bone to bone, and the cartilage that is a structural part of most joints. This chapter describes the anatomy of the skeleton and relates anatomy to the functioning of the skeleton within the body as a whole.

FUNCTIONS OF THE SKELETON

1. Some bones contain and protect the _____ , a hemopoietic tissue that produces the blood cells.

2. Bones are a storage site for excess _____ (mineral), which is essential for blood clotting as well as bone structure.

3. a) The skeleton is a framework that _____ the body.

   b) Attached to the skeleton are the _____ that move the bones.

4. a) Some bones protect internal organs from _____.

   b) State a specific example of this function. _____

BONE TISSUE

1. Match the following types and parts of bone tissue with the proper descriptive statements.

   Use each letter once. Two answer lines will have two correct letters.

   1) Compact bone _____

   2) Spongy bone _____

   3) Osteocytes _____

   4) Bone matrix _____

   A. Regulate the amount of calcium in the bone matrix
   B. Made of calcium carbonate and calcium phosphate
   C. Made of haversian systems, which are cylindrical arrangements of osteocytes within matrix
   D. Contains osteocytes and bone matrix, but these are not arranged in haversian systems
   E. Bone cells
   F. Often contains red bone marrow

CLASSIFICATION OF BONES

1. Match each type of bone with the proper example (a letter statement) and the proper aspects of its structure (a number statement).

   Use each letter once, and use each number as many times as it is correct. Each answer line will have one correct letter and two correct numbers.

   1) Long bones _____

   2) Short bones _____

   3) Flat bones _____

   4) Irregular bones _____

   Example

   A. Pelvic bone, cranial bones, ribs
   B. Vertebrae, facial bones
   C. Wrist and ankle bones
   D. Bones of the arms, legs, hands, and feet

   Structure

   1. Made of spongy bone covered with a thin layer of compact bone
   2. Each consists of a diaphysis made of compact bone and epiphyses made of spongy bone
   3. The spongy bone contains red bone marrow
   4. The marrow canal contains yellow bone marrow

2. The tissue that covers the joint surfaces of bones is _____ , which provides a smooth surface when joints are moved.

3. The membrane that covers the rest of a bone is called the _____ and is made of

   _____ connective tissue.

4. The periosteum contains _____ that enter the bone itself.

5. a) The periosteum anchors the _____ that connect muscle to bone, and the

   _____ that connect bone to bone.

   b) Both of these connecting structures are made of what type of tissue? _____

6. Below is a diagram of a long bone.

Label the parts indicated.

EMBRYONIC GROWTH OF BONE

1. a) The skeleton of the embryo is first formed of other tissues that are gradually replaced by bone. The process of bone replacement of another tissue is called _____.

   b) The production of bone matrix is accomplished by cells called _____.

2. a) In the embryo, the cranial and facial bones are first made of which tissue? _____

   b) The process of ossification begins in the _____ month of gestation when osteoblasts differentiate from _____ in the centers of ossification in these bones.

3. a) At birth, ossification of the bones of the skull is not complete, and areas of fibrous connective tissue called _____ remain between the bones.

b) Below is a diagram of an infant skull.

Label the bones and fontanels indicated.

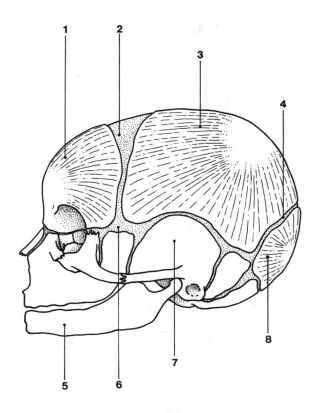

4. Explain the purpose of fontanels and when they become ossified.

_____

5. In the embryo, bones of the trunk and extremities are first made of which tissue?

_____

6. In a long bone, several centers of ossification develop: one in the _____ and one or more in each _____ of the bone.

7. At birth, ossification of these bones is not complete. In long bones, growth occurs at the sites of the _____, which are made of cartilage.

8. The diagram below shows a growing long bone. At each site indicated, state whether cartilage is being produced or whether bone is replacing cartilage.

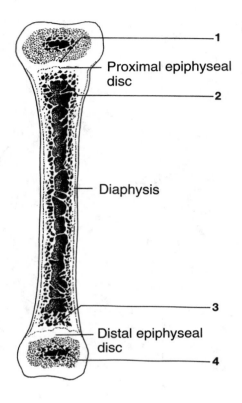

9. Closure of the epiphyseal discs means that all of the _____ of the discs has been

   replaced by _____ , and growth in length stops.

10. a) In long bones, the marrow canal is formed by cells called _____ that reabsorb
       bone matrix.

    b) After birth, the marrow canal contains _____ bone marrow, which is mostly

       _____ tissue.

FACTORS THAT AFFECT BONE GROWTH AND MAINTENANCE

1. Nutrients—Match each nutrient with its function related to bone growth.

   Two letters are used once only, and two letters are used twice. Each answer line will have only one correct letter.

   1) Vitamin D _____
   2) Vitamin C _____
   3) Vitamin A _____
   4) Calcium _____
   5) Phosphorus _____
   6) Protein _____

   A. Necessary for the *process* of bone formation
   B. Becomes part of the collagen in bone matrix
   C. Becomes part of the salts of bone matrix
   D. Necessary for the absorption of calcium and phosphorus in the small intestine

2. Hormones—Match each hormone with its specific function as related to bone growth.

   Use each letter once. In the space indicated, name the gland that secretes each hormone.

   1) Growth hormone _____

      Gland _____

   2) Insulin _____

      Gland _____

   3) Calcitonin _____

      Gland _____

   4) Thyroxine _____

      Gland _____

   5) Parathyroid hormone _____

      Gland _____

   6) Estrogen or testosterone _____

      Gland _____

      or _____

   A. Decreases the reabsorption of calcium from bones
   B. Increases protein synthesis and energy production from all food types
   C. Helps maintain a stable bone matrix and promotes closure of the epiphyses of long bones
   D. Increases protein synthesis and the rate of mitosis of chondrocytes in cartilage
   E. Increases the reabsorption of calcium by the small intestine and kidneys
   F. Increases energy production from glucose

   Name the hormone (from the list above) with each of these functions:

   7) Lowers the blood calcium level _____

   8) Raises the blood calcium level _____

   9) Causes long bones to stop growing _____

3. a) Heredity—A person's height is a genetic characteristic that is regulated by genes inherited from

      _____ and _____ .

b) You already know that genes are the genetic codes for proteins. The genes for height are probably

for the _____ that are needed for the production of _____ and

_____ (tissues).

4. a) Exercise or Stress—For bones, exercise or stress means _____.

b) Without this normal stress, bones will lose _____ faster than it is replaced.

c) Describe what may happen to affected bones. _____

THE SKELETON

1. The human skeleton has two divisions: a) the _____ skeleton, which consists of the

_____ , vertebrae, and _____ ; and b) the _____

skeleton, which consists of the bones of the _____ and _____ and
the shoulder and pelvic girdles.

2. a) Name the part of the skeleton that protects the heart, lungs, spleen, and liver from mechanical

injury. _____

b) Name the part of the skeleton that protects the brain from mechanical injury.

_____

c) Name the bones that attach the legs to the axial skeleton. _____

d) Name the bones that attach the arms to the axial skeleton. _____ and

_____

3. Below is a diagram of the full skeleton.

   Label the bones indicated.

○ Axial skeleton
○ Shoulder girdle
○ Pelvic girdle

THE SKULL

1. Below is a diagram with two views of the bones of the skull; label the bones indicated.

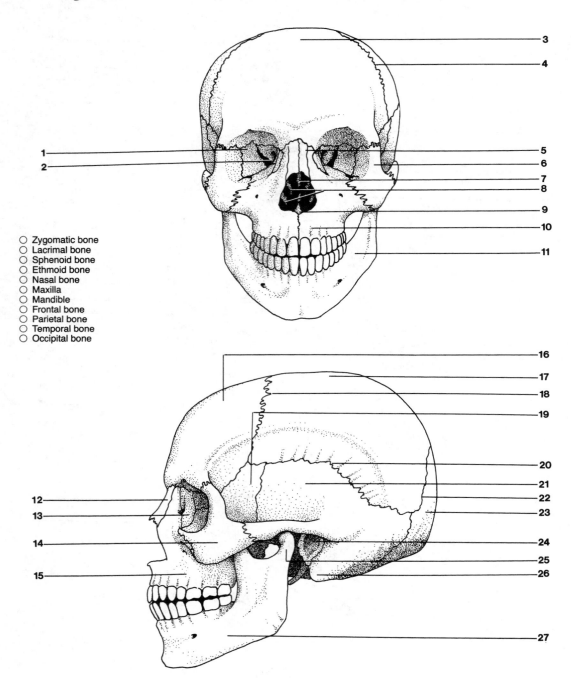

○ Zygomatic bone
○ Lacrimal bone
○ Sphenoid bone
○ Ethmoid bone
○ Nasal bone
○ Maxilla
○ Mandible
○ Frontal bone
○ Parietal bone
○ Temporal bone
○ Occipital bone

2. Name the bone or bones of the skull with each of these functions:

    1) Contain sockets for teeth. _____ and _____

    2) Contains the external auditory meatus. _____

    3) Forms the point of the cheek. _____

    4) Form the hard palate (roof of the mouth). _____ and _____

    5) Contains openings for the olfactory nerves. _____

    6) Form the nasal septum. _____ and _____

    7) Contains the nasolacrimal duct. _____

    8) Contains the foramen magnum _____ , which in turn contains the

    _____ .

    9) Protects the pituitary gland. _____

    10) Form the bridge of the nose. _____

    11) a) Contain paranasal sinuses. _____ , _____ ,

        _____ , and _____

       b) State the two functions of paranasal sinuses. _____

       _____

3. The squamosal suture is between the _____ and _____ bones.

4. The lambdoidal suture is between the _____ and _____ bones.

5. The coronal suture is between the _____ and _____ bones.

6. The sagittal suture is between the two _____ bones.

7. a) The three auditory bones in each middle ear cavity are the _____ ,

    _____ , and _____ .

   b) The vibrations of these bones are concerned with which sensation? _____

THE VERTEBRAL COLUMN

1. The functions of the vertebral column are to _____ the trunk and head and to protect the _____ from mechanical injury.

2. The vertebral column is shown in the diagram at the right.

   a) Label the parts indicated.

   b) State the number of each type of vertebrae.

      1) Cervical vertebrae _____

      2) Thoracic vertebrae _____

      3) Lumbar vertebrae _____

      4) Sacral vertebrae _____
         —fused into one bone

         called the _____

      5) Coccygeal vertebrae _____
         —fused into one bone

         called the _____

3. a) The first cervical vertebra is called the _____ , and the second cervical vertebra is

      called the _____ .

   b) These two vertebrae form a _____ joint that permits _____ movement of the head.

4. The _____ ends of the ribs articulate with the _____ vertebrae.

5. The two hipbones articulate with the _____ of the vertebral column.

6. a) The supportive part of each vertebra is called the _____ .

   b) The bodies of adjacent vertebrae are separated by discs of _____ .

   c) State the two functions of these discs. _____

      and _____

   d) Name the type of joint between two vertebrae. _____

THE RIB CAGE

1. The diagram below depicts the rib cage. Label the parts indicated.

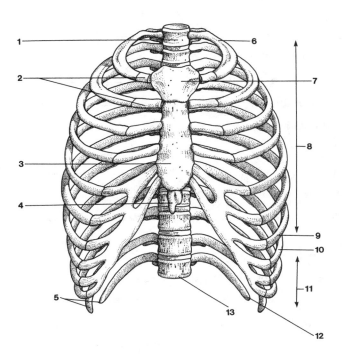

2. There are _____ pairs of true ribs, _____ pairs of false ribs, and _____ pairs of floating ribs.

3. Name two organs in the thoracic cavity that are protected from mechanical injury by the rib cage. _____ and _____

4. Name two organs in the upper abdominal cavity that are protected from mechanical injury by the rib cage. _____ and _____

5. During inhalation, the ribs are pulled _____ and _____ by the external intercostal muscles to _____ the chest cavity and bring about inflation of the _____ .

THE SHOULDER AND ARM

1. The shoulder girdle that attaches the arm to the axial skeleton consists of two bones, the _____ and the _____ .

2. Which of these two bones forms the socket for the humerus? _____

3. a) The clavicle articulates medially with the _____ of the sternum and laterally with

the _____ .

b) Explain the function of the clavicle. _____

4. The _____ of the humerus fits into the _____ of the scapula to form

a _____ joint at the shoulder.

5. a) The two bones of the forearm are the _____ and _____ .

b) Which of these is part of the elbow joint? _____

6. a) The elbow is the articulation of the _____ and _____ .

b) What type of joint is this? _____

7. a) At their proximal ends, the radius and ulna form a _____ joint.

b) This joint permits what motion of the hand? _____

8. a) At their distal ends, the radius and ulna articulate with the _____ , the bones of
the wrist.

b) How many carpals are found in each wrist? _____

c) What kind of joint is found between carpals? _____

9. In each hand there are _____ (number) metacarpals that articulate proximally with the

_____ and distally with the _____ .

10. a) The carpometacarpal joint of the thumb is what type of joint?

_____

b) The joint permits what type of motion of the thumb? _____

11. a) How many phalanges are present in the thumb? _____

b) How many phalanges are present in each other finger? _____

c) How many phalanges are present in one hand? _____

d) What type of joint is found between phalanges? _____

12. The diagram below depicts the bones of the shoulder and arm.

   Label the parts indicated.

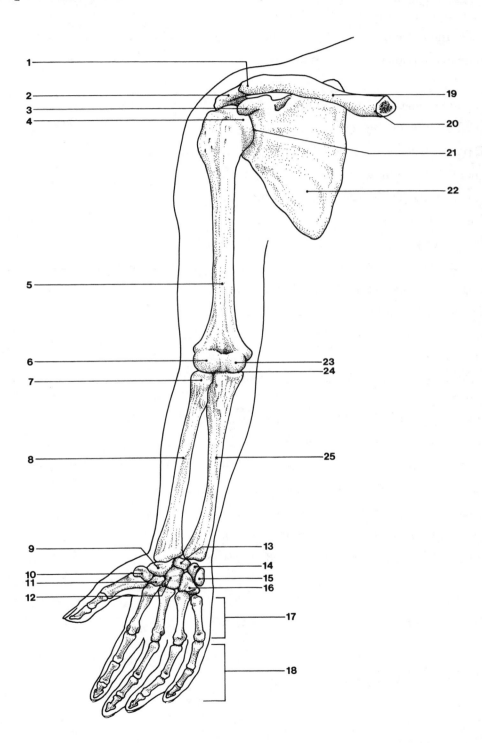

THE HIP AND LEG

1. The pelvic girdle that attaches the legs to the axial skeleton consists of one _____ on each side, that together may be called the pelvic bone.

2. The socket in the hipbone for the head of the femur is called the _____ .

3. a) The three major parts of each hipbone are the _____ , _____ , and

   _____ .

   b) Which part articulates with the sacrum? _____ .

   c) What name is this joint given? _____

   d) Which part articulates with the other hipbone? _____

   e) What name is this joint given? _____

   f) Which part supports the trunk when sitting? _____

4. a) The bone of the thigh is called the _____ .

   b) This bone forms what type of joint with the hipbone? _____

5. a) The two bones of the lower leg are the _____ and _____ .

   b) Which of these is part of the knee joint? _____

   c) What is the function of the fibula? _____

6. a) The knee is the articulation of the _____ and _____ .

   b) What type of joint is this? _____

7. a) At their distal ends, the tibia and fibula articulate with the _____ , the bones of the ankle.

   b) How many tarsals are found in each ankle? _____

   c) Name the tarsal that forms the heel. _____

8. In each foot there are _____ (number) metatarsals that articulate proximally with the

   _____ and distally with the _____ .

9. a) How many phalanges are present in each foot? _____

   b) How many phalanges are present in the big toe? _____

   c) How many phalanges are present in each other toe? _____

10. Below is a diagram of the pelvic bone.

   Label the parts indicated.

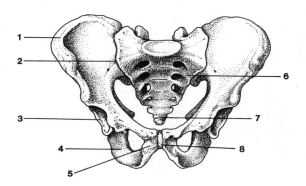

11. Below is a diagram of the bones of the hip and leg.

Label the parts indicated.

JOINTS (ARTICULATIONS)

1. The types of joints are listed in the chart below.

   For each, describe the movement possible at the joint, and give one or two examples by naming specific bones. Some answers have been filled in to get you started.

Name of Joint	Movement Possible	Examples (name two bones)
1) Suture		a. frontal and parietal bones b.
2) Symphysis	Slight movement	a. b.
3) Hinge		a. b.
4) Gliding	Sliding movement	a.
5) Saddle		a.
6) Ball and socket		a. scapula and humerus b.
7) Pivot		a. b.
8) Condyloid	Movement in one plane with some lateral movement	a.

SYNOVIAL JOINT STRUCTURE

1. Match each part of a synovial joint with the proper descriptive statement.

   Use each letter once.

   1) Articular cartilage _____

   2) Joint capsule _____

   3) Synovial membrane _____

   4) Synovial fluid _____

   5) Bursae _____

   A. Lines the joint capsule and secretes synovial fluid
   B. Prevents friction within the joint cavity
   C. Made of fibrous connective tissue; encloses the joint like a sleeve
   D. Sacs of synovial fluid that permit tendons to slide easily across a joint
   E. Provides a smooth surface on the joint surfaces of bones

2. The diagram below is of a typical synovial joint.

   Label the parts indicated.

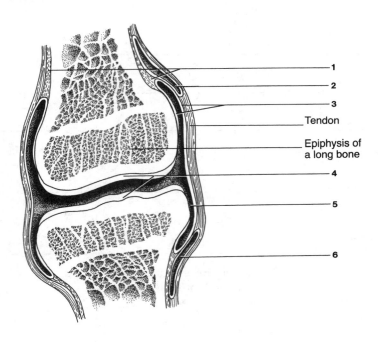

1 _____
2 _____
3 _____
Tendon
Epiphysis of a long bone
4 _____
5 _____
6 _____

CLINICAL APPLICATIONS

1. A 6-year-old boy has a compound fracture of the distal end of the humerus. A compound fracture means that the broken bone has pierced the skin.

   a) The boy's doctor orders antibiotics to prevent infection at the fracture site, because if the

      _____ were to be damaged by infection, the bone would cease to grow.

   b) To repair the fracture, new bone will be produced by cells called _____ .

2. A 76-year-old woman suffered a fractured hip upon getting out of bed one morning. Such a fracture is called a spontaneous fracture because there was no apparent trauma.

   In this case, the bones had become more fragile because of _____ , a degenerative bone disorder that often affects elderly women.

3. Mr. P. sees his doctor because of severe back and leg pain. He says that his symptoms began after he helped his sister's family move furniture.

   The doctor diagnoses a herniated lumbar disc, which means that an _____ disc has been compressed and has ruptured.

4. On patients' charts, fractures are indicated using the anatomically correct name of the broken bone, which may not be a familiar term for some people. How would you explain each of the fractures below to patients or their families?

   1) A fracture of the zygomatic bone _____

   2) A fracture of the occipital bone _____

   3) A fracture of the distal tibia _____

   4) A fracture of the patella _____

   5) A fracture of the clavicle and manubrium _____

   6) A fracture of the mandible _____

   7) A fracture of the phalanges (hand) _____

MULTIPLE CHOICE TEST # 1

Choose the correct answer for each question.

1. The largest bones of the arm and the leg are the:
   a) ulna/fibula   b) radius/femur   c) radius/tibia   d) humerus/femur

2. The nutrients that become part of the bone matrix are:
   a) calcium and vitamin C   c) phosphorus and vitamin A
   b) calcium and phosphorus   d) protein and vitamin D

3. The cells that produce bone matrix and those that reabsorb bone matrix are called:
   a) osteoclasts/fibroblasts   c) fibroblasts/osteoblasts
   b) osteoblasts/osteoclasts   d) osteoblasts/fibroblasts

4. Red bone marrow is found in the:
   a) compact bone in long bones   c) compact bone that covers flat bones
   b) marrow cavity of long bones   d) spongy bone in flat and irregular bones

5. Red bone marrow produces these cells:
   a) red blood cells   d) a, b, and c
   b) white blood cells   e) a and b only
   c) platelets   f) a and c only

6. All of these are irregular bones except:
   a) vertebrae   b) zygomatic bones   c) metacarpals   d) maxillae

7. The malleus, incus, and stapes are within the _____ bone and are concerned with
   _____
   a) occipital bone/vision
   b) temporal bone/hearing
   c) maxillae/chewing
   d) mandible/taste

8. Sutures are the _____ joints of the _____ .
   a) immovable/skull
   b) symphysis/vertebrae
   c) immovable/vertebrae
   d) gliding/skull

9. The fontanels of a baby's skull are made of:
   a) fibrous connective tissue   b) bone   c) cartilage   d) elastic connective tissue

10. The vitamin necessary for efficient absorption of calcium and phosphorus by the small intestine is:
    a) C   b) D   c) A   d) B_{12}

11. An example of a ball and socket joint is the one between the:
    a) femur and tibia   b) scapula and ulna   c) femur and hipbone   d) tibia and fibula

12. For bones, the terms "exercise" or "stress" mean:
    a) becoming fatigued
    b) bearing weight
    c) running 5 miles every day
    d) not having enough protein

13. These bones are all part of the axial skeleton except the:
    a) sternum   b) skull   c) hipbone   d) sacrum

14. In the embryo, the bones of the arms and legs are first made of:
    a) fibrous connective tissue   b) collagen fibers   c) bone   d) cartilage

15. Which bone is not part of the braincase that protects the brain?
    a) mandible   b) ethmoid   c) sphenoid   d) frontal bone

16. Which hormone increases the rate of mitosis in growing bones?
    a) thyroxine   b) insulin   c) growth hormone   d) parathyroid hormone

17. Which of these joints is not a freely movable joint (diarthrosis)?
    a) hinge   b) symphysis   c) saddle   d) pivot

18. In the long bones of a child, the part of the bone that is actually growing is the:
    a) articular cartilage   b) epiphyseal disc   c) diaphysis   d) synovial membrane

19. The hormones that regulate blood calcium level by regulating calcium intake or output from bones are:
    a) growth hormone and thyroxine
    b) calcitonin and parathyroid hormone
    c) insulin and parathyroid hormone
    d) calcitonin and growth hormone

20. The structure not directly involved in the functioning of a synovial joint is the:
    a) synovial membrane   b) marrow canal   c) joint capsule   d) articular cartilage

MULTIPLE CHOICE TEST # 2

Read each question and the four answer choices carefully. When you have made a choice, follow the instructions to complete your answer.

1. Which statement is NOT true of the tissues of the skeletal system?
   a) bone matrix provides strength and stores excess calcium
   b) the periosteum is made of fibrous connective tissue and anchors tendons and ligaments
   c) blood cells are produced by yellow bone marrow found in spongy bone
   d) ligaments are made of fibrous connective tissue and connect bone to bone

   Reword your choice to make it a correct statement.

   _____

2. Which statement is NOT true of hormones and bone growth?
   a) growth hormone increases mitosis and protein synthesis in growing bones
   b) thyroxine increases protein synthesis and energy production from all foods
   c) parathyroid hormone increases absorption of calcium by the small intestine
   d) calcitonin increases the reabsorption of calcium from bones

   For the hormone of your choice, state its correct function.

   _____

3. Which statement is NOT true of growing bones?
   a) estrogen or testosterone secretion stops the growth of long bones
   b) new bone matrix is produced by cells called osteoclasts
   c) a long bone grows as more cartilage is produced in the epiphyseal discs
   d) vitamins A and C are necessary for the production of bone matrix

   Reword your choice to make it a correct statement.

   _____

4. What statement is NOT true of the nutrients needed for bone growth?
   a) vitamin C is needed for the ossification process
   b) protein is needed for the synthesis of collagen in bone matrix
   c) calcium and phosphorus are needed to become part of the bone matrix
   d) vitamin D is necessary for the absorption of calcium by the kidneys

   For the nutrient of your choice, state the correct function.

   _____

5. Which statement is NOT true of the protective functions of bones?
   a) the vertebral column protects the spinal cord
   b) the rib cage protects the small and large intestines
   c) the skull protects the brain, eyes, and ears
   d) spongy bone in flat and irregular bones protects the red bone marrow

   Reword your choice to make it a correct statement.

   _____

6. Which statement is NOT true of synovial joints?
   a) joint surfaces are smooth because of the presence of articular cartilage
   b) synovial fluid increases friction within the joint cavity
   c) bursas permit tendons to slide easily as a joint is moved
   d) the fibrous connective tissue joint capsule encloses the joint

   Reword your choice to make it a correct statement.

   _____

7. Which statement is NOT true of types of joints?
   a) the hinge joint between femur and fibula permits movement in one plane at the knee
   b) the pivot joint between atlas and axis permits turning the head side to side
   c) the ball and socket joint between scapula and humerus permits movement in all planes at the shoulder
   d) the saddle joint of the carpometacarpal of the thumb permits the hand to grip

   Reword your choice to make it a correct statement.

   _____

8. Which statement is NOT true of the skull?
   a) sutures are the immovable joints between cranial bones and between facial bones
   b) the only movable joint is the condyloid joint between the temporal bone and the maxillae
   c) the spinal cord passes through the foramen magnum in the occipital bone
   d) sockets for the teeth are found in the mandible and the maxillae

   Reword your choice to make it a correct statement.

   _____

9. Which statement is NOT true of the vertebral column?
   a) discs of cartilage between vertebrae absorb shock and form symphysis joints
   b) the vertebral column supports the trunk and head
   c) thoracic vertebrae articulate with the posterior ends of the ribs
   d) the hipbones articulate with the lumbar vertebrae

   Reword your choice to make it a correct statement.

   _____

10. Which statement is NOT true of the bones of the leg and hip?
    a) the femur and tibia form a hinge joint at the knee
    b) the only weight-bearing bone in the lower leg is the fibula
    c) the calcaneus bears weight because it is the heel bone
    d) the hip, knee, and ankle joints are all weight-bearing joints

    Reword your choice to make it a correct statement.

    _____

11. Which statement is NOT true of the rib cage?
    a) the seven pairs of true ribs articulate with the thoracic vertebrae and sternum
    b) during inhalation, the ribs are pulled down and in to expand the lungs
    c) the rib cage protects the heart and liver from mechanical injury
    d) the two pairs of floating ribs articulate only with the thoracic vertebrae

    Reword your choice to make it a correct statement.

    _____

12. Which statement is NOT true of the bones of the arm and shoulder?
    a) the joints between phalanges are hinge joints
    b) the hinge joint between humerus and ulna permits movement in one plane at the elbow
    c) the clavicle braces the scapula and keeps the shoulder joint stable
    d) there are six carpals in each wrist and 16 phalanges in each hand

    Reword your choice to make it a correct statement.

    _____

Chapter 7

The Muscular System

This chapter presents the structure and functioning of the muscular system. Gross anatomy and physiology are discussed first, followed by microscopic anatomy and the biochemistry of muscle contraction. Also included are the locations and functions of the major skeletal muscles of the body.

MUSCLES AND MOVEMENT

1. Most of the more than 600 human skeletal muscles are attached to _____ by fibrous connective tissue structures called _____ .

2. a) The most obvious function of the muscular system is to _____ .
   b) State the other function of the skeletal muscles. _____

3. Name the other organ systems that contribute to movement with these functions:
   a) Exchanges oxygen and carbon dioxide between the air and blood _____
   b) Forms a framework with movable joints that are moved by muscles _____
   c) Transmits impulses to skeletal muscles to bring about contractions _____
   d) Transports oxygen to muscles and takes carbon dioxide away _____

MUSCLE STRUCTURE

1. One muscle is made of thousands of muscle fibers. A muscle fiber is simply another name for a

   _____ .

2. a) When muscle fibers contract, how does their length change? _____
   b) In a muscle, the more muscle fibers that contract, the _____ (more or less) work the muscle is able to do.

3. Tendons are made of fibrous connective tissue and anchor muscles to bones. The fibers of a tendon

   merge with the _____ , the fibrous connective tissue membrane around a muscle, and at the other end merge with the _____ , the fibrous connective tissue membrane that covers a bone.

4. a) A muscle usually has two points of attachment to two different bones, and the muscle itself crosses the _____ formed by the two bones.

   b) The more stationary attachment (bone) is called the _____ of the muscle.

   c) The more movable attachment (bone) is called the _____ of the muscle.

   d) When the muscle contracts, it pulls on the _____ and moves that bone at the joint.

MUSCLE ARRANGEMENTS

1. a) Antagonistic muscles have _____ functions.

   b) Synergistic muscles have _____ functions.

2. a) Antagonistic muscle arrangements are necessary because a contracting muscle can only _____ (pull or push) a bone in one direction.

   b) When the muscle relaxes and lengthens, it does not exert force and cannot _____ (pull or push) the bone the other way.

   c) Another muscle is needed to _____ (pull or push) the bone back to its original position.

3. For each muscle action listed below, define the term and state the term that has the opposite meaning.

   1) Flexion: _____

      Opposite: _____

   2) Abduction: _____

      Opposite: _____

   3) Pronation: _____

      Opposite: _____

   4) Plantar flexion: _____

      Opposite: _____

4. a) The parts of the brain that generate the nerve impulses that initiate voluntary movement are the _____ lobes of the _____ .

   b) The part of the brain that coordinates voluntary movement is the _____ .

5. Below is a diagram of the biceps brachii and triceps brachii.

   Label the parts and actions indicated.

MUSCLE TONE AND EXERCISE

1. Muscle tone is the state of _____ that is usually present in healthy muscles.

2. The maintenance of muscle tone requires ATP. When ATP is produced in cell respiration, _____ energy is also released, which contributes to normal _____ .

3. a) Isotonic exercise involves contraction of muscles and _____ of part of the body.

   b) During isometric exercise, muscles contract, but there is _____ of body parts.

   c) Which of these types of exercise (or both) will improve muscle tone? _____

   d) Which of these types of exercise (or both) may be considered aerobic? _____

   e) Besides strengthening skeletal muscles of the body, aerobic exercise also strengthens the _____ and the _____ muscles that enlarge the chest cavity.

4. State two reasons why good muscle tone is important.

   1) _____

   2) _____

MUSCLE SENSE

1. State a brief definition of muscle sense. _____
   _____

2. The stretching of muscles is detected by sensory receptors that may be called
   _____ or _____ .

3. When sensory impulses from proprioceptors are interpreted by the _____ , a mental picture is created of where the muscle is.

4. a) Conscious muscle sense is integrated by the _____ lobes of the cerebrum.

   b) Unconscious muscle sense is integrated by the _____ of the brain and is used to promote good _____ .

5. Briefly explain the importance of muscle sense. _____
   _____

ENERGY SOURCES FOR MUSCLE CONTRACTION

1. a) Name the three sources of energy for muscle contraction, in the order they are used.
   _____ , _____ , and _____

   b) The second and third energy sources are actually used to produce more _____ , which is the direct energy source for muscle contraction.

   c) The most abundant of the three energy sources is _____ .

2. When creatine phosphate is broken down to creatine plus phosphate plus energy, some of the creatine is converted to the waste product _____ , which is excreted by the _____ .

3. Glycogen is made of many molecules of which monosaccharide? _____

4. a) Complete the summary reaction of cell respiration:

   Glucose + _____ → _____ + H_2O + _____ + _____

   b) The energy product used for muscle contraction is _____ .

5. a) The oxygen needed for cell respiration comes from breathing, and muscles have two sources of oxygen, both of which are proteins. The protein in muscle cells that stores oxygen is

   _____ .

   b) The protein in red blood cells that transports oxygen to muscles is _____ .

   c) The mineral that both these proteins contain is _____ .

6. a) Muscles that lack sufficient oxygen are in a state called _____ .

   b) In this state, the intermediate molecule _____ is produced and causes

   _____ of the muscles.

7. The reversal of oxygen debt requires oxygen to enable the _____ (organ) to convert lactic acid back to _____ .

8. With respect to the other products of cell respiration (besides ATP), state what happens to, or the purpose of:

   a) Water: _____

   b) Heat: _____

   c) Carbon dioxide: _____

MUSCLE FIBER—MICROSCOPIC STRUCTURE

1. The neuromuscular junction is the junction of a _____ and a _____ (types of cells).

2. Match each part of the neuromuscular junction with the proper descriptions.

   Use each letter once. Each answer line will have two correct letters.

   1) Sarcolemma _____

   2) Axon terminal _____

   3) Synapse _____

   A. The space between the motor neuron and the muscle fiber
   B. The cell membrane of the muscle fiber
   C. Contains the inactivator cholinesterase
   D. The end of the motor neuron
   E. Contains the neurotransmitter acetylcholine
   F. An impulse is transmitted by the diffusion of acetylcholine

3. Match each internal structure of a muscle fiber with its proper function.

    Use each letter once.

    1) Sarcomeres _____

    2) Myosin and actin _____

    3) Troponin and tropomyosin _____

    4) Sarcoplasmic reticulum _____

    A. A reservoir for calcium ions
    B. The proteins that inhibit contraction when a muscle fiber is relaxed
    C. The proteins that contract when a muscle fiber receives a nerve impulse
    D. The structural units of contraction

4. Below is a diagram showing the neuromuscular junction and a sarcomere.

    Label the parts indicated.

Sarcomere

SLIDING FILAMENT THEORY

1. Match each part of the muscle contraction process with its proper function.

   Use each letter once.

   1) Acetylcholine _____

   2) Cholinesterase _____

   3) Sarcolemma _____

   4) Sarcoplasmic reticulum _____

   5) Myosin _____

   6) Actin _____

   7) Troponin and tropomyosin _____

   8) Calcium ions _____

   A. Releases energy from ATP, then pulls the actin filaments toward the center of the sarcomere
   B. Inhibit the sliding of myosin and actin when a muscle fiber is relaxed
   C. The cell membrane of the muscle fiber; carries electrical charges
   D. Bond to troponin to permit contraction to take place
   E. Released by the axon terminal; stimulates an electrical change at the sarcolemma
   F. Pulled by myosin toward the center of the sarcomere
   G. Found at the sarcolemma to inactivate acetylcholine
   H. Releases calcium ions when stimulated by the electrical change at the sarcolemma

2. A sustained muscle contraction is called a _____ .

3. Explain the relationship between nerve impulses and tetanus.

   _____

EXERCISE—HOMEOSTASIS

1. Match each response to exercise with the purpose(s) of each.

   Use each letter once. Two answer lines will have two correct letters.

   1) Increased heart rate _____

   2) Increased sweating _____

   3) Increased respiration _____

   4) Increased cell respiration _____

   5) Vasodilation in muscle _____

   A. Produces more ATP for the muscle contraction process
   B. Permits the loss of excess body heat
   C. Circulates oxygen more rapidly to the muscles
   D. Permits more oxygen to enter the blood
   A. Produces more ATP for the muscle contraction process
   B. Permits the loss of excess body heat
   C. Circulates oxygen more rapidly to the muscles
   D. Permits more oxygen to enter the blood
   E. Circulates excess carbon dioxide more rapidly to the lungs to be exhaled
   F. Permits excess carbon dioxide to be exhaled rapidly
   G. Increases the blood flow within muscles

MAJOR MUSCLES OF THE BODY

1. The accompanying diagrams show the body's muscles.

   Label the muscles indicated.

   a) Anterior view

b) Posterior view

2. List three antagonistic pairs of muscles among those you have labeled on the diagrams.

1) _____

2) _____

3) _____

3. Muscle Actions

Name each muscle action shown in the diagrams below. Several of these have been completed to get you started.

1) Flexion of head

2)

3) Flexion of arm

4)

5)

6)

7)

8) Extension of forearm

9)

10)

11)

12)

13) Abduction of thigh

14)

CLINICAL APPLICATIONS

1. a) Following a severe compound fracture of his leg, Mr. M. has difficulty extending his foot and

   moving his toes. It is possible that the extent of the fracture damaged the _____ to the leg muscles for these functions.

   b) When a muscle is unable to contract because it does not receive nerve impulses, the muscle is said

   to be _____ .

   c) How will paralyzed muscles change in size? _____

   d) What is the term for this? _____

2. Name the muscle in each of these situations:

   a) A baseball player pulls the muscles on the back of the thigh, and has difficulty extending the thigh.

   _____

   b) An elderly man, following prolonged bed rest, finds his calves painfully stretched when he first tries to walk. _____

   c) A friend says she has a "stiff neck," and she cannot raise the shoulder on that side.

   _____

MULTIPLE CHOICE TEST # 1

Choose the correct answer for each question.

1. The contracting proteins within a muscle fiber are:
    a) troponin and tropomyosin
    b) hemoglobin and myoglobin
    c) myosin and myoglobin
    d) myosin and actin

2. When a muscle contracts, it:
    a) shortens and pushes a bone
    b) lengthens and pulls a bone
    c) shortens and pulls or pushes a bone
    d) shortens and pulls a bone

3. Muscles are attached to bones by:
    a) ligaments   b) fascia   c) other muscles   d) tendons

4. Some oxygen may be stored within muscle fibers bonded to the protein:
    a) myosin   b) troponin   c) myoglobin   d) hemoglobin

5. An antagonist to a muscle that flexes the arm would be a muscle that:
    a) adducts the arm   b) abducts the arm   c) extends the arm   d) rotates the arm

6. The axon terminal of a motor neuron releases:
    a) myosin   b) cholinesterase   c) acetylcholine   d) calcium ions

7. The effect of acetylcholine on the sarcolemma is to:
    a) release oxygen
    b) cause an electrical change
    c) change lactic acid to glucose
    d) remove CO_2

8. The most abundant source of energy in a muscle fiber is:
   a) glycogen   b) ATP   c) fat   d) creatine phosphate

9. The part of the brain that coordinates voluntary movement is the:
   a) frontal lobe   b) cerebellum   c) parietal lobe   d) cerebrum

10. The neuromuscular junction refers to the:
    a) axon terminal, sarcolemma, and sarcomeres
    b) sarcolemma, synapse, and sarcomeres
    c) synapse, sarcomeres, and motor neuron
    d) axon terminal, synapse, and sarcolemma

11. Unconscious muscle sense is integrated by the:
    a) cerebellum, and we are unaware of it   c) parietal lobes, and we are unaware of it
    b) parietal lobes, and we are aware of it   d) cerebellum, and we are aware of it

12. The more movable attachment of a muscle to a bone is called the:
    a) origin   b) tendon   c) insertion   d) wobbly part

13. Good muscle tone is important to:
    a) be able to do strenuous exercise
    b) get rid of carbon dioxide
    c) know where our muscles are without looking at them
    d) maintain posture and produce body heat

14. Muscle fatigue is the result of the lack of _____ and the production of _____ :
    a) oxygen/lactic acid   c) glucose/oxygen
    b) lactic acid/oxygen   d) oxygen/glucose

15. The specific part of the brain that initiates muscle contraction is the:
    a) frontal lobe   b) cerebellum   c) cerebrum   d) parietal lobe

16. During exercise, the blood flow within a muscle is increased by:
    a) vasoconstriction   c) increased respiration
    b) more nerve impulses to the muscle   d) vasodilation

17. The product of cell respiration that is considered a waste product is:
    a) water   b) ATP   c) carbon dioxide   d) heat

18. The organ system that transports oxygen to muscles and removes carbon dioxide is the:
    a) skeletal system   c) respiratory system
    b) circulatory system   d) nervous system

19. The energy of ATP is released within muscle fibers by:
    a) calcium ions   b) troponin   c) actin   d) myosin

20. The unit of contraction within a muscle fiber is called a:
    a) myofibril   b) sarcoplasmic reticulum   c) troponin   d) sarcomere

MULTIPLE CHOICE TEST # 2

Read each question and the four answer choices carefully. When you have made a choice, follow the instructions to complete your answer.

1. Which statement is NOT true of the role of the brain in the functioning of muscles?
   a) the cerebellum coordinates voluntary movement
   b) the frontal lobes initiate voluntary movement
   c) conscious muscle sense is integrated by the parietal lobes
   d) unconscious muscle sense is integrated by the cerebrum

   Reword your choice to make it a correct statement.

   _____

2. Which statement is NOT true of muscles and bones?
   a) the more stationary attachment of a muscle to a bone is called the origin
   b) when a muscle contracts, it pulls a bone
   c) muscles are attached to bones by tendons, which are made of elastic connective tissue
   d) the tendon of a muscle merges with the periosteum that covers the bone

   Reword your choice to make it a correct statement.

   _____

3. Which statement is NOT true of muscle locations and functions?
   a) the deltoid is the shoulder muscle that adducts the arm
   b) the quadriceps femoris group is on the front of the thigh and extends the lower leg
   c) the triceps brachii extends the forearm; its antagonist is the biceps brachii
   d) the rectus abdominus is on the front of the abdomen and flexes the vertebral column

   Reword your choice to make it a correct statement.

   _____

4. Which statement is NOT true of muscle locations and functions?
   a) the gluteus maximus extends the thigh
   b) the hamstring group is on the back of the thigh and extends the thigh
   c) the pectoralis major is on the front of the chest and extends the arm
   d) the trapezius raises the shoulder

   Reword your choice to make it a correct statement.

   _____

5. Which statement is NOT true of muscle tone?
   a) muscle tone is a state of slight contraction
   b) good muscle tone improves coordination and helps maintain posture
   c) the cerebellum regulates muscle tone
   d) muscle tone does not depend on nerve impulses to muscle fibers

   Reword your choice to make it a correct statement.

   _____

6. Which statement is NOT true of the energy sources for muscle contraction?
   a) creatinine is a waste product formed when creatine phosphate is used for energy
   b) the direct energy source for contraction is glycogen
   c) when glycogen is used for energy, it is first broken down to glucose
   d) oxygen is required for the cell respiration of glucose to produce ATP

   Reword your choice to make it a correct statement.

7. Which statement is NOT true of the neuromuscular junction?
   a) the axon terminal is the end of the motor neuron
   b) acetylcholine stimulates an electrical change at the sarcolemma
   c) the sarcolemma contains myoglobin to inactivate acetylcholine
   d) the synapse is the small space between the axon terminal and the sarcolemma

   Reword your choice to make it a correct statement.

8. Which statement is NOT true of exercise?
   a) increased heart rate transports oxygen to muscles more rapidly
   b) isotonic exercise is aerobic because it involves contraction without movement
   c) increased cell respiration produces more heat, ATP, and carbon dioxide
   d) increased respiration is necessary to exhale excess carbon dioxide

   Reword your choice to make it a correct statement.

9. Which statement is NOT true of oxygen and muscle contraction?
   a) oxygen is brought to muscle fibers by hemoglobin in red blood cells
   b) some oxygen is stored in muscles by the protein myosin
   c) oxygen is needed for the complete breakdown of glucose in cell respiration
   d) in the absence of oxygen, lactic acid is formed and causes fatigue

   Reword your choice to make it a correct statement.

10. Which statement is NOT true of the sliding filament theory of muscle contraction?
    a) the sarcoplasmic reticulum releases calcium ions
    b) myosin filaments pull actin filaments toward the center of the sarcomere
    c) troponin and tropomyosin are inhibiting proteins
    d) within a muscle fiber, the sarcomeres contract one at a time

    Reword your choice to make it a correct statement.

Chapter 8

The Nervous System

This chapter describes the anatomy and physiology of the nervous system, one of the regulating systems of the body. The general functions of the nervous system are to detect changes and feel sensations, initiate appropriate responses to changes, and organize information for immediate or later use. These functions of the nervous system are directly related to the normal physiology of other organ systems and to homeostasis of the body as a whole.

NERVOUS SYSTEM DIVISIONS

1. The central nervous system (CNS) consists of the _____ and _____ .

2. The peripheral nervous system (PNS) consists of the _____ nerves and the _____ nerves.

3. The autonomic nervous system (ANS) is part of which division? _____

NERVE TISSUE

1. The term that means nerve cell is _____ .

2. Name the three major parts of a neuron.

   1) _____

   2) _____

   3) _____

3. On the following page is a diagram of two neurons.

   Label the major parts and put each with its proper function.

   a) _____

   b) _____ carries impulses away from the cell body

   c) _____ contains the nucleus of the neuron

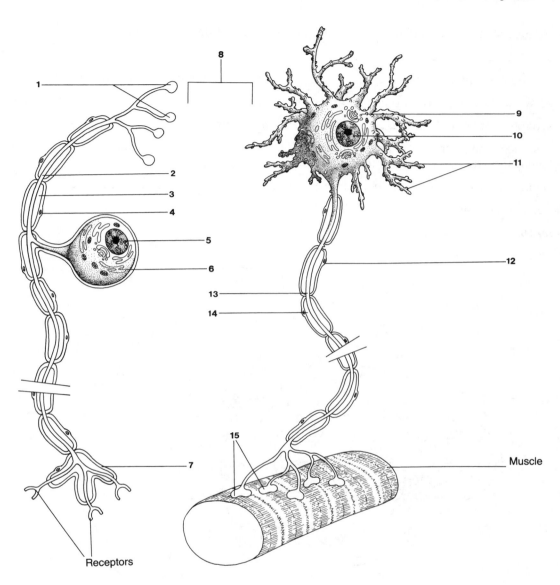

Receptors

Muscle

d) _____ carries impulses toward the cell body

e) The space between the axon of one neuron and the dendrites of cell body of the next neuron is called the _____ .

f) Label the neuron that is the sensory neuron and the one that is the motor neuron.

4. a) In the PNS, the myelin sheath is made by cells called _____ .

b) In the CNS, the myelin sheath is made by cells called _____ .

c) State the function of the myelin sheath. _____

5. a) In the PNS, the neurolemma is formed by which parts of the Schwann cells?

    _____ and _____

    b) The neurolemma permits _____ of damaged axons of dendrites in the PNS.

6. a) At synapses, the nerve impulse is carried by a _____ that is released by the synaptic knobs of the _____ of a neuron.

    b) The receiving neuron contains an _____ to prevent continuous impulses by inactivating the neurotransmitter.

    c) Name the inactivator for the neurotransmitter acetylcholine _____ .

7. The diagram below shows a synapse.

    Label the parts indicated.

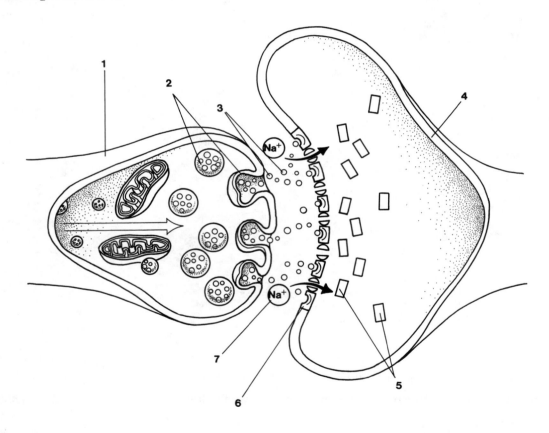

NEURONS, NERVES, AND NERVE TRACTS

1. Match each of the following structures with its proper description.

   Use each letter once. Two answer lines will have two correct letters.

   1) Sensory neurons _____

   2) Motor neurons _____

   3) Interneurons _____

   4) Mixed nerve _____

   5) Nerve tract _____

   A. Neurons found entirely within the CNS
   B. Carry impulses from receptors to the CNS
   C. Also called efferent neurons
   D. Also called afferent neurons
   E. A group of functionally related neurons within the CNS
   F. Carry impulses from the CNS to effectors
   G. Made of both sensory and motor neurons

THE NERVE IMPULSE

1. a) When a neuron is not carrying an impulse, its cell membrane has a _____ charge outside and a _____ charge inside.

   b) The ions that are more abundant outside the cell are _____ ions.

   c) The ions that are more abundant inside the cell are _____ and _____ ions.

   d) The name for this distribution of ions (and charges) is _____ .

2. a) Depolarization is brought about by a stimulus, which makes the neuron membrane very permeable to _____ ions, which rush _____ the cell.

   b) As a result, the membrane now has a _____ charge outside and a _____ charge inside.

3. a) Immediately following depolarization, the neuron membrane becomes very permeable to _____ ions, which rush _____ the cell.

   b) This is called _____ .

   c) As a result, the membrane now has a _____ charge outside and a _____ charge inside.

   d) The sodium and potassium ions are returned to their proper sites by the _____ .

THE SPINAL CORD AND SPINAL NERVES

1. State the two functions of the spinal cord.

   1) _____

   2) _____

2. a) The spinal cord is protected from mechanical injury by the _____ (bones).

   b) In length, the spinal cord extends from the _____ of the skull to the disc between

     the _____ vertebrae.

3. The diagram below shows a cross section of the spinal cord and spinal nerve roots.

   a) Label the parts indicated and complete the statements.

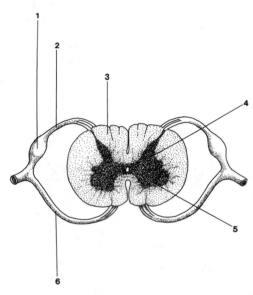

   b) The cell bodies of motor neurons and interneurons are located in the _____ .

   c) The cell bodies of sensory neurons are located in the _____ .

   d) The dorsal root may also be called the _____ root because it is made of

     _____ neurons.

   e) The ventral root may also be called the _____ root because it is made of

     _____ neurons.

   f) The ascending and descending tracts of the spinal cord are located in the _____ .

   g) Ascending tracts may be called _____ tracts because they carry impulses

     _____ the brain.

   h) Descending tracts may also be called _____ tracts because they carry impulses

     _____ the brain.

   i) Cerebrospinal fluid is found within the _____ .

4. There are 31 pairs of spinal nerves, which are named according to their locations. State the number of pairs of:

   1) cervical spinal nerves _____

   2) thoracic spinal nerves _____

   3) lumbar spinal nerves _____

   4) sacral spinal nerves _____

   5) coccygeal spinal nerves _____

5. Name the groups of spinal nerves that supply these parts of the body.

   1) trunk of the body _____

   2) hips, legs, and pelvic cavity _____

   3) neck, shoulders, and arms _____

   4) diaphragm _____

SPINAL CORD REFLEXES

1. Define reflex. _____

2. A reflex arc is the pathway nerve impulses travel during a reflex.

   Number the following parts of a reflex arc in proper sequence.

   ____1____ Receptors that detect a change and generate impulses

   _____ An effector, which performs the reflex action

   _____ Motor neurons that transmit impulses from the CNS to an effector

   _____ The central nervous system, with one or more synapses

   _____ Sensory neurons that transmit impulses from receptors to the CNS

3. Below is a diagram of the patellar reflex arc.

Label the parts indicated.

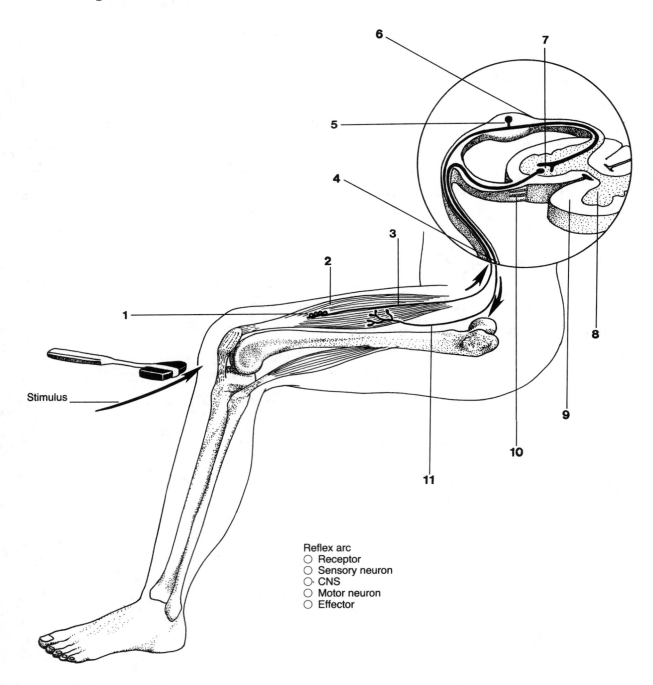

Stimulus

Reflex arc
○ Receptor
○ Sensory neuron
○ CNS
○ Motor neuron
○ Effector

4. The patellar reflex is an example of a stretch reflex, which means that the stimulus is _____ ,

   and the response is _____.

5. a) Explain the everyday importance of stretch reflexes. _____

   _____

   b) Explain the everyday importance of flexor reflexes. _____

   _____

   c) Explain why it is important that these are spinal cord reflexes that do not depend directly on the brain.

   _____

THE BRAIN

1. Match each part of the brain with its proper function(s).

   Use each letter once. Some answer lines will have two or more correct letters.

   1) Ventricles _____

   2) Medulla _____

   3) Pons _____

   4) Midbrain _____

   5) Cerebellum _____

   6) Hypothalamus _____

   7) Thalamus _____

   8) Basal ganglia _____

   9) Corpus callosum _____

   10) Cerebrum _____

   A. Regulates visual and auditory reflexes
   B. Regulates heart rate and respiration
   C. Coordinates voluntary movement
   D. Responsible for thinking and memory
   E. Produces ADH and oxytocin
   F. Connects the cerebral hemispheres
   G. Regulates accessory movements
   H. Four cavities within the brain
   I. Regulates body temperature and eating
   J. Regulates muscle tone and equilibrium
   K. Is anterior to the medulla and helps regulate respiration
   L. Regulates coughing and swallowing
   M. Integrates sensations before relaying them to the cerebral cortex
   N. Contain choroid plexuses that form cerebrospinal fluid
   O. Regulates blood pressure
   P. Encloses the cerebral aqueduct and helps maintain equilibrium
   Q. Integrates the functioning of the autonomic nervous system
   R. Suppresses unimportant sensations
   S. Regulates the secretions of the anterior pituitary gland

2. Match the lobes of the cerebral cortex with the functional areas they contain.

   Use each letter once. Three answer lines will have two correct letters.

   1) Frontal lobes _____

   2) Parietal lobes _____

   3) Temporal lobes _____

   4) Occipital lobes _____

   A. General sensory areas for cutaneous sensations
   B. Taste areas, which overlap the temporal lobes
   C. Motor areas that initiate voluntary movement
   D. Visual areas
   E. Auditory areas
   F. Motor speech area (left lobe only)
   G. Olfactory areas

3. Below is a diagram which shows a midsagittal section of the brain.

   Label the parts indicated.

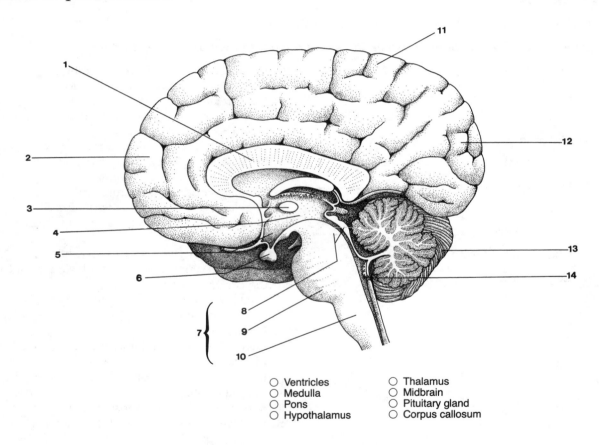

   ○ Ventricles   ○ Thalamus
   ○ Medulla   ○ Midbrain
   ○ Pons   ○ Pituitary gland
   ○ Hypothalamus   ○ Corpus callosum

4. The diagram below shows the brain from the left side.

   Label the parts indicated.

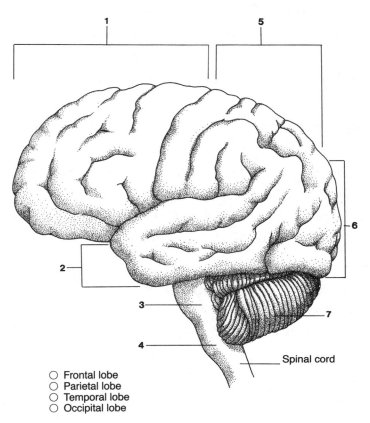

○ Frontal lobe
○ Parietal lobe
○ Temporal lobe
○ Occipital lobe

5. The gray matter on the surface of the cerebral hemispheres is called the _____ and is made of the _____ of neurons.

6. a) The two ventricles within the cerebral hemispheres are called _____ ventricles.

   b) The ventricle between the cerebellum and the medulla-pons is called the _____ ventricle.

   c) The ventricle within the hypothalamus and thalamus is called the _____ ventricle.

   d) The tunnel through the midbrain called the _____ connects the third to the fourth ventricle.

MENINGES AND CEREBROSPINAL FLUID

1. The meninges consist of how many layers of connective tissue? _____

2. a) The outermost of the meninges is called the _____ .

   b) This layer lines the _____ and _____ .

   c) The middle layer is called the _____ membrane.

   d) The innermost layer is the _____ , which is on the surface of the

      _____ and _____ .

3. The subarachnoid space is between the _____ and the _____ and

   contains _____ .

4. Cerebrospinal fluid is formed from blood plasma by capillary networks called _____

   that are found within the _____ of the brain.

5. Cerebrospinal fluid is the circulating tissue fluid of the CNS. Its locations are the:

   1) _____ within the brain

   2) _____ around the brain

   3) _____ within the spinal cord

   4) _____ around the spinal cord

6. State the two functions of cerebrospinal fluid.

   1) _____

   2) _____

7. a) Cerebrospinal fluid is reabsorbed from the cranial subarachnoid space through the _____

      _____ into the blood in the _____ .

   b) Normally, the rate of reabsorption is _____ (faster than, the same as, or slower
      than) the rate of production.

8. The diagram below shows the spinal cord and meninges.

   Label the parts indicated.

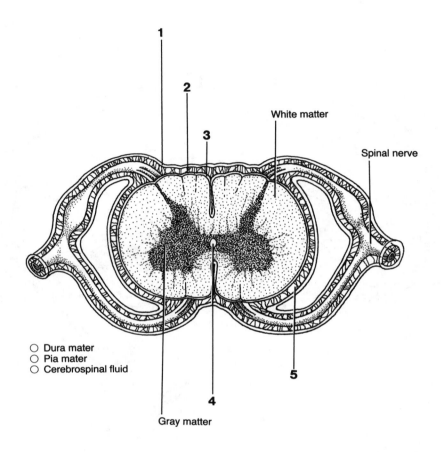

White matter

Spinal nerve

○ Dura mater
○ Pia mater
○ Cerebrospinal fluid

Gray matter

9. The diagram below shows the formation, circulation, and reabsorption of cerebrospinal fluid.
   Label the parts indicated.

CRANIAL NERVES

1. Name the cranial nerve(s) with each of the following functions. Choose your answers from this list.

abducens   glossopharyngeal   optic
accessory   hypoglossal   trigeminal
acoustic   oculomotor   trochlear
facial   olfactory   vagus

1) Vision _____

2) Hearing _____

3) Taste _____ and _____

4) Smell _____

5) Equilibrium _____

6) Secretion of saliva _____ and _____

7) Movement of eyeball _____ , _____ , and _____

8) Peristalsis of the intestine _____

9) Decreasing the heart rate _____

10) Speaking (larynx) _____ and _____

11) Movement of the tongue _____

12) Contraction of shoulder muscles _____

13) Constriction of pupil of eye _____

14) Sensory in cardiac and respiratory reflexes _____ and _____

15) Sensation in the face and teeth _____

16) Contraction of muscles of the face _____

17) Contraction of chewing muscles _____

2. The diagram below shows the cranial nerves by number and their destinations.

   Name each nerve.

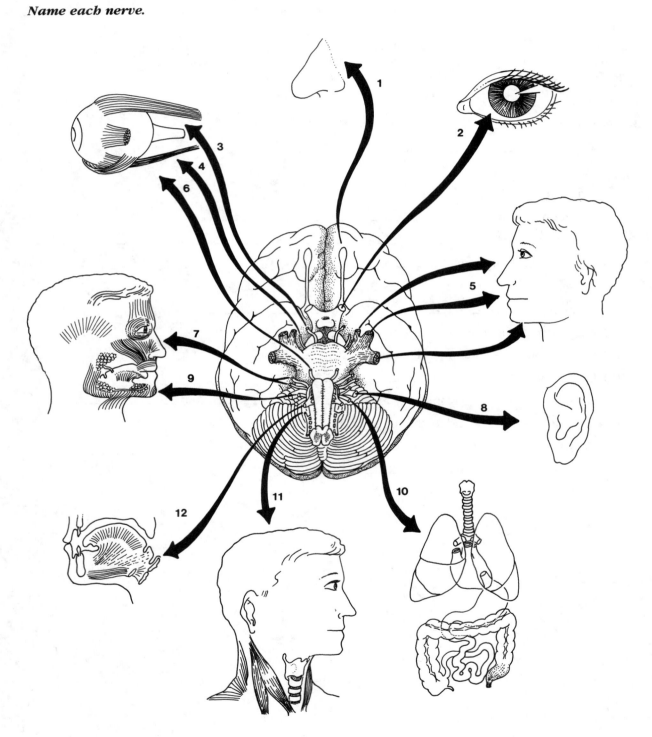

THE AUTONOMIC NERVOUS SYSTEM (ANS)

1. The autonomic nervous system (ANS) consists of motor neurons to visceral effectors, which are

   _____ muscle, _____ muscle, and _____ .

2. The part of the brain that integrates the functioning of the ANS is the _____ .

3. The two divisions of the ANS are the:

   a) _____ division, which dominates in _____ situations.

   b) _____ division, which dominates in _____ situations.

4. Each statement below refers to an aspect of the anatomy of the ANS.

   On the line before each statement, write "S" if it is true of the sympathetic division of the nervous system, or "P" if it is true of the parasympathetic division.

   1) _____ Preganglionic neuron cell bodies are in the brain and sacral spinal cord

   2) _____ Preganglionic neuron cell bodies are in the thoracic and lumbar spinal cord

   3) _____ Most ganglia are located in two chains outside the spinal column

   4) _____ Ganglia are located near or in the visceral effector

   5) _____ One preganglionic neuron synapses with only a few postganglionic neurons, which all go to one effector

   6) _____ One preganglionic neuron synapses with many postganglionic neurons, which go to many effectors

   7) _____ All neurons release the neurotransmitter acetylcholine

   8) _____ The neurotransmitters acetylcholine and norepinephrine are released

5. The diagram below illustrates the pathways of the autonomic nervous system (ANS).

   Label the parts indicated.

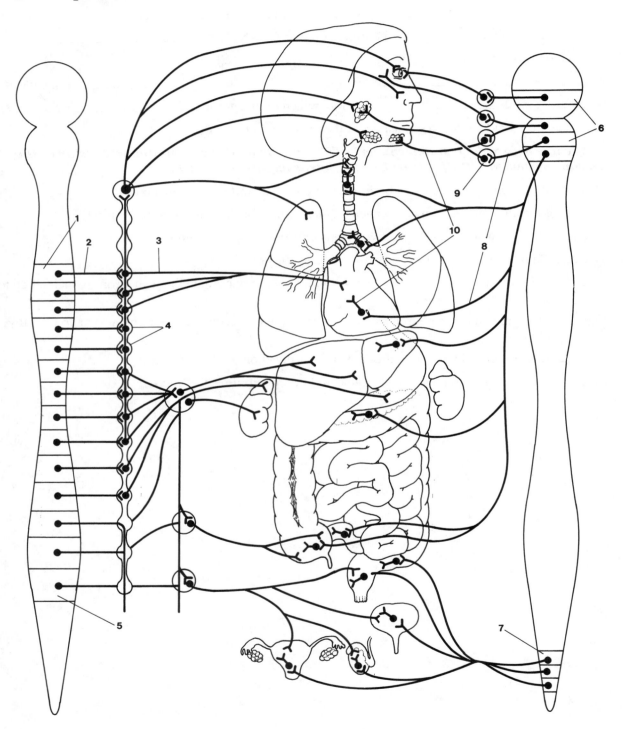

6. Complete the following chart by supplying the proper sympathetic and parasympathetic responses for the visceral effectors listed. Several have been included to get you started.

Visceral Effector	Parasympathetic Response	Sympathetic Response
1) Stomach and intestines (glands)		
2) Stomach and intestines (smooth muscle)		slow peristalsis
3) Heart		
4) Iris		
5) Urinary bladder	contracts	
6) Bronchioles		
7) Salivary glands		decrease secretion
8) Blood vessels in skeletal muscle	none	
9) Blood vessels in skin and viscera		
10) Sweat glands		
11) Liver	none	

CLINICAL APPLICATIONS

1. a) Mrs. C. brings her 5-year-old son to the hospital because he has a high fever and a severe headache. The doctor suspects that these symptoms are being caused by a bacterial infection of the meninges called _____ .

   b) The doctor orders a lumbar puncture. This procedure involves the removal of _____ from the meningeal sac.

2. a) Mr. H. is 70 years old and has suffered a stroke (CVA). He can neither move his right arm nor bend his head to the right. This indicates that the CVA is in the _____ lobe on the _____ side of the brain.

   b) Mr. H. understands everything said to him but has great difficulty speaking to answer questions. This indicates that the _____ was also partially damaged.

3. a) Ms. J. was in a car accident, and her spinal cord was severed at the level of the 12th thoracic vertebra. She will have loss of _____ below the level of the injury, because impulses cannot get from the lower body to the brain.

   b) What other consequence will there be? _____

   c) Explain why. _____

4. a) Mr. W. is a construction worker who is brought to the hospital after being struck on the back of the head by falling debris. He is awake and oriented, and the following assessments are performed to determine if any brain damage has occurred. Pulse, blood pressure, and respirations are all within normal limits. This indicates that the _____ is functioning properly.

   b) Vision is normal. This indicates that the _____ lobes have not been damaged.

   c) Coordination is good, and Mr. W. can touch his nose or ear when asked to do so. This indicates that the _____ is functioning normally.

MULTIPLE CHOICE TEST # 1

Choose the correct answer for each question.

1. The part of the brain that initiates voluntary movement is the:
   a) cerebellum   b) parietal lobes   c) frontal lobes   d) hypothalamus

2. Neurons that carry impulses from receptors to the CNS are called:
   a) sensory   b) mixed   c) motor   d) efferent

3. The cranial nerve that decreases heart rate is the:
   a) vagus   b) abducens   c) accessory   d) hypoglossal

4. The part of the brain that regulates heart rate and blood pressure is the:
   a) cerebrum   b) hypothalamus   c) cerebellum   d) medulla

5. Cerebrospinal fluid is formed by:
   a) dura mater   b) choroid plexuses   c) subarachnoid spaces   d) pia mater

6. The gray matter on the surface of the cerebral hemispheres is called the:
   a) cerebral cortex   b) interneurons   c) a nerve tract   d) gray stuff

7. Neurons are electrically insulated by the presence of the:
   a) white matter   b) myelin sheath   c) astrocytes   d) interneurons

8. The part of the brain that regulates body temperature and the autonomic nervous system is the:
   a) thalamus   b) cerebrum   c) medulla   d) hypothalamus

9. During depolarization of a neuron, sodium ions:
   a) stay outside the cell   c) stay inside the cell
   b) rush out of the cell   d) rush into the cell

10. The spinal nerve root that is made of sensory neurons is the:
    a) internal root   c) external root   b) ventral root   d) dorsal root

11. The part of a neuron that carries impulses away from the cell body is the:
    a) myelin sheath   b) dendrite   c) axon   d) Schwann cell

12. At a synapse, a nerve impulse is carried by:
    a) depolarization   b) the myelin sheath   c) a neurotransmitter   d) repolarization

13. Which of these is NOT a sympathetic response?
    a) decreased peristalsis   c) decreased heart rate
    b) dilation of the bronchioles   d) dilation of the pupils

14. The lobes of the cerebral cortex that contain the areas for cutaneous sensation are the:
    a) frontal lobes   b) parietal lobes   c) temporal lobes   d) occipital lobes

15. Within the spinal cord, the cell bodies of motor neurons are contained within the:
    a) dorsal root ganglion   b) white matter   c) ventral root   d) gray matter

16. A reflex is:
    a) an involuntary response to a stimulus
    b) a conscious decision to maintain homeostasis
    c) a sensation to be interpreted
    d) a stimulus to be felt

17. Keeping the body upright is the purpose of:
    a) brain reflexes   b) stretch reflexes   c) flexor reflexes   d) cerebrum reflexes

18. The two cerebral hemispheres are connected by the:
    a) frontal lobes   b) corpus callosum   c) hypothalamus   d) medulla

19. The correct description of the location of a layer of the meninges is:
    a) middle—dura mater   c) outer—arachnoid membrane
    b) inner—pia mater   d) middle—pia mater

20. Which part of the brain regulates muscle tone and coordination?
    a) frontal lobes   b) medulla   c) cerebellum   d) hypothalamus

21. The cranial nerve for hearing and equilibrium is the:
    a) abducens   b) trochlear   c) acoustic   d) vagus

22. Which of the following is NOT a parasympathetic response?
    a) decreased peristalsis   c) contraction of the urinary bladder
    b) constriction of the pupils   d) increased secretion of saliva

23. Which spinal nerve group is matched with its correct number of pairs?
    a) cervical—seven   b) thoracic—five   c) lumbar—five   d) sacral—twelve

24. The descending tracts of the spinal cord are:
    a) made of white matter and carry impulses away from the brain
    b) made of white matter and carry impulses toward the brain
    c) made of gray matter and carry impulses away from the brain
    d) made of gray matter and carry impulses toward the brain

MULTIPLE CHOICE TEST # 2

Read each question and the four answer choices carefully. When you have made a choice,
follow the instructions to complete your answer.

1. What statement is NOT true of cerebrospinal fluid (CSF)?
    a) CSF is formed by choroid plexuses in the ventricles of the brain
    b) CSF exchanges nutrients and wastes between the CNS and the blood
    c) CSF is reabsorbed into the blood in the cranial arteries
    d) CSF is a shock absorber around the brain and spinal cord

   Reword your choice to make it a correct statement.

2. Which part of the brain is NOT paired with its proper function?
    a) pons—helps regulate respiration
    b) thalamus—suppresses unimportant sensations
    c) basal ganglia—regulate accessory movements
    d) cerebellum—initiates voluntary movement

For your choice, state a correct function.

_____

3. Which statement is NOT true of peripheral nerves and neurons?
    a) motor neurons carry impulses from the CNS to effectors
    b) a mixed nerve contains both sensory and motor neurons
    c) peripheral nerves are in the arms, legs, and trunk of the body
    d) sensory neurons may also be called efferent neurons

Reword your choice to make it a correct statement.

_____

4. Which lobe of the cerebral cortex is NOT paired with its correct function?
    a) frontal lobe—initiates voluntary movement
    b) parietal lobe—cutaneous sensory area
    c) occipital lobe—hearing area
    d) temporal lobe—olfactory area

For your choice, state a correct function.

_____

5. Which statement is NOT true of a reflex arc?
    a) the effector responds and carries out the reflex act
    b) the stimulus is detected by motor neurons
    c) the CNS contains one or more synapses
    d) sensory neurons carry impulses from receptors to the CNS

Reword your choice to make it a correct statement.

_____

6. Which part of the brain is NOT paired with its correct function?
    a) midbrain—taste and smell reflexes
    b) hypothalamus—regulates secretions of the anterior pituitary gland
    c) medulla—regulates respiration and heart rate
    d) cerebellum—regulates coordination and muscle tone

For your choice, state a correct function.

_____

7. Which statement is NOT true of the spinal cord?
    a) the gray matter is shaped like the letter H and contains cell bodies of motor neurons and interneurons
    b) the white matter consists of myelinated neurons that form ascending and descending tracts

c) the spinal cord extends from the foramen magnum to the disc between the 1st and 2nd sacral vertebrae

d) the spinal cord is protected from mechanical injury by the backbone and by cerebrospinal fluid

Reword your choice to make it a correct statement.

_____

8. Which statement is NOT true of the spinal nerves?
   a) there are 12 thoracic pairs and 8 cervical pairs
   b) each spinal nerve has two roots; the dorsal root and the ventral, or sensory, root
   c) the cauda equina refers to the lumbar and sacral spinal nerves that extend below the end of the spinal cord
   d) the neck, shoulder, and arm are supplied by cervical spinal nerves

Reword your choice to make it a correct statement.

_____

9. Which statement is NOT true of neuron structure?
   a) the myelin sheath provides electrical insulation for neurons
   b) the axon carries impulses away from the cell body
   c) the nucleus is located within the end of the axon
   d) the neurolemma of the PNS is formed by Schwann cells and is necessary for regeneration of damaged axons or dendrites

Reword your choice to make it a correct statement.

_____

10. Which statement is NOT true of the meninges?
    a) the cranial dura mater has two layers and contains cranial venous sinuses
    b) the pia mater is the outermost layer and is on the surface of the brain and spinal cord
    c) the subarachnoid space is between the arachnoid membrane and the pia mater and contains cerebrospinal fluid
    d) arachnoid villi are the pathway for reabsorption of CSF back to the blood

Reword your choice to make it a correct statement.

_____

11. Which statement is NOT true of cranial nerve functions?
    a) vagus nerves—increasing peristalsis and decreasing heart rate
    b) facial and glossopharyngeal nerves—secretion of saliva
    c) hypoglossal nerves—movement of the tongue
    d) olfactory nerves—sense of taste

For your choice, state the correct function.

_____

12. Which statement is NOT true of the autonomic nervous system?
    a) the sympathetic division dominates in stress situations
    b) the parasympathetic division causes constriction of the bronchioles and decreased peristalsis

c) the sympathetic division causes the liver to change glycogen to glucose

d) the parasympathetic division includes four pairs of cranial nerves

Reword your choice to make it a correct statement.

_____

13. Which statement is NOT true of the nerve impulse?
    a) when not carrying an impulse, a neuron membrane has a positive charge outside and a negative charge inside
    b) during depolarization, potassium ions rush into the cell
    c) during depolarization, the neuron membrane has a negative charge outside and a positive charge inside
    d) during repolarization, potassium ions rush out of the cell

Reword your choice to make it a correct statement.

_____

Chapter 9

The Senses

The senses provide us with information about the constant changes that take place in the external and internal environments. This chapter describes the organs that contain sensory receptors and includes the role of the nervous system in sensation.

SENSORY PATHWAY

1. Name the four parts of a sensory pathway:

   1) _____

   2) _____

   3) _____

   4) _____

2. The purpose (or function) of receptors is to detect _____ and then to generate _____ .

3. Sensory neurons transmit impulses from _____ to the _____ .

4. Sensory tracts consist of white matter in the _____ that transmit sensory impulses to a specific part of the _____ .

5. Most sensory areas are located in the _____ of the brain. These areas feel, project, and interpret sensations.

CHARACTERISTICS OF SENSATIONS

1. Match each characteristic of sensations with the proper description.

   Use each letter once.

   1) Projection _____

   2) Intensity _____

   3) Contrast _____

   A. Some sensations are felt more strongly than are others

   B. The effect of a current sensation may be exaggerated when the brain compares it with a previous sensation

    4) Adaptation _____

    5) After-image _____

C. A stimulus is still present, but we become unaware of it

D. The sensation seems to come from the area where the receptors were stimulated

E. The stimulus stops, but we remain aware of the sensation

CUTANEOUS SENSES

1. a) State the location of the receptors for the cutaneous senses (be specific).

   _____

   _____

   b) These receptors give us information about _____.

2. a) For the sense of _____ , the receptors are free nerve endings.

   b) For the senses of _____ , _____ , _____ , and

   _____ , the receptors are encapsulated nerve endings.

3. The sensory areas for the cutaneous senses are in the _____ lobes of the cerebrum.

4. Referred pain means that pain that originates in an _____ may be felt as

   _____ pain.

5. Give a specific example of referred pain by naming the organ where the pain originates:

   _____ , and the area where the pain is felt: _____ .

MUSCLE SENSE

1. The receptors for muscle sense are called _____ , and they detect the

   _____ of muscles.

2. a) Name the lobe of the cerebral cortex that contains the sensory area for conscious muscle sense.

   _____

   b) Name the part of the brain that uses unconscious muscle sense to coordinate voluntary movement.

   _____

3. Briefly explain the importance of muscle sense.

   _____

   _____

   _____

HUNGER AND THIRST

1. Match each of these visceral sensations with the proper descriptive statements.

   Use each letter once. Each answer line will have three correct letters.

   1) Hunger _____

   2) Thirst _____

   A. Receptors in the hypothalamus detect changes in the water content of the body
   B. Receptors in the hypothalamus detect changes in the blood nutrient levels
   C. Projection is to the stomach
   D. Projection is to the mouth and pharynx
   E. Adaptation does occur
   F. Adaptation does not occur

TASTE AND SMELL

1. Match the senses of taste and smell with the proper descriptive statements.

   Use each letter once. One answer line will have six correct letters, and the other will have four correct letters.

   1) Taste _____

   2) Smell _____

   A. Chemoreceptors are in the upper nasal cavities
   B. Chemoreceptors are in taste buds on the tongue
   C. Impulses are interpreted in a sensory area in the temporal lobes only
   D. Impulses are interpreted in a sensory area that overlaps the temporal-parietal lobes
   E. A cranial nerve that is sensory is the facial nerve
   F. A cranial nerve that is sensory is the olfactory nerve
   G. A cranial nerve that is sensory is the glossopharyngeal nerve
   H. The receptors detect chemicals in solution in saliva
   I. The receptors detect vaporized chemicals
   J. Much of what we think of as this sense is really the other sense

2. Below is a diagram showing a midsagittal section of the head.

   Label the parts indicated.

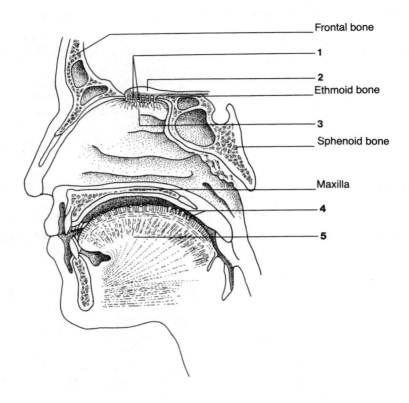

Frontal bone

1

2

Ethmoid bone

3

Sphenoid bone

Maxilla

4

5

THE EYE—STRUCTURES OUTSIDE THE EYEBALL

1. Match each structure or substance with the proper descriptive statement.

   Use each letter once.

   1) Lacrimal glands _____
   2) Eyelids _____
   3) Conjunctiva _____
   4) Eyelashes _____
   5) Nasolacrimal duct _____
   6) Lysozyme _____
   7) Tears _____

   A. Takes tears to the nasal cavity
   B. Mostly water, to wash the front of the eyeball
   C. Small hairs that help keep dust out of the eyes
   D. Within the orbits; secrete tears
   E. An enzyme in tears that inhibits the growth of bacteria on the front of the eyeball
   F. A thin membrane that lines the eyelids and covers the white of the eye
   G. Contain skeletal muscle; spread tears across the front of the eyeball

2. Below is a diagram of an anterior view of the eye's orbit.

   Label the parts indicated.

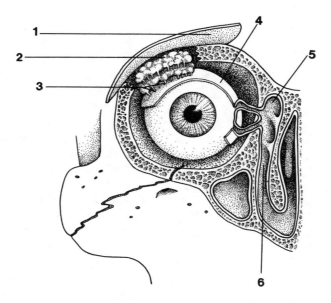

3. a) Also outside the eyeball are the extrinsic muscles of the eye. These are attached to the surface of

   the eyeball and to the _____ .

   b) How many of these muscles are there for each eye? _____

   c) Describe the general function of these muscles. _____

4. Name the cranial nerves involved in movement of the eyeball. The _____ nerve, the

   _____ nerve, and the _____ nerve

THE EYE—EYEBALL

1. a) The eyeball has three layers. The outer layer is the _____ , which is made of

   _____ tissue.

   b) The middle layer is the _____ .

   c) The inner layer is the _____ , which is made of nerve tissue.

2. Match each structure or substance of the eyeball with the proper descriptive statement.

Use each letter once.

1) Optic nerve _____

2) Rods _____

3) Cones _____

4) Optic disc _____

5) Choroid layer _____

6) Ciliary body _____

7) Cornea _____

8) Extrinsic muscles _____

9) Iris _____

10) Lens _____

11) Fovea _____

12) Posterior cavity _____

13) Anterior cavity _____

14) Aqueous humor _____

15) Vitreous humor _____

16) Sclera _____

17) Retina _____

18) Canal of Schlemm _____

A. Contains a dark blue pigment to absorb light and prevent glare within the eyeball

B. The only adjustable part of the light-refracting system

C. The receptors that detect color

D. The part of the retina that contains only cones

E. Regulates the size of the pupil

F. Formed by ganglion neurons, transmits impulses from the retina to the brain

G. Between the cornea and the lens, contains aqueous humor

H. The transparent part of the sclera that refracts light

I. The layer of the eyeball that contains the visual receptors

J. Small veins that reabsorb aqueous humor

K. Between the lens and the retina, contains vitreous humor

L. The area of the retina where the optic nerve passes through; no rods or cones are present

M. Helps hold the retina in place

N. The white of the eye

O. The tissue fluid of the eye; nourishes the lens and cornea

P. Move the eyeball side to side or up and down

Q. Contracts to change the shape of the lens

R. Contain rhodopsin and detect the presence of light

3. Below is a diagram showing a section through the eyeball.

   Label the parts indicated.

4. Name the following nerves that are involved in vision:

   1) The sensory nerve for sight _____

   2) The cranial nerve for constriction of the pupil _____

   3) The type of nerves that dilate the pupil _____

5. a) The lobes of the cerebral cortex that contain the sensory areas for vision are the

      _____ lobes.

   b) These visual areas put together the slightly different images from each eye to create one image.

      This is called _____ vision.

   c) Since the images on the retinas are upside down, the visual areas also turn the images

      _____ .

SUMMARY OF VISION

1. Number the following in the proper sequence as they are involved in the process of vision.

    Light rays $\longrightarrow$ ___1___ cornea

    _____ vitreous humor

    _____ optic nerve

    _____ aqueous humor

    _____ occipital lobe

    _____ lens

    _____ retina

THE EAR

1. The ear contains the receptors for the senses of _____ and _____ .
2. Name the three major portions of the ear. The _____ , the _____ , and the _____

OUTER EAR

1. a) The auricle, or pinna, is made of skin supported by _____ .

    b) Does the auricle have a significant function for humans? _____ Explain why or why not. _____

2. a) The ear canal is a tunnel into the _____ bone.

    b) Name the glands that are found in the dermis of the ear canal. _____

    c) What do these glands produce? _____

MIDDLE EAR

1. The middle ear is a cavity in the _____ bone that contains _____ (air or fluid).
2. Match each middle ear structure with its proper function.

    Use each letter once.

    1) Ear drum _____

    2) Malleus _____

    3) Eustachian tube _____

    A. Permits air to enter or leave the middle ear cavity to equalize pressure on both sides of the ear drum

    B. At the end of the ear canal; vibrates when sound waves strike it

4) Stapes _____

5) Incus _____

C. Transmits vibrations from the incus to the oval window of the inner ear

D. Transmits vibrations from the malleus to the stapes

E. Transmits vibrations from the ear drum to the incus

3. Below is a diagram of the ear.

   Label the parts indicated.

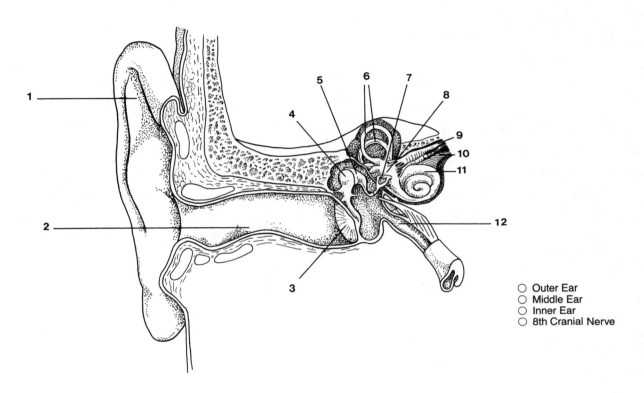

○ Outer Ear
○ Middle Ear
○ Inner Ear
○ 8th Cranial Nerve

INNER EAR

1. The inner ear is a cavity in the _____ bone that is lined with _____ and filled with _____ (air or fluid).

2. Within the inner ear are the structures that contain the receptors for hearing and for equilibrium. Name these structures.

   1) _____ contain receptors for the equilibrium of motion

   2) _____ contain receptors for hearing

   3) _____ contain receptors for equilibrium of position

3. a) All these receptors are called hair cells. Each group of hair cells responds to a different type of stimulus, bends, and generates _____ .

   b) Name the cranial nerve that carries these impulses to the brain. _____

4. a) In the cochlea, the hair cells are part of the _____ .

   b) Vibrations of the _____ within the cochlea bend the hair cells, which generate nerve impulses.

   c) The 8th cranial nerve transmits these impulses to the auditory areas in the _____ lobes of the cerebrum.

5. a) The utricle and saccule are two membranous sacs located in an area called the

   _____ .

   b) Their hair cells bend in response to the pull of _____ as the position of the

   _____ changes.

6. a) In each inner ear, there are _____ semicircular canals.

   b) Their hair cells bend in response to _____ .

7. a) The nerve impulses from the utricle and saccule and the semicircular canals are transmitted to these parts of the brain: the _____ and the _____ , which are concerned with the maintenance of equilibrium at a subconscious level.

   b) And the _____ , which is concerned with awareness of motion or changes in position.

8. Below is a diagram of the inner ear.

   Label the parts indicated.

SUMMARY OF HEARING

1. Number the following in the order that they function in the hearing process.

   Sound waves ⟶ __1__ ear drum   _____ stapes

   (vibrations)   _____ oval window   _____ fluid in the cochlea

        _____ incus   _____ hair cells in the organ of Corti

        _____ 8th cranial nerve

        _____ malleus   _____ temporal lobes

CLINICAL APPLICATIONS

1. a) Mr. G. is 58 years old and has come to his eye doctor to get a new prescription for his glasses. The doctor performs another test and tells Mr. G. that he has the condition called glaucoma. This means that there is excess _____ in the anterior cavity of the eye.

   b) Fortunately, Mr. G.'s glaucoma can be treated, but if untreated, it would eventually damage the _____ and result in blindness.

2. Mrs. A. is 63 years old and does not hear as well as she used to. Her doctor tells her that the auditory bones are not vibrating properly. These bones are the _____ .

3. Mrs. T. brings her 8-year-old daughter Sara to the doctor because Sara's eyes have suddenly become very red, watery, and itchy. The doctor diagnoses a bacterial infection of the membranes that line the eyelids and cover the white of the eye. This membrane is called the _____ , and the inflammation is called _____ .

4. Mr. S. tells his doctor that his vision seems cloudy, even with his glasses. Mr. S. thinks he needs new glasses. The doctor determines that new glasses are not needed but that Mr. S. does have cataracts. This means that the _____ of the eye has become opaque and is causing Mr. S.'s cloudy vision.

MULTIPLE CHOICE TEST # 1

Choose the correct answer for each question.

1. The receptors for vision are located in which part of the eye?
   a) cornea   b) lens   c) iris   d) retina

2. The receptors for hearing and equilibrium are located in the:
   a) outer ear   b) ear drum   c) middle ear   d) inner ear

3. The receptors for touch, cold, heat, and pressure are:
   a) stretch receptors in the epidermis   c) encapsulated nerve endings in the dermis
   b) free nerve endings in the dermis   d) free nerve endings in the epidermis

4. When holding a pencil, you experience the touch of it in the hand. This is an example of:
   a) contrast   b) after-image   c) projection   d) adaptation

5. Bacterial growth on the front of the eyeball is inhibited by:
   a) aqueous humor on the cornea   c) lysozyme in the lens
   b) lysozyme in tears   d) aqueous humor in tears

6. The lens and cornea have no capillaries and are nourished by:
   a) tears   b) aqueous humor   c) vitreous humor   d) intracellular fluid

7. The chemoreceptors that detect vaporized chemicals are the:
   a) olfactory receptors in the upper nasal cavities
   b) taste receptors in the taste buds

c) olfactory receptors in the taste buds
d) taste receptors in the upper nasal cavities

8. The part of a sensory pathway that detects changes is the:
   a) receptor   b) sensory neuron   c) sensory tract   d) sensory area in the brain

9. The shape of the lens of the eye is changed by the:
   a) retina   b) cornea   c) aqueous humor   d) ciliary muscle

10. The pain of a heart attack may be felt in the left shoulder; this is an example of:
    a) visceral pain   b) referred pain   c) adaptation pain   d) after-image pain

11. Which of these cranial nerves is not involved in movement of the eyeball?
    a) optic   b) oculomotor   c) abducens   d) trochlear

12. Becoming unaware of a continuing stimulus is called:
    a) after-image   b) adaptation   c) contrast   d) projection

13. The receptors that detect movement of the body are located in the:
    a) vestibule   b) organ of Corti   c) semicircular canals   d) middle ear

14. The receptors for hearing are part of the _____ within the _____ :
    a) stapes/cochlea   c) organ of Corti/middle ear
    b) cochlea/middle ear   d) organ of Corti/cochlea

15. The visual receptors that detect colors are the:
    a) rhodopsins   b) optic discs   c) cones   d) rods

16. The first part of the eye that refracts light rays is the:
    a) lens   b) retina   c) aqueous humor   d) cornea

17. The receptors for muscle sense are _____ that detect _____ :
    a) free nerve endings/contraction   c) proprioceptors/contraction
    b) proprioceptors/stretching   d) free nerve endings/stretching

18. The receptors for thirst are in the _____ , and they detect _____ :
    a) mouth/changes in saliva   c) hypothalamus/changes in saliva
    b) hypothalamus/changes in body water   d) mouth/changes in body water content
       content

19. The retina is kept in place by the:
    a) sclera   b) extrinsic muscles   c) vitreous humor   d) aqueous humor

20. Keeping dust off the front of the eyeball is a function of the:
    a) tears and lens   c) sclera and eyelids
    b) conjunctiva and aqueous humor   d) eyelids and eyelashes

MULTIPLE CHOICE TEST # 2

Read each question and the four answer choices carefully. When you have made a choice, follow the instructions to complete your answer.

1. Which statement is NOT true of the structure of the ear?
   a) the middle ear and inner ear structures are located within the temporal bone
   b) the auditory bones are the malleus, incus, and stapes

   c) the ear drum is at the end of the semicircular canal
   d) the auricle does not have an important function for people's hearing

Reword your choice to make it a correct statement.

_____

2. Which statement is NOT true of the brain and sensation?
   a) the visual areas are in the occipital lobes
   b) the auditory areas are in the parietal lobes
   c) subconscious equilibrium is integrated by the cerebellum and midbrain
   d) the olfactory areas are in the temporal lobes

Reword your choice to make it a correct statement.

_____

3. Which statement is NOT true of the physiology of vision?
   a) light rays are focused on the retina by the cornea, aqueous humor, lens, and vitreous humor
   b) the visual receptors are the rods and cones in the retina
   c) if too much light strikes the eye, the iris will dilate the pupil
   d) the only adjustable part of the focusing mechanism is the lens

Reword your choice to make it a correct statement.

_____

4. Which statement is NOT true of the physiology of hearing?
   a) the stapes transmits vibrations to the oval window of the inner ear
   b) vibrations in the fluid in the cochlea cause bending of the hair cells in the organ of Corti
   c) the ear drum transmits vibrations to the malleus, incus, and temporal bone
   d) the cranial nerves for hearing are the acoustic or 8th cranial nerves

Reword your choice to make it a correct statement.

_____

5. Which statement is NOT true of taste and smell?
   a) much of what we taste is actually the contribution of the sense of smell
   b) the receptors for taste are chemoreceptors that detect chemicals dissolved in saliva
   c) the cranial nerves for the sense of taste are the facial and glossopharyngeal nerves
   d) the cranial nerves for the sense of smell are the nasal nerves

Reword your choice to make it a correct statement.

_____

6. Which statement is NOT true of the cutaneous senses?
   a) the receptors for pain are free nerve endings in the epidermis
   b) the sensory tracts include white matter in the spinal cord
   c) the receptors for pressure and touch are encapsulated nerve endings in the dermis
   d) the sensory areas are in the parietal lobes of the cerebrum

Reword your choice to make it a correct statement.

_____

7. Which statement is NOT true of the characteristics of sensations?
   a) the degree to which a sensation is felt is called intensity
   b) an after-image is a sensation that continues after the stimulus stops
   c) the effect of a previous sensation on a current sensation is called adaptation
   d) projection is a function of the brain, and the sensation seems to come from the area of the stimulated receptors

   Reword your choice to make it a correct statement.

   _____

8. Which statement is NOT true of the structure of the eye?
   a) the vitreous humor in the posterior cavity helps keep the retina in place
   b) the sclera is the outermost layer of the eyeball
   c) aqueous humor is reabsorbed back to the blood at the Canal of Schlemm
   d) the eyeball is moved from side to side by the intrinsic muscles

   Reword your choice to make it a correct statement.

   _____

9. Which statement is NOT true of equilibrium?
   a) the utricle and saccule contain the receptors that detect changes in the position of the head
   b) the cerebellum and medulla regulate the reflexes that keep us upright
   c) the semicircular canals contain the receptors that detect motion
   d) the nerves for equilibrium are the acoustic or 8th cranial nerves

   Reword your choice to make it a correct statement.

   _____

Chapter 10

The Endocrine System

The endocrine system is one of the regulating systems of the body. This chapter describes the endocrine glands and the functions of their hormones. Each hormone has a role in a particular aspect of homeostasis.

ENDOCRINE GLANDS

1. a) The secretions of endocrine glands are called _____ , which enter capillaries and
    circulate in the _____ .

    b) The cells (organ) on which a hormone exerts its specific effects are called its
    _____ cells (organ).

    c) These cells respond to particular hormones because of the presence of _____ for
    these hormones, often on the cell membrane.

2. Hormones may be classified in three groups based on their chemical structure. These groups are

    _____ , _____ , and _____ .

3. a) The pituitary gland is enclosed and protected by the _____ bone.

    b) The thyroid gland is on the anterior side of the trachea just below the _____ .

    c) The parathyroid glands are located on the posterior sides of the lobes of the

    _____ .

    d) The pancreas is located in the upper abdominal cavity between the _____ and the

    _____ .

    e) The adrenal glands are located on top of the _____ .

    f) The ovaries are located in the pelvic cavity on either side of the _____ .

    g) The testes are located outside the abdominal cavity in the _____ .

4. Below is a diagram of the endocrine glands of the body.

   Label each.

THE PITUITARY GLAND

1. The two parts of the pituitary gland are the _____ and the _____ .

2. a) The posterior pituitary gland stores two hormones that are actually produced by the

   _____ .

   b) The anterior pituitary gland secretes its hormones in response to _____ factors

   from the _____ .

Posterior Pituitary Gland

1. Antidiuretic hormone (ADH)—Its target organs are the _____ .

2. a) The function of ADH is to _____ reabsorption of _____ by the
   kidneys.

   b) As a result of this function, urinary output _____ , and blood volume

   _____ , which helps maintain blood pressure.

3. The stimulus for secretion of ADH is _____ (increased or decreased) water within the
   body.

4. Oxytocin—a) Its target organs are the _____ and _____ .

   b) With respect to the uterus, oxytocin causes contractions of the _____ for delivery

   of the _____ and the _____ .

   c) With respect to the mammary glands, oxytocin causes the release of _____ .

   d) The stimulus for secretion of oxytocin is nerve impulses from the _____ during
   labor or when nursing a baby.

Anterior Pituitary Gland

1. Growth hormone (GH)—Has many target organs and tissues.

   a) Functions:

      1) Increases the transport of _____ into cells and the synthesis of

         _____ .

      2) Increases the rate of _____ , which results in more cells in growing organs.

      3) Increases the use of _____ for energy, by increasing its removal from adipose
         tissue.

   b) The stimulus for secretion of GH is _____ from the hypothalamus.

   c) The secretion of GH is inhibited by _____ from the hypothalamus.

2. Thyroid-stimulating hormone (TSH)—a) Its target organ is the _____ .

    b) Function:

       1) Stimulates the thyroid gland to secrete _____ and _____ .

    c) The stimulus for secretion of TSH is _____ from the hypothalamus.

3. Adrenocorticotropic hormone (ACTH)—a) Its target organs are the _____ .

    b) Function:

       1) Stimulates the adrenal cortex to secrete _____ .

    c) The stimulus for secretion of ACTH is _____ from the hypothalamus.

4. Prolactin—a) Its target organs are the _____ .

    b) Function:

       1) Causes production of _____ by the mammary glands.

    c) The secretion of prolactin is regulated by PRF and PRIF from the _____ .

5. Follicle-stimulating hormone (FSH)—a) Its target organs in women are the _____ and in men are the _____ .

    b) Functions in women:

       1) Initiates the development of _____ in ovarian follicles and increases the secretion of the hormone _____ by the follicle cells.

    c) Function in men:

       1) Initiates the production of _____ in the testes.

    d) The stimulus for secretion of FSH is _____ from the hypothalamus.

6. Luteinizing hormone (LH)—a) Its target organs in women are the _____ and in men are the _____ .

    b) Functions in women:

       1) Causes _____ , which is the release of a mature egg from an ovarian follicle.

       2) Causes the ruptured follicle to become the _____ and to secrete the hormone _____ .

    c) Function in men:

       1) Causes the testes to secrete the hormone _____ .

    d) The stimulus for secretion of LH is _____ from the hypothalamus.

    e) Both FSH and LH have their effects on the ovaries or testes and may therefore be called _____ hormones.

THYROID GLAND

1. Thyroxine (T_4) and triiodothyronine (T_3)—Have many target organs and tissues.

   a) Functions:

      1) Increases the synthesis of _____ within cells.

      2) Increases the rate of cell respiration of _____ , _____ , and _____ to produce ATP and heat.

      3) These functions are essential for _____ growth and _____ growth.

   b) The mineral necessary for the synthesis of thyroxine and T_3 is _____ .

   c) The stimulus for secretion of thyroxine and T_3 is _____ from the _____ .

2. Calcitonin—a) Its target organs are the _____ .

   b) Function:

      1) Decreases the reabsorption of _____ from bones.

   c) As a result of this function, the blood levels of calcium and phosphorus are _____ .

   d) The stimulus for secretion of calcitonin is _____ .

PARATHYROID GLANDS

1. Parathyroid hormone (PTH)—a) Its target organs are the _____ , _____ , and _____ .

   b) Functions:

      1) Increases the reabsorption of _____ from bones to the blood.

      2) Increases the absorption of Ca and P from food in the _____ .

      3) Increases the reabsorption of _____ by the kidneys.

   c) As a result of this function, the blood level of calcium is _____ , and the phosphate blood level is _____ .

   d) The stimulus for secretion of PTH is _____ .

PANCREAS

1. a) The endocrine glands of the pancreas are called _____ , which contain alpha cells and beta cells.

   b) Alpha cells produce the hormone _____ and beta cells produce the hormone _____ .

2. Glucagon—a) Its primary target organ is the _____ .

b) Functions:

    1) Causes the liver to convert stored _____ to glucose to be used for energy production.

    2) Increases the use of _____ and _____ for energy production.

c) As a result of these functions, the blood glucose level is _____ , and all three _____ types may be used to produce ATP.

d) The stimulus for secretion of glucagon is _____ .

3. Insulin—Has many target organs and tissues.

a) Functions:

    1) Causes the liver to change _____ to glycogen to be stored.

    2) Glycogen is also stored in _____ muscles.

    3) Enables other body cells to take in _____ from the blood to use for _____ production.

    4) Increases the intake of _____ and _____ by cells, to be used for the synthesis of _____ and _____ .

b) As a result of these functions, the blood glucose level is _____ .

c) The stimulus for secretion of insulin is _____ .

ADRENAL GLANDS

1. The two parts of an adrenal gland are the _____ and the _____ .

2. The term catecholamines is a collective term for the hormones _____ and _____ , which are secreted by the adrenal _____ .

3. The adrenal _____ secretes a group of hormones called mineralocorticoids, of which _____ is the most important.

4. The adrenal _____ secretes a group of hormones called glucocorticoids, of which _____ is the most important.

ADRENAL MEDULLA

1. Norepinephrine—a) Its primary target organs are _____ .

b) Function:

    1) Causes _____ throughout the body, which raises blood pressure.

2. Epinephrine—Has many target organs and tissues.

   a) Functions:

      1) Effect on the heart: _____

      2) Effect on blood vessels in skeletal muscle: _____

      3) Effect on blood vessels in skin and viscera: _____

      4) Effect on intestines: _____

      5) Effect on bronchioles: _____

      6) Effect on liver: _____

      7) Effect on use of fats for energy: _____

   b) Many of these functions mimic those of the _____ division of the autonomic nervous system.

   c) The stimulus for secretion of both norepinephrine and epinephrine is _____ impulses from the hypothalamus in _____ situations.

ADRENAL CORTEX

1. Aldosterone—a) Its target organs are the _____ .

   b) Functions:

      1) Increases the reabsorption of _____ ions and the excretion of _____ ions by the kidneys.

   c) As a result of this function:

      1) _____ ions are excreted in urine.

      2) _____ ions and _____ ions are returned to the blood.

      3) _____ is returned to the blood by osmosis following Na^+ ion reabsorption.

   d) Therefore, aldosterone helps maintain normal blood volume and _____ .

   e) The stimuli for secretion of aldosterone are decreased blood level of _____ ions, or increased blood level of _____ ions, or a decrease in _____ .

2. Cortisol—Has many target organs and tissues.

   a) Functions:

      1) Increases the use of _____ and _____ for energy production.

      2) Decreases the use of _____ for energy, so that this energy source is available for use by brain cells.

      3) Has an _____ effect, which prevents excessive tissue destruction when damage occurs.

b) The stimulus for secretion of cortisol is _____ from the _____ in situations of physiological stress.

OVARIES

1. Estrogen—a) Its target organs include the _____ and the _____ .

    b) Functions:

    1) Promotes maturation of the _____ in an ovarian follicle.

    2) Promotes growth of blood vessels in the _____ of the uterus, to prepare for a fertilized egg.

    3) Promotes the development of the female secondary sex characteristics, which include

    _____ .

    4) Stops growth in height by promoting _____ in long bones.

    c) The stimulus for secretion of estrogen is _____ from the _____ .

2. Progesterone—a) Its target organs are the _____ and _____ .

    b) Functions:

    1) Increases the growth of _____ and the storage of _____ in the endometrium of the uterus.

    2) Promotes the growth of the _____ of the mammary glands.

    c) The stimulus for secretion of progesterone is _____ from the

    _____ .

TESTES

1. Testosterone—a) Its target organs include the _____ and _____ .

    b) Functions:

    1) Promotes maturation of _____ in the testes.

    2) Promotes the development of the male secondary sex characteristics, which include

    _____ .

    3) Stops growth in height by promoting _____ in long bones.

    c) The stimulus for secretion of testosterone is _____ from the

    _____ .

2. Inhibin—a) Its target organ is the _____ .

   b) Function:

     1) Decreases the secretion of _____ , which helps maintain _____ at a constant rate.

   c) The stimulus for secretion of inhibin is _____ .

PROSTAGLANDINS

1. a) Prostaglandins are hormone-like substances made by cells from the _____ of their cell membranes.

   b) In contrast to hormones, whose site of action is often distant from the site of production,

   prostaglandins usually exert their effects _____ .

2. There are many different prostaglandins with many functions. State three different functions of prostaglandins.

   1) _____

   2) _____

   3) _____

STIMULUS FOR SECRETION—SUMMARY

1. Match each hormone with the proper stimulus for secretion.

   Each letter is used once, and two letters are used twice. Each answer line will have only one correct letter.

   1) ADH _____

   2) Aldosterone _____

   3) Calcitonin _____

   4) Cortisol _____

   5) Estrogen _____

   6) Epinephrine and norepinephrine _____

   7) FSH _____

   8) Glucagon _____

   9) Growth hormone _____

   10) Insulin _____

A. Decreased sodium ion concentration in the blood
B. GHRH
C. Impulses from the hypothalamus during labor or nursing
D. ACTH
E. Decreased water content in the body
F. FSH
G. Sympathetic impulses from the hypothalamus during stressful situations
H. Hyperglycemia
I. Hypoglycemia
J. Hypercalcemia
K. Hypocalcemia
L. LH

11) LH _____   M. GnRH

12) Oxytocin _____   N. TSH

13) PTH _____

14) Progesterone _____

15) Thyroxine and T$_3$ _____

16) Testosterone _____

CLINICAL APPLICATIONS

1. An abnormally high blood calcium level may be caused by an oversecretion of which hormone?

   _____

2. Symptoms of weight gain and fatigue, which indicate an inability of cells to use nutrients for energy, may be caused by a deficiency of which hormone? _____

3. a) The organ that produces insulin is the _____.

   b) Without insulin, the nutrient _____ cannot be used by most cells for energy.

   c) Lack of insulin is characteristic of the disease called _____.

4. A 13-year-old boy is much shorter than everyone else in his 7th-grade class. It is possible that his short stature is caused by a deficiency of which hormone? _____

MULTIPLE CHOICE TEST # 1

Choose the correct answer for each question.

1. The hormone that lowers blood glucose level by enabling cells to take in glucose is:
   a) glucagon   b) cortisol   c) insulin   d) growth hormone

2. The hormone that increases the rate of cell division is:
   a) thyroxine   b) calcitonin   c) insulin   d) growth hormone

3. The two hormones that regulate blood calcium level are:
   a) insulin and glucagon   c) calcitonin and growth hormone
   b) parathyroid hormone and calcitonin   d) parathyroid hormone and thyroxine

4. The hormone that initiates egg or sperm production is:
   a) FSH   b) LH   c) estrogen   d) testosterone

5. In men, the hormone necessary for maturation of sperm is:
   a) testosterone   b) FSH   c) LH   d) aldosterone

6. In women, the hormone that causes ovulation is:
   a) FSH   b) LH   c) estrogen   d) progesterone

7. Two hormones that cause the liver to change glycogen to glucose are:
   a) insulin and cortisol
   b) glucagon and epinephrine
   c) thyroxine and insulin
   d) insulin and epinephrine

8. The hormone that increases protein synthesis and the use of all three food types for energy is:
   a) insulin   b) glucagon   c) growth hormone   d) thyroxine

9. The hormone that slows peristalsis and dilates the bronchioles is:
   a) glucagon   b) cortisol   c) epinephrine   d) thyroxine

10. The hormone that has an anti-inflammatory effect is:
    a) epinephrine   b) aldosterone   c) cortisol   d) calcitonin

11. The hormone that increases water reabsorption by the kidneys is:
    a) PTH   b) oxytocin   c) thyroxine   d) ADH

12. The hormone that increases calcium reabsorption by the kidneys is:
    a) aldosterone   b) ADH   c) calcitonin   d) PTH

13. The hormone that increases sodium reabsorption by the kidneys is:
    a) aldosterone   b) ADH   c) PTH   d) cortisol

14. In women, the two hormones that promote growth of blood vessels in the endometrium are:
    a) FSH and estrogen
    b) estrogen and progesterone
    c) LH and progesterone
    d) FSH and LH

15. In women, the hormone that promotes growth of the corpus luteum is:
    a) progesterone   b) estrogen   c) LH   d) FSH

16. The hormone that stimulates milk production in the mammary gland is:
    a) oxytocin   b) estrogen   c) progesterone   d) prolactin

17. The hormone that causes strong contractions of the uterus during labor is:
    a) estrogen   b) prolactin   c) oxytocin   d) progesterone

18. The hormone that increases the use of fats and excess amino acids for energy while sparing glucose for use by the brain is:
    a) epinephrine   b) cortisol   c) thyroxine   d) insulin

19. Two hormones that help maintain normal blood pressure by maintaining normal blood volume are:
    a) ADH and aldosterone
    b) aldosterone and thyroxine
    c) insulin and cortisol
    d) ADH and oxytocin

20. Localized hormones that are synthesized from the phospholipids of cell membranes are called:
    a) steroids   b) amines   c) prostaglandins   d) proteins

MULTIPLE CHOICE TEST # 2

Read each question and the four answer choices carefully. When you have made a choice, follow the instructions to complete your answer.

1. Which statement is NOT true of hormone effects on the liver?
   a) insulin causes the liver to change glycogen to glucose
   b) cortisol causes the liver to store glucose as glycogen

c) glucagon causes the liver to change glycogen to glucose
d) epinephrine causes the liver to change glycogen to glucose

Reword your choice to make it a correct statement.

_____

2. Which statement is NOT true of hormone effects on bones?
   a) GH decreases the rate of mitosis in growing bones
   b) PTH increases the reabsorption of calcium from bones
   c) calcitonin decreases the reabsorption of calcium from bones
   d) GH and thyroxine increase the rate of protein synthesis in growing bones

   Reword your choice to make it a correct statement.

_____

3. Which statement is NOT true of the hormones of the anterior pituitary gland?
   a) TSH stimulates the thyroid gland to secrete thyroxine and T_3
   b) ACTH stimulates the adrenal cortex to secrete cortisol
   c) these hormones are secreted in response to releasing hormones from the hypothalamus
   d) FSH and LH are called gonadotropic hormones because their target organs are the kidneys

   Reword your choice to make it a correct statement.

_____

4. Which hormone is NOT paired with its correct stimulus for secretion?
   a) calcitonin—hypercalcemia
   b) insulin—hypoglycemia
   c) PTH—hypocalcemia
   d) glucagon—hypoglycemia

   For your choice, state the correct stimulus for secretion. _____

5. Which statement is NOT true of the functions of hormones in stress situations?
   a) cortisol has an anti-inflammatory effect
   b) norepinephrine causes vasoconstriction throughout the body and raises blood pressure
   c) epinephrine increases heart rate and decreases peristalsis
   d) epinephrine causes the liver to change glucose to glycogen

   Reword your choice to make it a correct statement.

_____

6. Which statement is NOT true of hormone effects on the kidneys?
   a) PTH increases reabsorption of calcium ions
   b) ADH increases reabsorption of water
   c) aldosterone decreases the reabsorption of sodium ions
   d) aldosterone increases the excretion of potassium ions

   Reword your choice to make it a correct statement.

_____

7. Which statement is NOT true of the hormones of the posterior pituitary gland?
   a) ADH is secreted during states of dehydration
   b) oxytocin causes release of milk from the mammary glands

c) the target organs of ADH are the kidneys
d) these hormones are actually produced by the thalamus

Reword your choice to make it a correct statement.

_____

8. Which statement is NOT true of the locations of endocrine glands?
   a) the pancreas is located between the duodenum and the spleen
   b) the thyroid gland is superior to the larynx on the front of the trachea
   c) the adrenal glands are superior to the kidneys
   d) the pituitary gland hangs by a stalk from the hypothalamus

Reword your choice to make it a correct statement.

_____

9. Which statement is NOT true of hormone effects on reproduction?
   a) FSH initiates production of ova or sperm cells
   b) LH stimulates ovulation in women
   c) LH stimulates secretion of testosterone in men
   d) secondary sex characteristics in men and women are regulated by testosterone and progesterone, respectively

Reword your choice to make it a correct statement.

_____

Chapter 11

Blood

The blood consists of blood plasma and the blood cells, which are red blood cells, white blood cells, and platelets. As blood circulates, each component carries out specific functions that are essential for homeostasis. This chapter describes the components of blood and their functions.

GENERAL FUNCTIONS OF BLOOD

1. Match each function of blood with the proper examples.

   Use each letter once. Each answer line will have more than one correct letter.

   1) Transportation _____
   2) Regulation _____
   3) Protection _____

   A. Acid-base balance
   B. Blood clotting
   C. Destroys pathogens
   D. Nutrients and waste products
   E. Body temperature
   F. Fluid-electrolyte balance
   G. Gases and hormones

CHARACTERISTICS OF BLOOD

1. The amount of blood within the body varies with the size of the person; this amount is in the range of _____ liters.

2. a) The blood cells make up _____ % to _____ % of the total blood.

   b) The blood plasma makes up _____ % to _____ % of the total blood.

3. a) The normal pH range of blood is _____ to _____ .

   b) This pH range is slightly _____ .

4. a) The viscosity of blood refers to its _____ .

   b) The presence of _____ and _____ make blood more viscous than water.

BLOOD PLASMA

1. Blood plasma is approximately _____ % water.

2. a) The water of plasma is a solvent, which means that substances may _____ in this water and be transported.

   b) Name two types of substances that are transported in dissolved form in the plasma. _____ and _____

3. a) Carbon dioxide is carried in the plasma in the form of _____ ions.

   b) State the chemical formula of this ion. _____

4. Match each plasma protein with the proper descriptive statements.

   One letter is used twice, and each other letter is used once. Each answer line will have three correct letters.

   1) Albumin _____

   2) Clotting factors _____

   3) Globulins _____

   A. Synthesized only by the liver
   B. Synthesized by lymphocytes or by the liver
   C. Include fibrinogen and prothrombin
   D. Pulls tissue fluid into capillaries to maintain blood volume
   E. Include antibodies
   F. The most abundant plasma protein
   G. Help prevent blood loss when blood vessels rupture
   H. Include carrier molecules for fats in the blood

HEMOPOIETIC TISSUES

1. The term hemopoietic tissue means a tissue in which _____ are formed.

2. The two types of hemopoietic tissues are _____ and _____ .

3. a) Red bone marrow is found in _____ and _____ bones.

   b) Lymphatic tissue is found in lymphatic organs such as the _____ and _____ .

4. a) Name the two types of WBCs formed in lymphatic tissue. _____ and _____

   b) Name the types of cells formed in red bone marrow. _____ , _____ , and _____

5. Below is a diagram of hemopoietic tissues.

   Label each one.

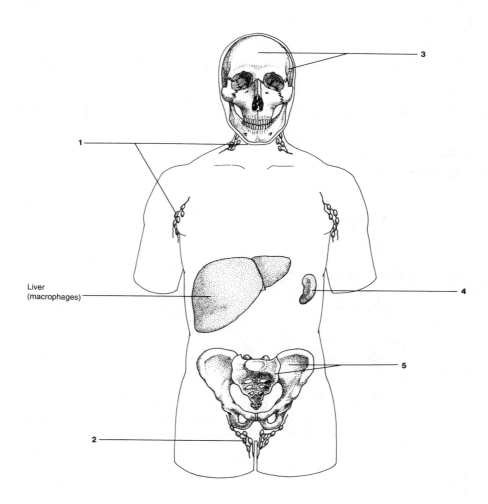

Liver
(macrophages)

RED BLOOD CELLS

1. a) Red blood cells (RBCs) are also called _____ and are formed in

   _____ .

   b What major cellular structure do mature RBCs lack? _____

   c) Describe the appearance of RBCs. _____

2. a) The oxygen-carrying protein in RBCs is _____ .

   b) The oxygen-carrying mineral in hemoglobin is _____ .

3. a) RBCs pick up oxygen when they circulate through the _____ capillaries (in the

_____), and this hemoglobin is now called _____ .

   b) RBCs release oxygen in _____ capillaries, and their hemoglobin is then called

_____ .

4. a) In the red bone marrow, the precursor cell for all the types of blood cells is called the

_____ .

   b) These cells constantly undergo the process of _____ to produce new cells, most
   of which will become RBCs.

5. Below is a diagram of blood cell types.

   Label the cells indicated.

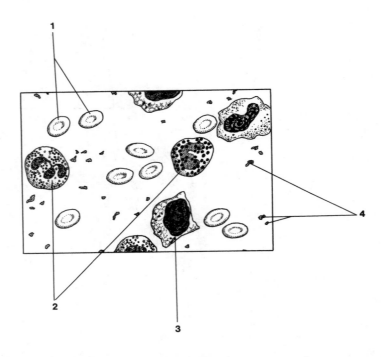

6. a) The major regulating factor for RBC production is the amount of _____ in the
   blood.

   b) The term "hypoxia" means _____ .

   c) When hypoxia occurs, the kidneys produce a hormone called _____ , which

   stimulates the red bone marrow to increase the rate of _____ .

7. a) In RBC formation, the last stage with a nucleus is called a _____ .

   b) The stage in which fragments of the ER are present is called a _____ .

c) When these immature RBCs are present in large numbers in circulating blood, it means that there are not enough _____ to transport sufficient _____ throughout the body.

8. a) The nutrients needed for RBC formation include _____ and _____ , which will become part of the hemoglobin molecule.

   b) The extrinsic factor is _____ that is needed for the synthesis of _____ by the stem cells in the red bone marrow.

   c) The intrinsic factor is produced by the lining of the _____ (organ).

   d) The function of intrinsic factor is to prevent the digestion of _____ and promote its absorption in the small intestine.

9. a) The lifespan of RBCs is approximately _____ days.

   b) The organs that contain macrophages (RE cells) to phagocytize old RBCs are the _____ , the _____ , and the _____ .

   c) The iron from old RBCs may be stored in the _____ or transported to the red bone marrow for the synthesis of new _____ .

10. a) The heme portion of the hemoglobin of old RBCs is converted to _____ by RE cells.

    b) Since it has no usefulness, bilirubin is considered a waste product. It is removed from circulation by the _____ (organ) and excreted into _____ .

    c) The colon eliminates bilirubin in _____ .

11. a) If the blood level of bilirubin rises, perhaps because of liver disease, the _____ may appear yellow.

    b) This is called _____ .

12. CBC values:

    1) The range of a normal RBC count is _____ to _____ cells/mm^3.

    2) The range of a normal hematocrit (Hct) is _____ % to _____ %.

    3) The range of normal hemoglobin (Hb) level is _____ to _____ grams/100 ml.

RED BLOOD CELL TYPES

1. The two most important RBC types are the _____ group and the _____ factor.

2. The ABO group contains four blood types, which are _____ , _____ , _____ , and _____ .

3. Complete the following chart with respect to RBC antigens and plasma antibodies for the four ABO group blood types.

	Type A	Type B	Type AB	Type O
Antigens present on RBCs				
Antibodies present in plasma				

4. Below is a diagram of RBCs representing each of the above blood types.

   Label the antigens and antibodies indicated.

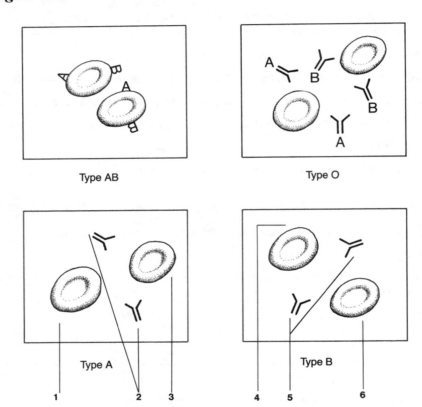

Type AB

Type O

Type A

Type B

1   2   3   4   5   6

5. a) The Rh factor is another RBC antigen; it is often called D. A person who is Rh

   _____ has this antigen on the RBCs. A person who is Rh _____
   does not have this antigen on the RBCs.

   b) Are anti-Rh antibodies naturally present in the plasma of a person who is Rh negative? _____

   c) When would such antibodies be formed? _____

6. a) If a patient receives a transfusion of an incompatible blood type, the donated RBCs will rupture;

   this is called _____ .

b) The most serious effects of such a transfusion reaction occur in the _____

(organ), when the capillaries there become clogged by _____ from the ruptured RBCs.

WHITE BLOOD CELLS

1. a) White blood cells (WBCs) are also called _____ .

   b) The five kinds of WBCs are in two groups called _____ and

   _____ .

2. a) The granular WBCs are produced in the _____ .

   b) The three kinds are _____ , _____ , and _____ .

   c) The agranular WBCs are produced in _____ tissue as well as in the red bone marrow.

   d) The two kinds are _____ and _____ .

3. In appearance, WBCs differ from RBCs in that all WBCs have _____ present when the cells are mature.

4. The general function of WBCs is to protect the body from _____ and to provide

   _____ to certain infectious diseases.

5. Match each kind of WBC with its proper functions.

   Use each letter once. Two answer lines will have two correct letters.

   1) Neutrophils _____

   2) Monocytes _____

   3) T lymphocytes _____

   4) B lymphocytes _____

   5) Basophils _____

   6) Eosinophils _____

   A. The most abundant phagocytes
   B. Become macrophages to phagocytize pathogens or damaged tissue
   C. Contain heparin to prevent abnormal blood clotting
   D. Detoxify foreign proteins
   E. Help recognize foreign antigens
   F. Become plasma cells that produce antibodies
   G. Contain histamine, which contributes to inflammation
   H. Important in allergic reactions and parasitic infections

6. CBC values:

   1) The range of a normal WBC count is _____ to _____ cells/mm^3.

   2) A high WBC count is called _____ and often indicates _____ .

   3) A low WBC count is called _____ . State one cause. _____

PLATELETS

1. Platelets are also called _____ and are formed in _____ .

2. Platelets are fragments of the large bone marrow cells called _____ .

3. a) The function of platelets is hemostasis, which means _____ .

   b) The three mechanisms of hemostasis are _____ , _____ , and

   _____ .

4. Vascular spasm is the mechanism of hemostasis necessary in large vessels that are ruptured or cut.

   a) What tissue in arteries and veins permits them to constrict? _____

   b) This tissue contracts in response to _____ released by platelets or to the

   _____ caused when the vessel ruptures.

   c) As a result, the opening in the vessel is made _____ and may then be covered by

   a _____ .

5. a) Platelet plugs are the only effective mechanism of hemostasis for rupture of

   _____ (type of vessel).

   b) The rough surface of a ruptured capillary causes platelets to _____ and form a
   mechanical barrier over the opening.

6. The range of a normal platelet count is _____ to _____ cells/mm³.

7. The term for a low platelet count is _____ .

CHEMICAL BLOOD CLOTTING

1. The stimulus for chemical clotting is a _____ surface within a vessel or a break in a

   vessel that also creates a _____ surface.

2. The clotting factors such as prothrombin and fibrinogen are synthesized by the

   _____ and circulate in the _____ until activated in the clotting
   mechanism.

3. a) The vitamin necessary for prothrombin synthesis is _____ .

   b) Most of a person's supply of this vitamin is produced by the _____ in the person's

   own _____ .

4. The mineral necessary for chemical clotting is _____ , which the body stores in

   _____ .

5. a) Stage 1 of clotting involves chemical factors released by _____ and other

   chemicals from _____ .

b) The result of stage 1 is the formation of _____ .

c) In stage 2, _____ converts prothrombin to _____ .

d) In stage 3, _____ converts fibrinogen to _____ .

e) The clot itself is made of _____ , which forms a mesh over the break in the vessel.

6. a) The process of clot _____ pulls the edges of the break in the vessel together,
which makes _____ of the area easier.

b) Once a clot has accomplished its function, it is dissolved in a process called
_____ .

7. Abnormal clotting within vessels is prevented in several ways.

a) The _____ epithelium that lines blood vessels is very smooth and repels platelets.

b) An anticoagulant produced by basophils is _____ .

c) Antithrombin is produced by the _____ to inactivate excess
_____ .

8. a) The term for an abnormal clot in an intact vessel is _____ .

b) The term for a clot that dislodges and travels to another vessel is _____ .

CLINICAL APPLICATIONS

1. The lab results for a particular patient show these CBC values:

   RBCs—4.9 million/mm^3 Hb—14 grams/100 ml
   Hct—42%   WBCs—23,000/mm^3
                                    platelets—190,000/mm^3

   Based on these values, you would expect that this patient _____. (choose one answer)
   a) is anemic
   b) has an infection
   c) is experiencing bruising and bleeding
   d) is in good health, because all these values are within normal ranges

2. Mr. and Mrs. R.'s first child has been diagnosed with hemophilia A. The parents have been very worried about the episodes of prolonged bleeding their son has experienced, but they are assured by their doctor that this form of hemophilia can be controlled. The missing clotting factor is _____ ,
   which is usually produced by the _____

3. a) Mrs. C. has just given birth to her second child, and the baby is severely jaundiced. She is told that
   the baby has Rh disease of the newborn, which may also be called _____ .

   b) Based on this information, you can now say that Mrs. C. is Rh _____ , Mr. C. is Rh
   _____ , Baby C. is Rh _____ , and the first child was probably Rh _____ .

c) If this were Mrs. C.'s first pregnancy, she could have been given RhoGam to prevent this from happening again in a later pregnancy. Explain what RhoGam would have done.

_____

MULTIPLE CHOICE TEST #1

Choose the correct answer for each question.

1. Lymphatic tissue produces:
   a) monocytes and neutrophils
   b) lymphocytes and monocytes
   c) basophils and neutrophils
   d) all five types of WBCs

2. A person with type AB blood has:
   a) A and B antigens on the RBCs and neither anti-A nor anti-B antibodies in the plasma
   b) A antigens on the RBCs and anti-B antibodies in the plasma
   c) B antigens on the RBCs and anti-A antibodies in the plasma
   d) A and B antibodies on the RBCs and no antigens in the plasma

3. The plasma protein that helps maintain blood volume by pulling tissue fluid into capillaries is:
   a) prothrombin b) albumin c) gamma globulin d) hemoglobin

4. The WBCs that recognize foreign antigens and produce antibodies are:
   a) monocytes b) neutrophils c) lymphocytes d) eosinophils

5. When old RBCs are destroyed, the waste product _____ is formed and then excreted by the _____.
   a) iron/kidneys, in urine
   b) bilirubin/liver, in bile
   c) hemoglobin/liver, in bile
   d) bilirubin/kidneys, in urine

6. The red bone marrow produces:
   a) RBCs only
   b) RBCs and platelets only
   c) RBCs and WBCs only
   d) all the types of blood cells

7. The cells in the hemopoietic tissues that undergo mitosis to produce all the types of blood cells are called:
   a) normoblasts b) stem cells c) reticulocytes d) megakaryocytes

8. Plasma makes up _____ % of the total blood and is itself _____ % water.
   a) 52%–62%/91% b) 91%–92%/55% c) 65%–75%/80% d) 50%–60%/50%

9. The extrinsic factor needed for DNA synthesis in the red bone marrow is:
   a) calcium b) vitamin B_{12} c) vitamin K d) iron

10. The organ that produces erythropoietin during hypoxia is the:
    a) liver b) red bone marrow c) spleen d) kidney

11. The oxygen-carrying protein of RBCs is:
    a) prothrombin b) hemoglobin c) myoglobin d) erythropoietin

12. A blood clot is made of:
    a) thrombin b) fibrinogen c) fibrin d) prothrombin activator

13. The mineral needed for chemical clotting is:
    a) sodium b) calcium c) iron d) potassium

14. The normal pH range of blood is:
    a) 7.15–7.25, slightly alkaline
    b) 7.35–7.45, slightly alkaline
    c) 7.00–7.15, neutral
    d) 7.45–7.55, slightly acidic

15. A large artery that is cut can contract in vascular spasm because its wall contains:
    a) smooth muscle
    b) elastic connective tissue
    c) blood
    d) simple squamous epithelium

16. The stimulus for the formation of a platelet plug or a blood clot is:
    a) a rough surface
    b) a smooth surface
    c) a very smooth surface
    d) an intact vessel lining

17. Lymphatic tissue is found in all of these except the:
    a) lymph nodes   b) thymus gland   c) liver   d) spleen

18. A hematocrit is a measure of the:
    a) percent of WBCs in the total blood
    b) percent of blood in the body fluids
    c) percent of plasma in total blood
    d) percent of RBCs in the total blood

19. An abnormal clot that forms on a rough surface in an intact vessel is called:
    a) a thrombus   b) an embolism   c) a platelet plug   d) inflammation

20. The Rh factor is an antigen that is found on the:
    a) WBCs of people who are Rh negative
    b) RBCs of people who are Rh negative
    c) WBCs of people who are Rh positive
    d) RBCs of people who are Rh positive

MULTIPLE CHOICE TEST #2

Read each question and the four answer choices carefully. When you have made a choice, follow the instructions to complete your answer.

1. Which of the following is NOT transported by blood plasma?
   a) carbon dioxide   b) nutrients   c) hormones   d) oxygen

   For your choice, state how it is transported in the blood.

   _____

2. Which statement is NOT true of the functions of WBCs?
   a) lymphocytes produce antibodies
   b) neutrophils help detoxify foreign proteins
   c) monocytes become macrophages that phagocytize pathogens
   d) basophils contain heparin and histamine

   For your choice, state the type of WBC that does have this function.

   _____

3. Which statement is NOT true of RBC formation?
   a) red bone marrow is found in flat and irregular bones
   b) the nutrients iron and protein are needed to become part of hemoglobin

c) the intrinsic factor is produced by the liver to prevent digestion of vitamin B_{12}
d) erythropoietin increases the rate of RBC production in the red bone marrow

Reword your choice to make it a correct statement.

___

4. Which statement is NOT true of chemical blood clotting?
   a) the mineral necessary is calcium
   b) prothrombin, fibrinogen, and other clotting factors are synthesized by the spleen
   c) the second stage of clotting results in the formation of thrombin
   d) the clot itself is made of fibrin

Reword your choice to make it a correct statement.

___

5. Which statement is NOT true of the ABO blood types?
   a) type O has neither A nor B antigens on the RBCs
   b) a person has antibodies in the plasma for those antigens NOT present on the person's own RBCs
   c) type B has A antigens on the RBCs
   d) this blood type is a hereditary characteristic

Reword your choice to make it a correct statement.

___

6. Which of these is NOT a normal value in a CBC?
   a) RBCs—5.1 million/mm³
   b) Hb—8 grams/100 ml
   c) WBCs—9000/mm³
   d) platelets—210,000/mm³

For your choice, state the correct normal range.

___

7. Which statement is NOT true of the destruction of old RBCs?
   a) the normal lifespan of RBCs is 90 days
   b) the organs that contain macrophages are the liver, spleen, and red bone marrow
   c) the iron may be stored in the liver or returned to the red bone marrow
   d) the bilirubin formed is excreted by the liver into bile

Reword your choice to make it a correct statement.

___

8. Which statement is NOT true of the plasma proteins?
   a) the presence of albumin in plasma helps maintain blood volume
   b) gamma globulins are antibodies produced by basophils
   c) alpha and beta globulins are carriers for molecules such as fats
   d) fibrinogen and prothrombin are clotting factors synthesized by the liver

Reword your choice to make it a correct statement.

___

9. Which statement is NOT true of RBC formation?
   a) a normoblast is the last stage with a cell membrane
   b) small numbers of reticulocytes are often found in circulating blood
   c) the precursor cells are stem cells
   d) vitamin B$_{12}$ may also be called the extrinsic factor

   Reword your choice to make it a correct statement.

   _____

10. Which statement is NOT true of the prevention of abnormal clotting?
   a) antithrombin inactivates excess thrombin
   b) heparin is a natural anticoagulant that blocks chemical clotting
   c) the simple squamous epithelium that lines blood vessels is smooth to prevent abnormal clotting
   d) heparin is produced by monocytes

   Reword your choice to make it a correct statement.

   _____

11. Which statement is NOT true of the prevention of blood loss in ruptured vessels?
   a) vascular spasm in a large vessel will make the size of the ruptured area smaller
   b) platelet plugs are useful only in medium-sized vessels
   c) chemical clotting is stimulated by damage to a vessel
   d) if a large vessel did not first constrict, the clot that forms would be washed out by the flow of blood

   Reword your choice to make it a correct statement.

   _____

12. Which term is NOT paired with its correct meaning?
   a) leukocytosis—increased WBC count
   b) thrombus—abnormal blood clot
   c) thrombocytopenia—decreased platelet count
   d) anemia—increased RBC count

   For your choice, state the correct meaning of this term.

   _____

Chapter 12

The Heart

This chapter describes the heart, which is the pump of the circulatory system. The anatomy of the heart includes the chambers and their vessels and the coronary blood vessels. The physiology of the heart includes the generation and regulation of the heartbeat and the relationship between cardiac output and the functioning of the body as a whole.

FUNCTION AND LOCATION

1. The function of the heart is to _____ .

2. a) The heart is located in the mediastinum, which is the area between the _____ in

   the _____ cavity.

   b) Name the organ directly below the heart. _____

PERICARDIAL MEMBRANES

1. How many layers of pericardial membranes are around the heart? _____

2. The outermost layer is called the _____ pericardium and is made of _____

   _____ tissue.

3. a) The serous membrane that lines the fibrous pericardium is called the _____
   pericardium.

   b) The serous membrane that is on the surface of the heart muscle is called the

   _____ pericardium, or the _____ .

4. The function of the serous fluid produced by the serous layers is to _____
   as the heart beats.

CHAMBERS OF THE HEART

1. The heart has _____ chambers: two upper chambers called _____ and two lower chambers called _____ .

2. Name the tissue that forms the walls of these chambers: _____ , or its other name _____

3. a) The chambers of the heart are lined with simple squamous epithelium called the _____ , which also covers the _____ of the heart.

   b) The most important physical characteristic of the endocardium is that it is very _____ , which prevents abnormal _____ in the chambers of the heart.

4. a) Which pair of chambers have the thicker walls? _____

   b) The wall of myocardium between the two atria is the _____ .

   c) The wall of myocardium between the two ventricles is the _____ .

CHAMBERS—VESSELS AND VALVES

1. Match each chamber of the heart with its proper vessel (a letter) and the function of the vessel (a number).

   Use each letter and number once.

   1) Right atrium _____

   2) Left atrium _____

   3) Right ventricle _____

   4) Left ventricle _____

   Vessel(s)
   A. Pulmonary veins
   B. Pulmonary artery
   C. Aorta
   D. Superior and inferior caval veins

   Function of Vessel(s)
   1. Returns blood from the body
   2. Takes blood to the body
   3. Takes blood to the lungs
   4. Returns blood from the lungs

2. Below is a diagram of an anterior view of the exterior of the heart.

   Label the parts indicated.

3. Match each heart valve with its proper location (a letter statement) and its function (a number statement).

   Use each letter and number once.

   1) Tricupsid valve _____

   2) Mitral valve _____

   3) Pulmonary semilunar valve _____

   4) Aortic semilunar valve _____

   Location
   A. At the junction of the right ventricle and the pulmonary artery
   B. Between the left atrium and left ventricle
   C. Between the right atrium and right ventricle
   D. At the junction of the left ventricle and the aorta

   Function
   1. Prevents backflow of blood to the left ventricle when the ventricle relaxes
   2. Prevents backflow of blood to the left atrium when the left ventricle contracts

3. Prevents backflow of blood to the right atrium when the right ventricle contracts
4. Prevents backflow of blood to the right ventricle when the ventricle relaxes

4. Below is a diagram of the interior of the heart (anterior view).

Label the parts indicated.

1 ——
2 ——
3 ——
4 ——
5 ——
6 ——
7 ——

8 ——
9 ——
10 ——
11 ——
12 ——
13 ——
14 ——
15 ——
16 ——
17 ——

○ Semilunar valves
○ AV valves

19
20   18

5. a) The papillary muscles are columns of _____ that project into each _____ (chamber) of the heart.

   b) The chordae tendineae are strands of _____ tissue that extend from the papillary muscles to the _____ .

   c) The function of these structures is to prevent inversion of the AV valves when the ventricles _____ . (AV valves is the term for the mitral and tricuspid valves.)

6. a) The atria secrete a hormone called _____ when blood volume or blood pressure _____ .

   b) ANH causes the _____ to excrete sodium ions and water, which will _____ blood pressure.

CIRCULATION THROUGH THE HEART

1. a) The heart is actually a double pump, and both pumps work simultaneously. The left side of the
      heart receives blood from the _____ and pumps this blood to the
      _____ .

   b) The right side of the heart receives blood from the _____ and pumps this blood to
      the _____ .

2. Number the following in proper sequence with respect to the flow of blood through the heart to and
   from the body and lungs.

   Begin at the left atrium.

   _____1_____ Left atrium   _____ Lungs

   _____ Left ventricle   _____ Pulmonary artery

   _____ Right atrium   _____ Pulmonary veins

   _____ Right ventricle   _____ Aorta

   _____ Body   _____ Superior and inferior caval veins

CORONARY VESSELS

1. a) The purpose of the coronary vessels is to supply the _____ with blood.

   b) The most important substance in the blood is _____ .

2. a) The right and left coronary arteries are branches of the _____ .

   b) The coronary sinus is formed by the union of coronary veins and returns blood from the
      myocardium to the _____ (chamber).

3. a) What will happen to a part of the heart muscle that is deprived of its blood supply? _____

      _____

   b) State one possible cause of this. _____

CARDIAC CYCLE AND HEART SOUNDS

1. The cardiac cycle is the term for the sequence of events in one _____ .

2. a) The term "systole" means _____ .

   b) The term "diastole" means _____ .

3. In the cardiac cycle, when the atria are in systole, the ventricles are in _____ , and
   when the ventricles are in systole, the atria are in _____ .

4. Number the events of one cardiac cycle in the proper sequence. Two events have been properly numbered to get you started.

1) ___1___ Blood continuously flows into both atria

2) _____ Two thirds of the atrial blood flows passively into the ventricles

3) _____ The right and left AV valves are closed, and the aortic and pulmonary semilunar valves are opened

4) _____ The pressure of incoming blood opens the right and left AV valves

5) _____ The atria contract to pump the remaining blood into the ventricles

6) _____ Ventricular contraction pumps blood into the arteries

7) ___5___ The atria relax, and the ventricles begin to contract

8) _____ The ventricles relax, and the semilunar valves are closed

5. From atria to ventricles, most blood _____ (flows passively or is pumped).

6. From ventricles to arteries, all blood _____ (flows passively or is pumped).

7. a) The cardiac cycle normally creates _____ (how many) heart sounds.

   b) The first sound is caused by the closure of the _____ valves.

   c) The second sound is caused by the closure of the _____ valves.

   d) An extra sound heard during the cardiac cycle is called a _____ .

CARDIAC CONDUCTION PATHWAY

1. a) The cardiac conduction pathway is the pathway of electrical _____ throughout the heart during each heartbeat.

   b) Must the heart receive nerve impulses to cause contraction? _____

   c) Nerve impulses regulate only the _____ of contraction.

2. Name the parts of the conduction pathway in order.

1) ___SA node___ In the wall of the right atrium

2) _____ In the lower interatrial septum

3) _____ In the upper interventricular septum

4) _____ Extend through the interventricular septum

5) _____ To the rest of the myocardium of the ventricles

3. Below is a diagram of the heart.

   Label the parts of the conduction pathway.

1

Right atrium _____

2 _____

Left ventricle

3

5

○ Impulse pathway in the atria
○ Impulse pathway in the ventricles

4

4. The SA node initiates each heartbeat because it has the most _____ rate of contraction.

5. Name the parts of the conduction pathway that bring about atrial systole. _____ and

   _____

6. Name the parts of the conduction pathway that bring about ventricular systole. _____ ,

   _____ , and _____

7. a) The electrical activity of the heart can be recorded and depicted in an _____ .

   b) The term for irregular heartbeats is _____ .

   c) The most serious arrhythmia is _____ , which is very rapid and uncoordinated.

HEART RATE

1. a) State a normal range of resting heart rate for a healthy adult. _____

   b) Name the vital sign that is a measure of heart rate. _____

2. Children and infants usually have _____ (higher or lower) heart rates than do adults,

   because children are _____ (younger or smaller) than adults.

3. Athletes in good physical condition often have _____ (higher or lower) heart rates
   than do other adults.

CARDIAC OUTPUT

1. Cardiac output is the amount of blood pumped by a ventricle in _____ (time).

2. Cardiac output is important to maintain normal _____ and to provide for the transport

   of _____ to tissues.

3. a) Stroke volume is the amount of blood pumped by a ventricle in _____ .

   b) State a normal range of resting stroke volume. _____ ml per beat

4. State the formula used to determine cardiac output:

   cardiac output = _____ × _____

5. Problem: Pulse is 60 bpm and stroke volume is 75 ml. What is the cardiac output?

6. Problem: An athlete's resting cardiac output is 6000 ml per minute and her stroke volume is 100 ml
   per beat. What is her pulse?

7. Problem: During exercise, pulse is 120 bpm and stroke volume is 100 ml. What is the cardiac output?

REGULATION OF HEART RATE

1. a) The cardiac centers are located in the _____ of the brain.

   b) Name the two centers. The _____ and the _____

2. a) Sympathetic nerves to the heart transmit impulses that _____ heart rate and force
      of contraction.

   b) The parasympathetic nerves to the heart are the _____ nerves, which transmit

      impulses that _____ heart rate.

3. In order to bring about changes in heart rate, the medulla must receive sensory information.

a) The receptors that detect changes in blood pressure are called _____ , and they are

located in the _____ sinus and the _____ sinus.

b) The receptors that detect changes in the oxygen level of the blood are called

_____ , and they are located in the _____ body and the

_____ body.

4. a) The sensory nerves for the carotid sinus and body are the _____ nerves.

b) The sensory nerves for the aortic sinus and body are the _____ nerves.

5. Below is a diagram of the heart and the nervous system.

Label the parts indicated.

6. The regulation of heart rate is a reflex, that is, an automatic motor response stimulated by sensory information. Complete the following description of the reflex arc that is started when blood pressure decreases.

1) When blood pressure to the brain decreases, the decrease is detected by _____ located in the carotid _____ .

2) Sensory impulses travel along the _____ nerves to the medulla of the brain.

3) The _____ center is stimulated and generates impulses that are carried by _____ nerves to the heart.

4) The effect of these impulses is to _____ heart rate and force of contraction in order to _____ blood pressure back to normal.

CLINICAL APPLICATIONS

1. a) Mr. N. has been hospitalized following a mild heart attack. His ECG is being monitored to detect possible ventricular fibrillation, which means _____ .

   b) Ventricular fibrillation is a medical emergency, because if the ventricles are fibrillating, they are not _____ blood, and cardiac output will _____ .

2. a) Mr. W. is 55 years old and has been hospitalized for surgery to implant an artificial pacemaker for his heart. The heart's own natural pacemaker, which is not functioning properly, is the _____ .

   b) Without an artificial pacemaker to maintain a normal heart rate, the remainder of Mr. W.'s heart would continue to beat but at a _____ (faster or slower) rate.

   c) What would then happen to Mr. W.'s cardiac output? _____

3. Name the disorder suggested by each statement.

   a) an abnormal extra sound heard during the cardiac cycle _____

   b) death of heart muscle due to lack of oxygen _____

   c) lipid deposits within the coronary arteries _____

MULTIPLE CHOICE TEST #1

Choose the correct answer for each question.

1. During one cardiac cycle:
   a) the atria contract first, followed by contraction of the ventricles
   b) the ventricles contract first, followed by contraction of the atria
   c) the atria and ventricles contract simultaneously
   d) there is no specific pattern of contraction

2. Backflow of blood from the ventricles to the atria is prevented by the:
   a) aortic and pulmonary semilunar valves
   b) tricuspid and pulmonary semilunar valves
   c) mitral and aortic semilunar valves
   d) mitral and tricuspid valves

3. The outermost of the pericardial membranes is the:
   a) visceral pericardium
   b) fibrous pericardium
   c) parietal pericardium
   d) epicardium

4. Each normal heartbeat is initiated by the:
   a) AV node   b) Bundle of His   c) SA node   d) ventricles

5. Backflow of blood from the arteries to the ventricles is prevented by the:
   a) aortic and pulmonary semilunar valves
   b) tricuspid and pulmonary semilunar valves
   c) mitral and aortic semilunar valves
   d) mitral and tricuspid valves

6. The vessel into which the left ventricle pumps blood is the:
   a) superior vena cava
   b) pulmonary artery
   c) inferior vena cava
   d) aorta

7. The veins that return blood to the right atrium are the:
   a) thoracic veins
   b) superior and inferior caval veins
   c) pulmonary veins
   d) visceral veins

8. The heart is located:
   a) lateral to the lungs and superior to the diaphragm
   b) medial to the lungs and inferior to the diaphragm
   c) medial to the lungs and superior to the diaphragm
   d) lateral to the lungs and inferior to the diaphragm

9. The function of the serous fluid of the pericardial membranes is to:
   a) prevent friction as the heart beats
   b) prevent abnormal clotting in the chambers of the heart
   c) keep blood flowing through the heart
   d) nourish the myocardium

10. The term systole means:
    a) rapid heart rate   b) slow heart rate   c) relaxation   d) contraction

11. The purpose of the coronary vessels is to:
    a) supply the brain with oxygenated blood
    b) supply the heart with oxygenated blood
    c) supply the lungs with oxygenated blood
    d) supply the body with oxygenated blood

12. A normal range of heart rate for a healthy adult is _____ beats per minute.
    a) 90–100   b) 70–100   c) 60–80   d) 50–60

13. The chambers of the heart that receive blood from veins are the:
    a) right and left ventricles
    b) right and left atria
    c) right atrium and ventricle
    d) left atrium and ventricle

14. The endocardium lines the chambers of the heart and:
    a) prevents friction when the heart beats
    b) is smooth to prevent abnormal clotting within the heart
    c) prevents backflow of blood
    d) helps pump blood

15. The centers that regulate heart rate are located in the:
    a) medulla   b) carotid sinus   c) cerebral cortex   d) wall of the right atrium

16. The nerves that transmit impulses to decrease the heart rate are the:
    a) sympathetic nerves   c) glossopharyngeal nerves
    b) coronary nerves   d) vagus nerves

17. The electrical activity of the heart may be depicted in an:
    a) EEG   b) EGG   c) ECG   d) ECC

18. The amount of blood pumped by a ventricle in 1 minute is called:
    a) stroke volume   b) pulse   c) coronary blood flow   d) cardiac output

19. The normal heart sounds are caused by:
    a) relaxation of the atria   c) opening of the valves
    b) relaxation of the ventricles   d) closure of the valves

20. Changes in blood pressure are detected by:
    a) pressoreceptors in the carotid and aortic sinuses
    b) pressoreceptors in the ventricles
    c) pressoreceptors in the medulla
    d) blood vessels in the medulla

21. The hormone ANH increases the loss of _____ in urine to decrease blood volume and blood pressure.
    a) calcium ions   b) sodium ions and water   c) potassium ions   d) water only

MULTIPLE CHOICE TEST #2

Read each question and the four answer choices carefully. When you have made a choice, follow the instructions to complete your answer.

1. Which statement is NOT true of the pericardial membranes?
   a) serous fluid prevents friction between the serous layers as the heart beats
   b) the fibrous pericardium is the thick, outermost layer
   c) the parietal pericardium lines the fibrous pericardium
   d) the visceral pericardium may also be called the endocardium

   Reword your choice to make it a correct statement.

   _____

2. Which statement is NOT true of the chambers and vessels of the heart?
   a) both ventricles pump blood into arteries
   b) the left ventricle pumps blood into the pulmonary artery
   c) the left atrium receives blood from the pulmonary veins
   d) the right atrium receives blood from the superior and inferior caval veins

   Reword your choice to make it a correct statement.

   _____

3. Which statement is NOT true of the valves of the heart?
   a) the mitral valve prevents backflow of blood from the right ventricle to the right atrium
   b) the right and left AV valves are anchored by papillary muscles and chordae tendineae
   c) the semilunar valves prevent backflow of blood from the arteries to the ventricles
   d) the valves are made of endocardium reinforced with connective tissue

   Reword your choice to make it a correct statement.

   _____

4. Which statement is NOT true of the cardiac cycle?
   a) most blood flow from the atria to the ventricles flows passively
   b) all blood flow from ventricles to arteries is actively pumped
   c) the atria contract first; then the ventricles contract
   d) when the atria are in systole, the ventricles are in systole

   Reword your choice to make it a correct statement.

   _____

5. Which statement is NOT true of the cardiac conduction pathway?
   a) the Purkinje fibers carry impulses to the ventricular myocardium
   b) the Bundle of His is located in the upper interventricular septum
   c) the AV node initiates each heartbeat
   d) the SA node and AV node promote contraction of the atria

   Reword your choice to make it a correct statement.

   _____

6. Which statement is NOT true of cardiac output?
   a) cardiac output is the amount of blood pumped by a ventricle in one beat
   b) a normal cardiac output is necessary to maintain normal blood pressure
   c) cardiac output equals stroke volume times pulse rate
   d) a normal cardiac output is necessary to maintain oxygenation of tissues

   Reword your choice to make it a correct statement.

   _____

7. Which statement is NOT true of the regulation of heart rate?
   a) the cardiac centers are located in the medulla
   b) sympathetic impulses to the heart decrease the heart rate
   c) pressoreceptors detect changes in blood pressure to supply sensory information
      to the medulla
   d) the parasympathetic nerves to the heart are the vagus nerves

   Reword your choice to make it a correct statement.

   _____

8. Which statement is NOT true of the heart's response to exercise?
   a) Starling's law permits the heart to contract more forcefully in response to increased
      venous return
   b) the heart rate will increase in response to parasympathetic impulses

c) stroke volume increases during exercise as the heart pumps more forcefully

d) cardiac output increases to supply more oxygen to the body

Reword your choice to make it a correct statement.

9. Which statement is NOT true of coronary circulation?
   a) the two major coronary arteries are branches of the aorta
   b) the coronary sinus empties blood from the myocardium into the left atrium
   c) for the myocardium, the most important substance in the blood is oxygen
   d) myocardium that is deprived of oxygen becomes ischemic

   Reword your choice to make it a correct statement.

10. Which statement is NOT true of heart rate?
    a) the normal range of heart rate for a healthy adult is 60–80 beats per minute
    b) an infant may have a normal heart rate as high as 120 beats per minute
    c) an athlete's heart rate may range from 40–60 beats per minute
    d) an athlete's heart rate is low because the heart's stroke volume is lower

    Reword your choice to make it a correct statement.

Chapter 13

The Vascular System

The vascular system consists of the arteries, capillaries, and veins that transport blood throughout the body. This chapter describes these vessels, the pathways of circulation, and the importance and regulation of blood pressure.

BLOOD VESSELS—STRUCTURE AND FUNCTIONS

1. a) The vessels that carry blood from arterioles to venules are _____ .

   b) The vessels that carry blood from the heart to capillaries are _____ .

   c) The vessels that carry blood from capillaries to the heart are _____ .

2. a) The tunica intima is the _____ of arteries and veins and is made of

   _____ tissue.

   b) This tissue is very smooth and has what function? _____

3. a) The tunica media is the middle layer of arteries and veins and is made of these tissues:

   _____ and _____ .

   b) What is the function of these tissues? _____

4. a) The tunica externa is the _____ layer of arteries and veins and is made of this

   tissue: _____

   b) What is the function of this tissue? _____

5. Match each type of vessel with the proper descriptive statements.

   Use each letter once. Each answer line will have three correct letters.

   1) Arteries _____

   2) Veins _____

   A. The lining is not folded into valves.
   B. The outer layer is thin, since blood pressure is low.
   C. The lining is folded into valves to prevent backflow of blood.
   D. The middle layer is thin, since these vessels are not as important in the maintenance of blood pressure.
   E. The middle layer is thick, since these vessels are important in the maintenance of blood pressure.
   F. The outer layer is thick, to prevent rupture by the high blood pressure in these vessels.

6. a) Direct connections between arteries or between veins are called _____ .

   b) Their purpose is to provide _____ for the flow of blood if one vessel becomes blocked or obstructed.

7. a) Capillaries are made of what type of tissue? _____

   b) Besides being smooth to prevent abnormal clotting, this tissue is thin to permit _____ _____ of materials between the blood and surrounding cells.

8. a) Blood flow through capillary networks is regulated by smooth muscle cells called _____ at the beginning of each network.

   b) Precapillary sphincters are not regulated by nerve impulses but by tissue needs. In an active tissue, precapillary sphincters will _____ (constrict or dilate) to _____ (increase or decrease) blood flow to supply the tissue with more _____ .

9. a) Large, very permeable capillaries are called _____ .

   b) Proteins and blood cells can enter or leave sinusoids, which are found in these organs (tissues): _____ and _____ .

10. Below is a diagram of the three types of blood vessels.

Label the parts indicated.

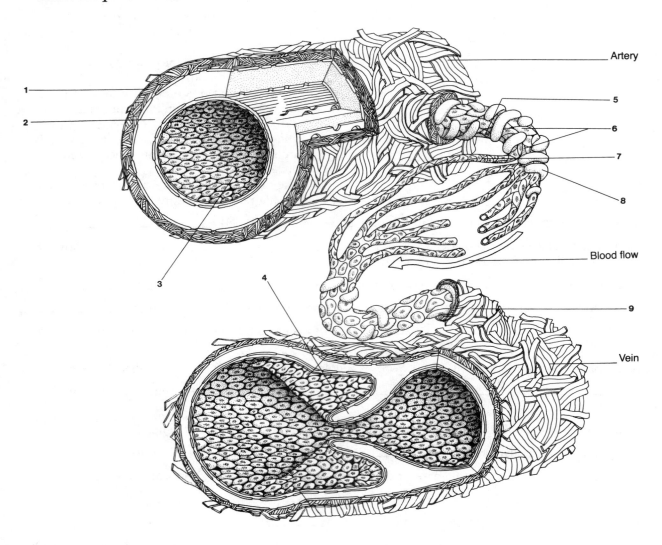

EXCHANGES IN CAPILLARIES

1. Match each process that occurs in capillaries with the proper descriptive statements.

   Use each letter once. Each answer line will have more than one correct letter.

   1) Diffusion _____

   2) Filtration _____

   3) Osmosis _____

   A. Molecules move from an area of greater concentration to an area of lesser concentration.
   B. The albumin in the blood creates a colloid osmotic pressure that pulls water and dissolved materials.
   C. The high blood pressure at the arterial end of capillary networks forces plasma out of capillaries.
   D. Nutrients move from the blood into tissue fluid.
   E. CO_2 moves from tissue fluid into the blood.
   F. Waste products move from tissue fluid into the blood.
   G. Oxygen moves from the blood to tissue fluid.

2. Below is a diagram of a capillary in a body tissue.

   Label the substances that move in the direction of the arrows by the means of the processes indicated.

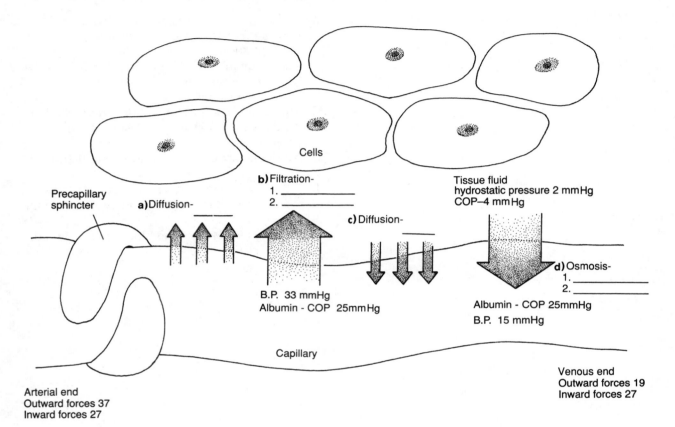

PATHWAYS OF CIRCULATION

Pathway—Pulmonary Circulation

1. a) This pathway begins at the _____ ventricle, which pumps blood through the

   pulmonary artery to the _____ .

   b) Blood in the pulmonary veins returns to the _____ atrium.

2. The purpose of this pathway of circulation is to exchange _____ and

   _____ between the blood in the pulmonary _____ and the air in the

   _____ of the lungs.

Pathway—Systemic Circulation

1. a) The pathway begins at the _____ ventricle, which pumps blood through the aorta

   to the _____ .

   b) Blood in the superior and inferior caval veins returns to the _____ atrium.

2. The purpose of this pathway of circulation is to exchange materials between the blood in the systemic

   _____ and the _____ throughout the body.

3. The parts of the aorta are named according to their locations. Name each part described:

   1) Below the level of the diaphragm _____

   2) Emerges from the left ventricle _____

   3) Passes through the chest cavity to the level of the diaphragm _____

   4) Curves over the top of the heart _____

4. Name the part of the body supplied by each of these arteries.

   1) Coronary a. _____

   2) Femoral a. _____

   3) Brachial a. _____

   4) Bronchial a. _____

   5) Internal carotid a. _____

   6) Renal a. _____

   7) Hepatic a. _____

   8) Intercostal a. _____

   9) Anterior tibial a. _____

   10) Subclavian a. _____

   11) Radial a. _____

   12) Superior mesenteric a. _____

   13) Esophageal a. _____

   14) Vertebral a. _____

   15) Celiac a. _____

   16) Popliteal a. _____

   17) Common iliac a. _____

   18) Plantar arches _____

5. Below is a diagram of the body in anterior view.

   Label the arteries indicated.

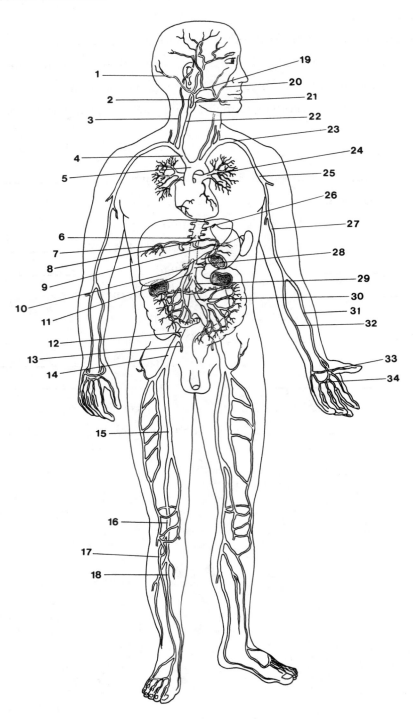

6. Name the part of the body drained of blood by each of these veins.

1) External jugular v. _____

2) Axillary v. _____

3) Great saphenous v. _____

4) Inferior vena cava _____

5) Common iliac v. _____

6) Ulnar v. _____

7) Cranial venous sinuses _____

8) Superior vena cava _____

9) Renal v. _____

10) Subclavian v. _____

11) Brachial v. _____

12) Femoral v. _____

7. Below is a diagram of the body in anterior view.

   Label the veins indicated.

Hepatic Portal Circulation

1. In this specialized pathway of systemic circulation, blood from the _____ and _____ circulates through the liver before returning to the heart.

2. The portal vein is formed by the union of two large veins, the _____ vein and the _____ vein.

3. From the portal vein, blood flows into the _____ in the liver and then to the hepatic veins to the _____ , which returns blood to the right atrium.

4. a) This pathway differs from the rest of systemic circulation in that there are two sets of _____ in which exchanges take place.

   b) The first set of capillaries is in the _____ , and the second set of capillaries is the sinusoids in the _____ .

5. Use a specific example to describe the purpose of portal circulation:

   1) Substance in the blood: _____

   2) Absorbed or produced by which organ: _____

   3) Function of the liver with respect to this substance: _____ .

Fetal Circulation

1. The site of exchanges of materials between fetal blood and maternal blood is the _____ .

2. a) Name the kinds of materials exchanged: _____ , _____ , and _____ .

   b) Name the mechanisms (processes) of exchange: _____ and _____ .

3. The fetus is connected to the placenta by the umbilical cord, which contains two _____ and one _____ .

4. a) The umbilical arteries carry blood from the _____ to the _____ .

   b) In this blood are _____ and _____ , which will be eliminated in the placenta.

5. a) The umbilical vein carries blood from the _____ to the _____ .

   b) In this blood are _____ and _____ obtained in the placenta.

6. Within the body of the fetus, the umbilical vein branches into two vessels. One branch takes blood to the fetal liver. The other branch is called the _____ and takes blood to the _____ , which returns blood to the right atrium of the fetal heart.

7. a) Within the fetal heart, the _____ is an opening in the interatrial septum that permits some blood to flow from the _____ atrium to the

    _____ atrium.

    b) This blood, therefore, bypasses the fetal _____ , which are still deflated and non-functional.

8. a) Just outside the fetal heart, the ductus arteriosus is a short vessel that permits blood to flow from the _____ to the _____ .

    b) State the purpose of the ductus arteriosus. _____

9. a) After birth, the ductus venosus _____ and becomes non-functional.

    b) The foramen ovale is _____ by a flap on the left side, and the ductus arteriosus

    _____ .

    c) This ensures that normal _____ circulation will be established.

10. Below is a diagram of fetal circulation.

Label the parts indicated.

BLOOD PRESSURE

1. Blood pressure (BP) is the force exerted by the blood against the walls of the _____ .

2. BP is measured in units called _____ .

3. a) Systemic BP is created by the pumping of the _____ of the heart.

   b) Systolic BP is the pressure when the left ventricle is _____ .

   c) Diastolic BP is the pressure when the left ventricle is _____ .

4. In systemic circulation, BP is highest in the _____ , then decreases in the arterioles and capillaries, and is lowest in the _____ .

5. a) In systemic capillaries, BP is 30–35 mmHg at the _____ end and decreases to 12–15 mmHg at the _____ end.

   b) This pressure is high enough to permit the process of _____ , but it is low enough to prevent _____ of the capillaries.

   c) The process of filtration in capillaries is important to bring _____ to tissues.

6. a) Pulmonary BP is always very low, because the _____ pumps less forcefully than does the left ventricle.

   b) The low BP in the pulmonary capillaries is important to _____ filtration, to prevent the accumulation of tissue fluid in the alveoli.

Maintenance of Systemic Blood Pressure

1. a) Venous return is the amount of blood that returns to the _____ .

   b) Venous return is essential to maintain cardiac output, and if venous return decreases, cardiac output will _____ , and BP will _____ .

   c) 1) Constriction of the veins helps increase venous return. The tissue in the wall of a vein that is capable of contraction is _____ .

      2) The skeletal muscle pump contributes to venous return in veins in which part of the body? _____ Contractions of skeletal muscles _____ these veins and force blood toward the heart.

      3) The respiratory pump contributes to venous return in veins in which part of the body? _____ The pressure changes during _____ alternately compress and expand these veins, and force blood toward the _____ .

2. If heart rate and force increase, BP will _____ .

3. a) Peripheral resistance is the resistance of the blood vessels to the flow of blood. Normal diastolic BP is maintained by slight _____ of arteries and veins.

   b) Greater vasoconstriction will _____ BP.

   c) Vasodilation will _____ BP.

4. a) The elastic walls of the large arteries are stretched during ventricular _____ and recoil during ventricular _____ .

   b) Therefore, normal elasticity _____ (increases or decreases) systolic BP and _____ (increases or decreases) diastolic BP.

5. a) The viscosity of blood depends upon the presence of _____ and

   _____ .

   b) Decreased blood viscosity will _____ BP.

   c) This may occur when there is a decrease in RBCs, called _____ , or when the

   _____ does not produce sufficient _____ .

6. a) Following severe hemorrhage, BP will _____ .

   b) Following a small loss of blood, certain compensating mechanisms will prevent a sharp decrease

   in BP. State one of these compensating mechanisms. _____

7. Several hormones have effects on BP.

   1) Norepinephrine raises BP because it stimulates _____ .

   2) Epinephrine raises BP because it stimulates _____ and _____ .

   3) ADH raises BP by increasing the reabsorption of water by the _____ , which

   increases blood _____ .

   4) Aldosterone raises BP by increasing the reabsorption of Na^+ ions by the _____ ,

   which is followed by the reabsorption of _____ to increase blood volume.

   5) ANH lowers BP by increasing urinary excretion of _____ , which

   _____ blood volume.

Regulation of Blood Pressure

1. Intrinsic Mechanisms:

   1) The heart responds to increased venous return by pumping more _____ .

   a) This will _____ cardiac output and BP and depends on the characteristic of

   cardiac muscle called _____ of the heart.

   2) Decreased blood flow to the kidneys will result in decreased _____ (process),
   which will decrease urinary output to maintain blood volume.

2. Nervous Mechanisms for Peripheral Resistance:

   1) The vasomotor center is located in the _____ of the brain.

   a) This center consists of two areas: the _____ area and the

   _____ area.

   b) The medulla receives sensory information about the need for changes in vessel diameter from

   the _____ in the carotid and aortic sinuses.

2) The division of the autonomic nervous system that regulates the diameter of arteries and veins is the _____ division.

   a) Several impulses per second maintain normal vasoconstriction of arteries and veins. More vasoconstriction is brought about by _____ impulses per second and will _____ BP.

   b) Vasodilation is brought about by _____ impulses per second and will _____ BP.

CLINICAL APPLICATIONS

1. Mr. T. has just been diagnosed with hypertension. This means that his systolic BP is consistently above _____ mmHg, and his diastolic BP is consistently above _____ mmHg.

2. a) As a person ages, the walls of the arteries begin to deteriorate. This is called _____ .

   b) Arteries may also be affected by _____ , in which deposits of cholesterol narrow the lumen.

MULTIPLE CHOICE TEST #1

Choose the correct answer for each question.

1. The fetal blood vessel that carries blood from the pulmonary artery to the aorta is the:
   a) ductus arteriosus
   b) ductus venosus
   c) pulmonary duct
   d) ductus pulmonarus

2. The fetal blood vessel that carries blood from the placenta to the fetus is the:
   a) umbilical vein
   b) ductus venosus
   c) ductus arteriosus
   d) umbilical artery

3. The layer of the walls of arteries and veins that is smooth to prevent abnormal clotting is the:
   a) middle layer, made of smooth muscle
   b) lining, made of smooth muscle
   c) lining, made of simple squamous epithelium
   d) outer layer, made of simple squamous epithelium

4. The layer of the walls of arteries that helps maintain diastolic blood pressure is made of:
   a) fibrous connective tissue and elastic connective tissue
   b) smooth muscle and fibrous connective tissue
   c) smooth muscle and elastic connective tissue
   d) fibrous connective tissue and simple squamous epithelium

5. Backflow of blood within veins is prevented by:
   a) smooth muscle
   b) valves
   c) precapillary sphincters
   d) the middle layer

6. In capillaries, nutrients are transported from the blood to tissues by the process of:
   a) osmosis
   b) diffusion
   c) active transport
   d) filtration

7. In capillaries, O_2 and CO_2 are exchanged between the blood and tissue fluid by the process of:
   a) osmosis   b) filtration   c) active transport   d) diffusion

8. A systemic blood pressure reading always consists of two numbers, which are called:
   a) systemic/systolic   c) diastolic/systolic
   b) systolic/diastolic   d) diastolic/systemic

9. Pulmonary blood pressure is always low and thereby prevents:
   a) osmosis of tissue fluid into pulmonary capillaries
   b) filtration of tissue fluid into the alveoli
   c) filtration of tissue fluid into pulmonary capillaries
   d) osmosis of blood plasma into the alveoli

10. Systemic circulation begins at the:
    a) right atrium   b) right ventricle   c) left ventricle   d) left foot

11. In hepatic portal circulation, blood from the digestive organs and spleen circulates through the _____ before returning to the _____ .
    a) brain/liver   b) liver/heart   c) liver/brain   d) heart/liver

12. Venous return in veins that pass through the thoracic cavity is increased by the:
    a) skeletal muscle pump   c) pumping of the left ventricle
    b) pumping of the right ventricle   d) respiratory pump

13. Venous return in the deep veins in the legs is increased by the:
    a) low pressure in the right atrium   c) low pressure in the left atrium
    b) respiratory pump   d) skeletal muscle pump

14. Following a large loss of blood, as in severe hemorrhage, blood pressure will:
    a) increase   b) decrease   c) remain the same   d) increase then decrease

15. Epinephrine increases blood pressure because it:
    a) causes vasodilation
    b) decreases heart rate and force
    c) increases heart rate and force
    d) increases water reabsorption by the kidneys

16. The vasomotor center is located in which part of the brain?
    a) medulla   b) hypothalamus   c) frontal lobes   d) cerebellum

17. ADH increases blood pressure because it:
    a) causes vasodilation
    b) increases heart rate and force
    c) decreases water reabsorption by the kidneys
    d) increases water reabsorption by the kidneys

18. The nerves that carry impulses to regulate the diameter of arteries and veins are:
    a) sympathetic nerves   c) somatic motor nerves
    b) parasympathetic nerves   d) visceral sensory nerves

19. Connections between arteries or between veins that provide alternate pathways for blood flow are called:
    a) capillary networks   b) venous sinuses   c) sinusoids   d) anastomoses

20. Large, very permeable capillaries that permit cells or proteins to enter or leave the blood are called:
    a) sinusoids   b) venous sinuses   c) anastomoses   d) precapillary sphincters

MULTIPLE CHOICE TEST #2

Read each question and the four answer choices carefully. When you have made a choice, follow the instructions to complete your answer.

1. Which statement is NOT true of hepatic portal circulation?
   a) blood from the digestive organs flows through the liver before returning to the heart
   b) the liver regulates the blood levels of nutrients such as glucose
   c) the vein that takes blood into the liver is the hepatic vein
   d) blood from the spleen circulates through the liver first, before returning to the heart

   Reword your choice to make it a correct statement.

   _____

2. Which statement is NOT true of fetal circulation?
   a) the foramen ovale permits blood to flow from the left atrium to the right atrium to bypass the fetal lungs
   b) the umbilical arteries carry blood from the fetus to the placenta
   c) the site of exchanges between maternal blood and fetal blood is the placenta
   d) the fetus depends upon the mother for oxygen and nutrients

   Reword your choice to make it a correct statement.

   _____

3. Which statement is NOT true of the structure of arteries and veins?
   a) veins have valves to prevent the backflow of blood
   b) the lining of both arteries and veins is very smooth to permit exchanges of materials between the blood and tissues
   c) the outer layer of arteries is thick and made of fibrous connective tissue to prevent rupture
   d) the smooth muscle of arteries and veins permits vasoconstriction or vasodilation

   Reword your choice to make it a correct statement.

   _____

4. Which statement is NOT true of venous return?
   a) the constriction of veins helps increase venous return
   b) the skeletal muscle pump is especially important for deep veins of the legs
   c) the respiratory pump depends on pressure changes during breathing
   d) decreased venous return will result in increased cardiac output

   Reword your choice to make it a correct statement.

   _____

5. Which artery is NOT paired with the part of the body it supplies with blood?
   a) common carotid artery—neck and head
   b) renal artery—liver

c) femoral artery—thigh
d) brachial artery—arm

For the artery of your choice, state its correct location.

_____

6. Which statement is NOT true of exchanges in capillaries?
   a) oxygen diffuses from the blood to tissues
   b) waste products dissolved in the tissue fluid are returned to the blood by osmosis
   c) carbon dioxide diffuses from the blood to tissues
   d) by the process of filtration, tissue fluid is formed, and nutrients are brought to tissues

Reword your choice to make it a correct statement.

_____

7. Which statement is NOT true of the pulse and pulse sites?
   a) in healthy people, the pulse rate equals the heart rate
   b) the radial pulse is felt on the thumb side of the wrist
   c) the temporal pulse is felt in front of the ear
   d) the carotid pulse is felt at the elbow

Reword your choice to make it a correct statement.

_____

8. Which statement is NOT true of the regulation of blood pressure (BP)?
   a) the vasomotor center is located in the medulla
   b) vasoconstrictor nerve fibers are part of the sympathetic division of the ANS
   c) fewer sympathetic impulses to an artery result in vasodilation
   d) the tissue in arteries and veins that constricts or dilates is fibrous connective tissue

Reword your choice to make it a correct statement.

_____

9. Which statement is NOT true of the effects of hormones on BP?
   a) epinephrine increases cardiac output, which raises BP
   b) norepinephrine causes vasoconstriction, which lowers BP
   c) ADH increases the reabsorption of water by the kidneys, which raises blood volume and BP
   d) aldosterone increases the reabsorption of sodium ions by the kidneys, and water follows to maintain (or raise) blood volume and BP

Reword your choice to make it a correct statement.

_____

10. Which statement is NOT true of systemic circulation?
    a) the left ventricle pumps blood throughout the body
    b) the superior and inferior caval veins return blood to the right atrium
    c) BP is highest in the aorta and lowest in the caval veins
    d) BP in the veins is higher than BP in the capillaries

Reword your choice to make it a correct statement.

_____

Chapter 14

The Lymphatic System and Immunity

The lymphatic system has two very different functions. It returns tissue fluid to the blood to maintain normal blood volume, and it protects the body from microorganisms that might cause disease. This chapter describes both of these functions, which are essential for homeostasis, the continued proper functioning of the body.

LYMPH AND LYMPH VESSELS

1. The fluid found in lymph vessels is called _____ .

2. a) In (blood) capillaries, the process of _____ forces some plasma out into tissue

   spaces, and this fluid is now called _____ .

   b) Tissue fluid becomes lymph when it enters _____ .

3. Match each lymph vessel or structure with its proper function.

   Use each letter once.

   1) Lymph capillaries _____
   2) Valves _____
   3) Smooth muscle layer _____
   4) Cisterna chyli _____
   5) Thoracic duct _____
   6) Right lymphatic duct _____

   A. Contracts to keep lymph moving through larger lymph vessels
   B. Empties lymph from the lower body and upper left quadrant into the left subclavian vein
   C. Empties lymph from the upper right quadrant into the right subclavian vein
   D. Collect tissue fluid from intercellular spaces
   E. The vessel formed by the union of lymph vessels from the lower body
   F. Prevent backflow of lymph in larger lymph vessels

LYMPH NODES AND NODULES

1. Lymph nodes and nodules are both made of _____ tissue, which produces the WBCs

   called _____ and _____ .

2. a) The fixed cells in lymph nodes and nodules that produce antibodies are called

   _____ .

   b) The fixed cells that phagocytize pathogens are called _____ .

3. Match the lymph nodes and nodules with their proper locations (letter statements) and functions
   (number statements).

   Use each letter and number once. Each answer line will have two correct letters and two correct numbers.

   1) Lymph nodes _____

   2) Lymph nodules _____

   Location

   A. Below the epithelium of all mucous membranes
   B. Along the pathways of lymph vessels
   C. The major paired groups are cervical, axillary, and inguinal
   D. In the pharynx, they are called tonsils

   Function

   1. Destroy pathogens in the lymph from the extremities before the lymph is returned to the blood
   2. Plasma cells produce antibodies that will enter the blood
   3. Destroy pathogens that penetrate mucous membranes
   4. Plasma cells produce antibodies that act locally in mucous membranes

4. Below is a diagram of the lymphatic system.

   Label the parts indicated.

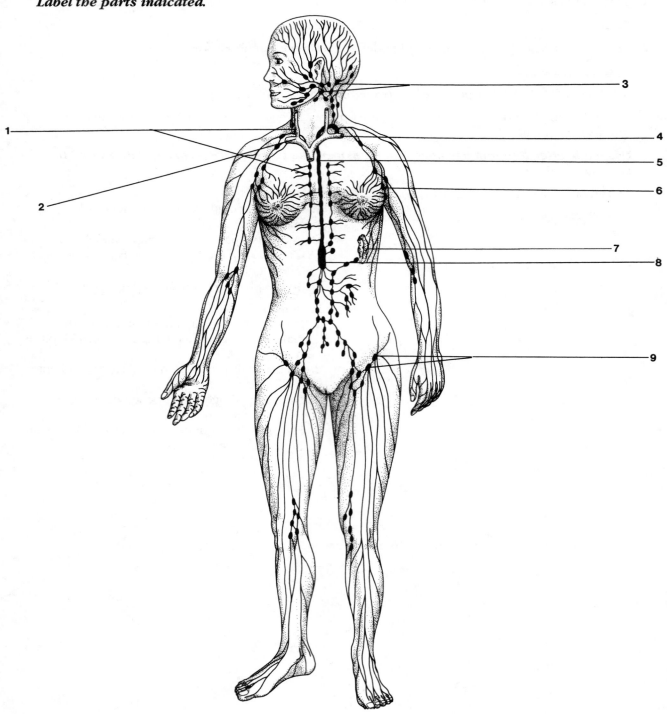

SPLEEN

1. a) The spleen is located in the _____ cavity below the _____ and
      behind the _____ .

   b) The spleen is protected from mechanical injury by which bones? _____

2. The two types of WBCs produced by the spleen are _____ and
   _____ , which enter the _____ (blood or lymph).

3. The spleen contains fixed macrophages that _____ pathogens in the blood and fixed
   plasma cells that produce _____ to foreign antigens.

4. The macrophages of the spleen may also be called reticuloendothelial cells because they phagocytize
   old _____ and form _____ , which will be excreted by the liver.

5. a) If the spleen must be removed, other organs will compensate for its functions. The
      _____ will produce lymphocytes and monocytes.

   b) The _____ and _____ will remove old RBCs from circulation.

6. The fetal spleen has a temporary function, which is the production of _____ .

THYMUS

1. The thymus is large and functional in which age group? _____

2. The thymus is located _____ the thyroid gland.

3. T cells is the name for the _____ produced by the thymus.

4. a) Thymosin and other thymic hormones enable the T cells to participate in the recognition of
      foreign _____ and to provide _____ for certain diseases.

   b) This capability of the T cells may be called immunological _____ .

IMMUNITY—ANTIGENS AND ANTIBODIES

1. Immunity includes the ability to destroy _____ and to _____ future
   cases of certain infectious diseases.

2. Immunity involves both types of lymphocytes, which are called _____ and
   _____ .

3. a) In the embryo, B cells are produced in the _____ .

   b) T cells are also produced in the _____ as well as in the _____ .

   c) Both T cells and B cells migrate to the _____ and _____ , where
      they are produced after birth.

4. Antigens are chemical markers, and there are two general types: _____ antigens that are found in the body's own cells and _____ antigens, which may also be called "non-self."

5. a) Antibodies are molecules made of _____ .

    b) When an antibody is produced, it is _____ for a foreign antigen and will label it for destruction.

    c) Antibodies may also be called _____ or _____ .

MECHANISMS OF IMMUNITY

1. The two mechanisms of immunity are called _____ immunity and _____ immunity.

2. a) The first step in both immune mechanisms is the recognition of an antigen as _____ .

    b) One way this is accomplished is by _____ , which phagocytize the foreign antigen and present it and self-antigens to _____ , to activate them specifically for this particular foreign antigen.

3. The purpose of both immune mechanisms is to _____ the foreign antigen and, if that foreign antigen is a microorganism, to provide _____ to the disease.

CELL-MEDIATED IMMUNITY

1. Match each aspect of cell-mediated immunity with its proper function.

    Use each letter once.

    1) Helper T cells _____

    2) Suppressor T cells _____

    3) Cytotoxic T cells _____

    4) Memory T cells _____

    5) Macrophages _____

    6) Cytokines _____

    A. Stop the immune response when the foreign antigen has been destroyed.
    B. Chemically destroy foreign antigens by disrupting their cell membranes
    C. Chemicals produced by cytotoxic T cells that attract macrophages
    D. Phagocytize foreign antigens
    E. Initiate a rapid immune response if the antigen enters the body again
    F. Compare the foreign antigen to the self-antigens on the macrophage and are activated and antigen specific

2. Below is a diagram of the events of cell-mediated immunity.

   Label the parts indicated.

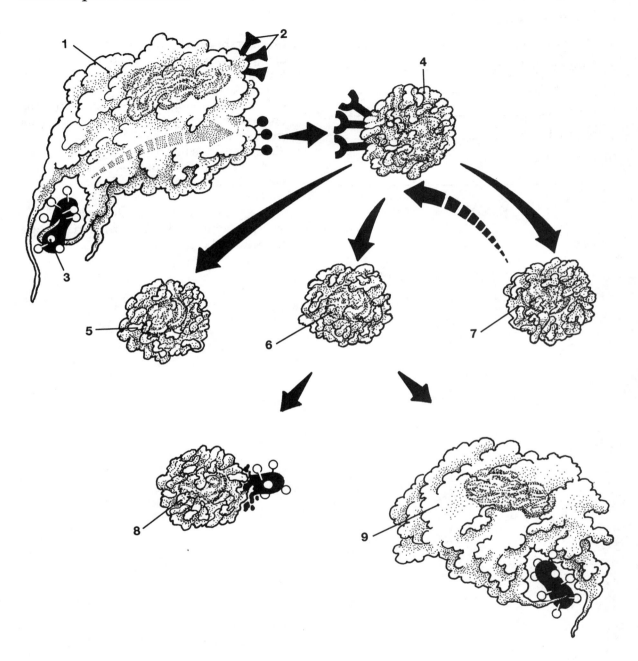

HUMORAL IMMUNITY

1. Match each aspect of humoral immunity with its proper function.

   Use each letter once.

   1) Helper T cells _____

   2) Suppressor T cells _____

   3) Memory B cells _____

   4) Plasma cells _____

   5) Macrophages _____

   6) Antibodies _____

   7) Complement _____

   A. Initiate rapid antibody production if the antigen enters the body again
   B. Proteins produced by plasma cells that bind to a specific foreign antigen
   C. Compare the foreign antigen to self-antigens on the macrophages; are antigen specific and strongly activate B cells
   D. Plasma proteins that are activated by antigen-antibody complexes and lyse cellular antigens
   E. Produce antibodies specific for one foreign antigen
   F. Phagocytize antigen-antibody complexes
   G. Stop the immune response when the foreign antigen has been destroyed

2. Below is a diagram of humoral immunity.

   Label the parts indicated.

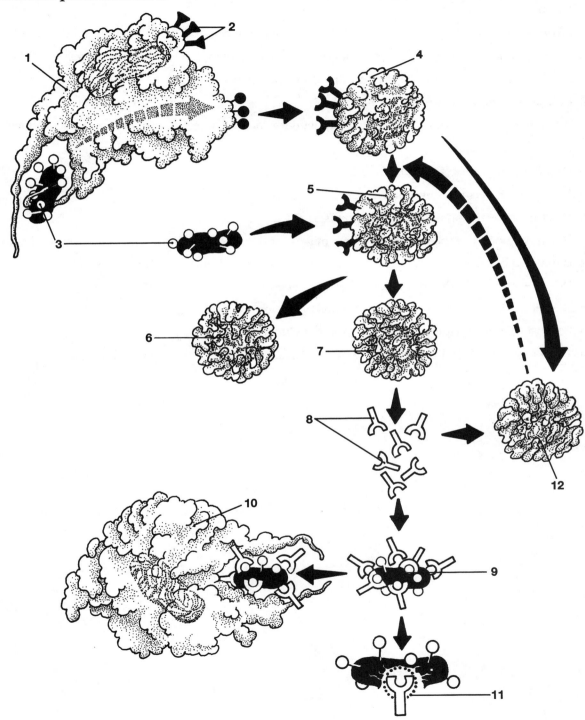

3. a) The term "opsonization" literally means "to buy food." As part of humoral immunity, opsonization is accomplished by _____ that bond to a specific foreign antigen and label it as "food."

   b) Opsonization attracts _____ that will phagocytize the antigen-antibody complex.

4. a) Complement fixation may be partial or complete. Partial complement fixation attracts _____ to phagocytize the foreign antigen.

   b) Complete complement fixation causes the _____ of cellular antigens.

5. a) When the body is exposed to a foreign antigen for the first time, is there any antibody production? _____

   b) Describe it in terms of speed. _____

   c) Describe it in terms of amount. _____

   d) What may then happen to the individual? _____ .

6. a) When the body is exposed to a foreign antigen for the second or third time, antibody production is initiated by _____ cells that were formed during the first exposure.

   b) Describe this antibody production in terms of speed. _____

   c) Describe this antibody production in terms of amount. _____

   d) Because of this, what is often true for the individual? _____ .

   e) This knowledge is utilized in our use of _____ to prevent certain diseases.

TYPES OF IMMUNITY

1. Match each type of immunity with its proper description (a letter statement) and its duration (a number statement).

   Use each letter once. Two numbers are used twice. Each answer line will have one correct letter and one correct number.

   1) Genetic immunity _____

   2) Naturally acquired passive immunity _____

   3) Artificially acquired passive immunity _____

   4) Naturally acquired active immunity _____

   5) Artificially acquired active immunity _____

   Description

   A. The injection of immune globulins after exposure to certain diseases
   B. A vaccine stimulates antibody production
   C. Does not involve antibodies
   D. Recovery from a disease provides antibodies and memory cells
   E. Antibodies are acquired by placental transmission or from breast milk

   Duration

   1. Always lasts a lifetime because it is programmed in DNA
   2. Is always temporary, since antibodies from another source break down within a few months
   3. Varies with the particular disease or vaccine

CLINICAL APPLICATIONS

1. a) AIDS is caused by a _____ called _____ .

   b) This virus infects which type of T cells? _____

2. a) A vaccine contains a non-pathogenic antigen that stimulates the immune system to produce

   specific _____ and _____ cells that will stimulate a more rapid response to the pathogen if it enters the body.

   b) How would you explain how a vaccine works to a mother whose infant has just received its first vaccination for measles?

3. a) Six-year-old Kenisha has a strep throat, and her mother tells the doctor that her daughter has "swollen glands" in her neck. These "glands" are the _____ which have become enlarged.

   b) Within these lymph nodes, _____ are attempting to phagocytize the bacteria that have entered the lymph from the pharynx.

MULTIPLE CHOICE TEST #1

Choose the correct answer for each question.

1. The lymphatic vessel that returns lymph to the left subclavian vein is the:
   a) right lymphatic duct   b) cisterna chyli   c) left cisterna   d) thoracic duct

2. Tissue fluid is called lymph when it enters:
   a) the thoracic duct   b) lymph capillaries   c) the cisterna chyli   d) veins

3. In larger lymph vessels, backflow of lymph is prevented by:
   a) smooth muscle   b) dilation   c) valves   d) expansion

4. An important function of the lymphatic system is to return tissue fluid to the:
   a) cells   b) liver   c) spleen   d) blood

5. The masses of lymphatic tissue located below the epithelium of mucous membranes are called:
   a) lymph nodules   b) lymph capillaries   c) lymph nodes   d) axillaries

6. The lymph nodes that remove pathogens in the lymph coming from the legs are called:
   a) thoracic nodes   b) cervical nodes   c) axillary nodes   d) inguinal nodes

7. Lymph nodes and nodules and the spleen produce the WBCs called:
   a) macrophages and neutrophils   c) lymphocytes and monocytes
   b) basophils and lymphocytes   d) T cells and eosinophils

8. The fixed macrophages of the spleen phagocytize old RBCs and form:
   a) more hemoglobin   b) bilirubin   c) bile   d) myoglobin

9. The spleen is located below which organ?
   a) the liver   b) the stomach   c) the colon   d) the diaphragm

10. The production of hormones by the thymus is important in which age group?
    a) old age   b) adolescence   c) fetal life   d) middle age

11. In the embryo, both T cells and B cells are produced in the:
    a) thymus   b) red bone marrow   c) liver   d) kidney

12. Antibodies are _____ molecules that may also be called _____ .
    a) inorganic/immune globulins   c) lipid/immune globulins
    b) carbohydrate/enzymes   d) protein/gamma globulins

13. The two general kinds of antigens, from the perspective of the immune system, are:
    a) self-antigens and foreign antigens   c) A antigens and B antigens
    b) T antigens and B antigens   d) gamma antigens and beta antigens

14. The return of tissue fluid to the blood is important to maintain normal:
    a) blood volume   b) blood pressure   c) both of these   d) neither of these

15. Plant viruses do not cause disease in people, which is an example of:
    a) passive acquired immunity   c) a vaccine
    b) natural acquired immunity   d) genetic immunity

16. In both immune mechanisms, the cells that remember a foreign antigen and initiate its rapid destruction upon a second exposure are:
    a) plasma cells   b) memory cells   c) suppressor T cells   d) macrophages

17. In both immune mechanisms, the cells that participate in the recognition of foreign antigens are:
    a) helper T cells and cytotoxic T cells
    b) B cells and cytotoxic T cells
    c) B cells and macrophages
    d) macrophages and helper T cells

18. Recovery from a disease may provide the type of immunity called:
    a) naturally acquired passive immunity
    b) artificially acquired passive immunity
    c) naturally acquired active immunity
    d) artificially acquired active immunity

19. Which of these organs does NOT compensate for any function of the spleen if the spleen must be removed?
    a) liver   b) thoracic duct   c) lymph nodes   d) red bone marrow

20. A baby is born temporarily immune to the diseases its mother is immune to; this is an example of:
    a) naturally acquired passive immunity
    b) artificially acquired passive immunity
    c) naturally acquired active immunity
    d) artificially acquired active immunity

MULTIPLE CHOICE TEST #2

Read each question and the four answer choices carefully. When you have made a choice, follow the instructions to complete your answer.

1. Which statement is NOT true of the spleen?
   a) the fetal spleen produces RBCs
   b) antibodies are produced in the spleen by cells called fixed monocytes
   c) the spleen is located in the upper left abdominal quadrant
   d) fixed macrophages in the spleen phagocytize pathogens in the blood

   Reword your choice to make it a correct statement.

   _____

2. Which statement is NOT true of lymph nodes?
   a) they are located along the pathway of lymph vessels
   b) during a serious infection they may become swollen
   c) they contain fixed macrophages and plasma cells
   d) the three major paired groups are the cervical, axillary, and plantar nodes

   Reword your choice to make it a correct statement.

   _____

3. Which statement is NOT true of lymph nodules?
   a) they are found below the epithelium of serous membranes
   b) they produce lymphocytes and monocytes
   c) they destroy pathogens that penetrate mucous membranes
   d) they are found in the digestive and respiratory tracts

   Reword your choice to make it a correct statement.

   _____

4. Which statement is NOT true of lymph?
   a) lymph is tissue fluid that has entered lymph capillaries
   b) lymph flows through lymph nodes as it travels back to the blood

c) lymph contains the neutrophils produced by the lymph nodes
d) lymph may contain pathogens that have entered breaks in the skin

Reword your choice to make it a correct statement.

5. Which statement is NOT true of lymph vessels?
   a) the right lymphatic duct returns lymph to the inferior vena cava
   b) the valves in larger lymph vessels prevent the backflow of lymph
   c) the return of lymph to the blood is assisted by the respiratory pump and the skeletal muscle pump
   d) the thoracic duct returns lymph to the left subclavian vein

Reword your choice to make it a correct statement.

6. Which statement is NOT true of the types of immunity?
   a) in passive immunity, antibodies come from another person or source
   b) genetic immunity is the result of the DNA makeup of a species
   c) in active immunity, a person produces his or her own antibodies
   d) a vaccine provides naturally acquired passive immunity

Reword your choice to make it a correct statement.

7. Which statement is NOT true of the thymus and immunity?
   a) the thymus is most active in the fetus and infant
   b) the thymus is located below the thyroid gland
   c) T cells are the monocytes produced by the thymus
   d) the hormones of the thymus are necessary for T cells to become immunologically competent

Reword your choice to make it a correct statement.

8. Which statement is NOT true of antigens and antibodies?
   a) when an antibody is produced, it will bond to the nearest foreign antigen
   b) self-antigens are found on all the cells of an individual
   c) foreign antigens stimulate antibody production
   d) antibodies are protein molecules

Reword your choice to make it a correct statement.

9. Which statement is NOT true of cell-mediated immunity?
   a) cytotoxic T cells chemically disrupt the cell membranes of foreign antigens
   b) the foreign antigen is recognized by macrophages and helper B cells
   c) suppressor T cells stop the immune response when the pathogen has been destroyed
   d) memory T cells remember a specific foreign antigen

Reword your choice to make it a correct statement.

10. Which statement is NOT true of humoral immunity?
    a) plasma cells come from activated B cells and produce antibodies
    b) opsonization is the labeling of foreign antigens by self-antigens
    c) memory B cells remember a specific foreign antigen
    d) macrophages phagocytize antigen-antibody complexes

    Reword your choice to make it a correct statement.

    _____

Chapter 15

The Respiratory System

This chapter describes the structure and functions of the respiratory system. The lungs provide a site for the exchange of oxygen and carbon dioxide between the air and the blood. The other organs of the respiratory system contribute to the movement of air into and out of the lungs. The two divisions of the respiratory system are the upper respiratory tract and the lower respiratory tract.

NOSE, NASAL CAVITIES, AND PHARYNX

1. The nose is the usual passageway for air into and out of the respiratory tract. The _____ just inside the nostrils help block the entry of dust.

2. a) Within the skull are the two nasal cavities, which are separated by the _____ .

   b) The nasal mucosa (lining) is made of _____ epithelium.

   c) State the three functions of the nasal mucosa.

   1) _____

   2) _____

   3) _____

   d) In the upper nasal cavities are the receptors for the sense of _____ .

3. a) The paranasal sinuses are air cavities that open into the _____ .

   b) Name two of the four bones that contain paranasal sinuses.

   1) _____

   2) _____

   c) State one function of these sinuses. _____

4. Match each part of the pharynx with the proper descriptive statements.

   Use each letter once. One answer line will have five correct letters; each other answer line will have two correct letters.

   1) Nasopharynx _____

   2) Oropharynx _____

   3) Laryngopharynx _____

   A. An air and food passage that opens into the larynx and esophagus
   B. Covered by the soft palate during swallowing
   C. An air passage only
   D. An air and food passage behind the mouth
   E. The palatine tonsils are on the lateral walls
   F. The adenoid is on the posterior wall
   G. The eustachian tubes open into this part
   H. The swallowing reflex involves contraction of the oropharynx and this part
   I. The only part lined with ciliated epithelium

5. From the pharynx, incoming air enters the _____ and then the trachea, both of which are part of the upper respiratory tract.

LARYNX

1. a) The larynx is an air passage between the _____ and the _____ .

   b) The other function of the larynx is _____ .

2. Match each part of the larynx with its proper description.

   Use each letter once. One answer line will have two correct answers.

   1) Epiglottis _____

   2) Vocal cords _____

   3) Ciliated epithelium _____

   4) Thyroid cartilage _____

   5) Glottis _____

   A. Two folds on either side of the glottis
   B. Sweeps mucus and pathogens upward
   C. The air passage between the vocal cords
   D. The largest, most anterior cartilage of the larynx
   E. The cartilage that covers the larynx during swallowing
   F. Vibrate to produce speech sounds

3. The cranial nerves that are the motor nerves to the larynx are the _____ and

   _____ nerves.

4. Speech sounds are produced when the intrinsic muscles of the larynx pull the vocal cords

   _____ (together or apart) across the glottis. The vocal cords are then vibrated by

   _____ air.

5. Below is a diagram of the anterior view and midsagittal section of the larynx.

   Label the parts indicated.

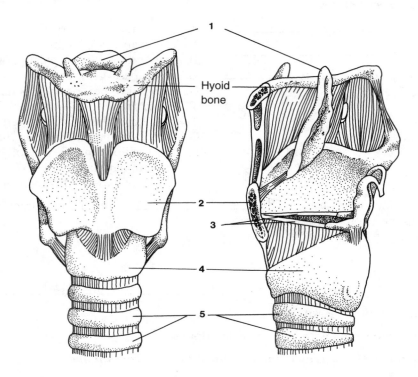

TRACHEA AND BRONCHIAL TREE

1. The trachea is an air passage that extends from the _____ to the

   _____ .

2. a) The tissue that forms C-shaped rings in the wall of the trachea is _____ .

   b) State the function of these incomplete rings. _____

   c) The tissue of the tracheal mucosa that sweeps mucus and pathogens upward is

      _____ .

3. a) The right and left primary bronchi are branches of the _____ .

   b) The secondary bronchi are within the lungs. There are _____ in the left lung and

      _____ in the right lung.

4. a) The smaller branches of the bronchial tree are called _____ , and they differ in

      structure from the bronchi in that there is no _____ in their walls to keep them
      open.

   b) The smallest bronchioles end in the clusters of _____ in the lungs.

5. Below is a diagram of the respiratory system.

   Label the parts indicated.

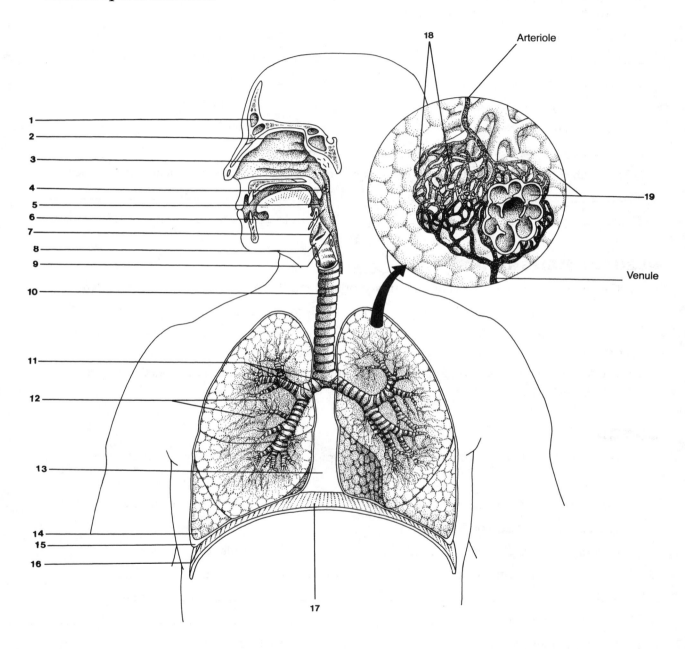

18
Arteriole

1
2
3
4
5
6
7
8
9
10

11
12
13
14
15
16

17

19

Venule

THE PATHWAY OF AIR

1. With respect to the flow of inhaled air, number the following in the proper sequence. The first and last have been indicated to get you started.

    ____1____ nose   _____ bronchioles

    _____ larynx   _____ nasopharynx

    _____ primary bronchi   _____ trachea

    _____ laryngopharynx   _____ secondary bronchi

    _____ nasal cavities   ____11____ alveoli

    _____ oropharynx

2. Which of the above structures are part of the lower respiratory tract? (Do not include the trachea.)

    1) _____   3) _____

    2) _____   4) _____

PLEURAL MEMBRANES

1. a) The serous membrane that is on the surface of the lungs is the _____ pleura.

    b) The serous membrane that lines the thoracic cavity is the _____ pleura.

2. a) The serous fluid _____ between the pleural membranes as the lungs expand and recoil.

    b) The serous fluid also keeps the pleural membranes _____ (together or apart) during breathing.

LUNGS

1. a) The lungs are within the thoracic cavity and are protected from mechanical injury by the

    _____ .

    b) Medial to the lungs is the area called the _____ , which contains the

    _____ (organ).

    c) Inferior to the lungs is the _____ , one of the respiratory muscles.

2. a) The indentation on the medial side of each lung is called the _____ .

    b) At this site, the _____ and the _____ enter the lung.

3. a) The alveoli of the lungs are made of what type of tissue? _____

    b) The pulmonary capillaries around the alveoli are made of what type of tissue?

    _____

c) The important characteristic of this tissue is that it is _____ to permit

_____ .

d) The tissue in the spaces between the alveoli important for normal exhalation is

_____ .

4. a) Each alveolus is lined with a thin layer of tissue fluid that is important to permit

_____ .

b) This tissue fluid is coated with _____ that decreases the surface tension of the

tissue fluid and permits _____ of the alveolus.

MECHANISM OF BREATHING

1. a) The movement of air into and out of the lungs is called _____ .

   b) The two phases of this movement are _____ and _____ .

2. The respiratory centers are located in the brain, in the _____ and

_____ .

3. The respiratory muscles are the:

   1) external and internal _____ muscles, which are supplied by the

   _____ nerves.

   2) the _____ , which is supplied by the _____ nerves.

4. Contractions of the respiratory muscles produce changes in _____ within the
   bronchial tree and alveoli to bring about ventilation.

5. Match each air pressure with the statements that apply to each.

   Use each letter once. Each answer line will have two correct letters.

   1) Atmospheric pressure _____

   2) Intrapleural pressure _____

   3) Intrapulmonic pressure _____

   A. The pressure in the bronchial tree and alveoli
   B. The pressure of the air around us
   C. The pressure within the potential pleural space
   D. 760 mmHg at sea level
   E. Fluctuates below and above atmospheric
      pressure during breathing
   F. Always slightly below atmospheric pressure

INHALATION (INSPIRATION)

1. With respect to normal inhalation, number these events in proper sequence.

   ___1___   The medulla generates motor impulses.

   _____   The chest cavity is enlarged in all directions.

   _____   The diaphragm and external intercostal muscles contract.

_____   Intrapulmonic pressure decreases.

_____   Motor impulses travel along the phrenic and intercostal nerves.

_____   The chest wall expands the parietal pleura, which expands the visceral pleura, which in turn expands the lungs.

_____   Air enters the lungs until intrapulmonic pressure equals atmospheric pressure.

2. A deep breath (more than normal) requires a more forceful _____ of the respiratory

muscles, which in turn would bring about greater expansion of the _____ .

EXHALATION (EXPIRATION)

1. With respect to normal exhalation, number these events in proper sequence.

____1____   Motor impulses from the medulla decrease.

_____   The chest cavity becomes smaller, and the elastic connective tissue around the alveoli recoils.

_____   Intrapulmonic pressure rises above atmospheric pressure.

_____   The lungs are compressed.

_____   The diaphragm and external intercostal muscles relax.

_____   Air is forced out of the lungs until intrapulmonic pressure equals atmospheric pressure.

2. Normal exhalation is considered a passive process because it does not require the

_____ of the respiratory muscles.

3. A forced exhalation requires contraction of the _____ muscles to pull the ribs

_____ or contraction of the _____ muscles to compress the

abdominal organs and push the diaphragm _____ .

EXCHANGE OF GASES

1. a) External respiration is the exchange of gases between the air in the _____ and the

_____ in the pulmonary capillaries.

   b) Internal respiration is the exchange of gases between the blood in the _____ and
   the tissue fluid (cells).

2. The two respiratory gases are _____ and _____ .

3. a) Inhaled air (the atmosphere) is approximately _____ % oxygen and _____ % CO_2.

   b) Exhaled air is approximately _____ % oxygen and _____ % CO_2.

4. The value that is used to express the concentration of O_2 and CO_2 in the air or in body fluids is called

_____ and is abbreviated _____ .

5. The diagram below depicts one alveolus and a pulmonary capillary. The presence of each respiratory gas in each site is shown, indicated as P_{O_2} or P_{CO_2}.

   a) For each gas in each site, indicate whether the partial pressure is "high" or "low," then use an arrow to show the direction of diffusion of each gas.

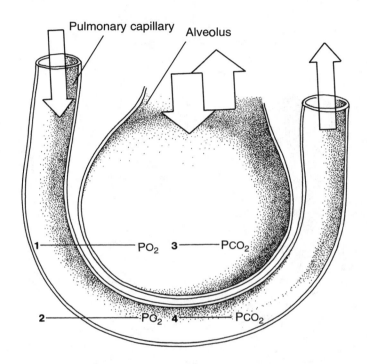

   b) This exchange of gases is called _____ respiration.

   c) The blood that leaves the pulmonary capillaries will return to the _____ and then be pumped by the _____ ventricle to the _____ .

6. The diagram below depicts a systemic capillary around cells in a body tissue. The presence of each respiratory gas in each site is shown, indicated as Po_2 or Pco_2.

   a) For each gas in each site, indicate whether the partial pressure is "high" or "low," then use an arrow to show the direction of diffusion of each gas.

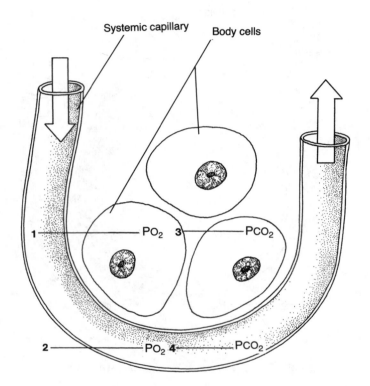

   b) This exchange of gases is called _____ respiration.

   c) The blood that leaves the systemic capillaries will return to the _____ and then be pumped by the _____ ventricle to the _____ .

TRANSPORT OF GASES IN THE BLOOD

1. a) Oxygen is carried in the blood by which cells? _____

   b) Within these cells, the oxygen is bonded to the mineral _____ in the protein _____ .

   c) The oxygen-hemoglobin bond is formed when blood circulates through the _____, where the Po_2 in the alveoli is high.

2. As blood circulates through the systemic capillaries, the O_2—Hb bond tends to break. State the three factors that will increase the release of oxygen from hemoglobin.

   a) _____

   b) _____

   c) _____

3. Most CO_2 is carried in the blood in the form of _____ ions in the

   _____ (part of blood).

4. The function of hemoglobin with respect to CO_2 transport is to act as a buffer for

   _____ ions in the RBCs.

PULMONARY VOLUMES

1. Match each pulmonary volume with its proper definition.

   Use each letter once.

   1) Tidal volume _____

   2) Vital capacity _____

   3) Inspiratory reserve _____

   4) Expiratory reserve _____

   5) Minute respiratory volume _____

   6) Residual air _____

   The Volume of Air
   A. Inhaled and exhaled in 1 minute
   B. Beyond tidal, in the most forceful exhalation
   C. Involved in the deepest inhalation followed by the most forceful exhalation
   D. That remains in the lungs after the most forceful exhalation
   E. Beyond tidal, in the deepest inhalation
   F. In one normal inhalation and exhalation

2. Residual air is important to provide air in the lungs at all times so that _____ is a continuous process.

NERVOUS REGULATION OF RESPIRATION

1. Within the brain, the respiratory centers are located in the _____ and

   _____ .

2. a) In the medulla, the _____ center generates impulses that travel to the respiratory muscles.

   b) The _____ center periodically depresses the inspiration center.

3. In the pons, the _____ center prolongs inhalation, and the _____

   center interrupts the apneustic center to help bring about _____ .

4. The normal rate of respirations ranges from _____ to _____ per minute.

5. The Hering-Breuer inflation reflex also contributes to a normal rate and rhythm of breathing. In this reflex, _____ in the lungs detect the stretching during inflation and generate impulses that depress the _____ center in the medulla to help bring about exhalation.

6. a) The hypothalamus may influence the rate or rhythm of breathing during _____ situations.

   b) The cerebral cortex may bring about _____ changes in breathing.

   c) State one example. _____

7. a) With respect to the cough reflex, the cough center is located in the _____ of the brain.

   b) The stimulus for a cough is irritation of the mucosa of the _____ , _____ , or _____ .

   c) The response is an _____ exhalation out the _____ to remove the irritation.

8. a) With respect to the sneeze reflex, the sneeze center is located in the _____ of the brain.

   b) The stimulus for a sneeze is irritation of the mucosa of the _____ .

   c) The response is an _____ exhalation out the _____ to remove the irritation.

CHEMICAL REGULATION OF RESPIRATION

1. a) Changes in the blood levels of the gases _____ and _____ may have an effect on the rate of breathing.

   b) A change in the _____ of the blood may also have an effect on respiration.

2. Match each change in blood-gas level with the proper descriptive statements.

   Use each letter once. Each answer line will have two correct letters.

   1) Decreased blood O_2 _____

   2) Increased blood CO_2 _____

   A. Detected by chemoreceptors in the carotid and aortic bodies

   B. The stimulus to increase respirations to inhale more oxygen

   C. Detected by chemoreceptors in the medulla

   D. The stimulus to increase respirations to exhale more carbon dioxide

3. a) Which of the two respiratory gases is the major regulator of respiration? _____

   b) This is so because a decrease in respirations will permit this gas to accumulate in the body and lower the _____ of the blood and other body fluids.

c) In contrast, decreased respirations will not have a great effect on the blood level of oxygen. This is so because of the _____ air that remains in the lungs after exhalation and because most of the oxygen in inhaled air _____ (does or does not) enter the blood but is available to do so if needed.

RESPIRATION AND ACID-BASE BALANCE

1. The respiratory system affects the pH of the blood and other body fluids because it regulates the amount of _____ present in these fluids.

2. Match each respiratory pH imbalance with proper cause and effects.

   Use each letter once. Each answer line will have three correct letters.

   1) Respiratory alkalosis _____

   2) Respiratory acidosis _____

   A. Caused by a decrease in the rate or efficiency of respiration
   B. Fewer H^+ ions are formed
   C. CO_2 accumulates in the body
   D. CO_2 is exhaled more rapidly
   E. Caused by an increase in the rate of respiration
   F. More H^+ ions are formed

3. State one specific cause of respiratory acidosis. _____

4. State one specific cause of respiratory alkalosis. _____

5. a) State one possible cause of metabolic acidosis. _____

   b) To compensate, respirations will _____ in order to _____ (exhale or retain) CO_2.

6. a) State one possible cause of metabolic alkalosis. _____

   b) To compensate, respirations will _____ in order to _____ (exhale or retain) CO_2.

CLINICAL APPLICATIONS

1. a) Mr. D. has mild emphysema and tells his doctor that he "can't seem to get enough air in." As Mr. D. will learn, his problem is not directly with inhalation but rather with exhalation. The deterioration of the _____ tissue around the alveoli has changed exhalation from a _____ process to an active process.

   b) Mr. D. will have to expend energy to _____ , in order to empty his lungs sufficiently to be able to inhale.

2. In asthma, an allergic reaction may cause constriction of the bronchioles. These small air passages may close completely because they have no _____ in their walls to keep them open.

3. The presence of excess tissue fluid in the alveoli is called _____ , and is often related to the weakening of what other organ? _____

4. a) Infection of the lungs is called _____ .

   b) Pathogens usually do not reach the alveoli because the _____ that line the respiratory passages sweep them toward the pharynx.

MULTIPLE CHOICE TEST #1

Choose the correct answer for each question.

1. The upper respiratory tract includes all of these except the:
   a) nasal cavities   b) larynx   c) primary bronchi   d) nasopharynx

2. During swallowing, the larynx is covered by the:
   a) soft palate   b) epiglottis   c) vocal cords   d) thyroid cartilage

3. During swallowing, the nasopharynx is covered by the:
   a) hard palate   b) oropharynx   c) epiglottis   d) soft palate

4. The trachea is kept open by which tissue?
   a) fibrous connective tissue   c) ciliated epithelium
   b) cartilage   d) elastic connective tissue

5. In the nasal cavities and trachea, mucus and pathogens are swept to the pharynx by:
   a) ciliated epithelium   c) cartilage
   b) simple squamous epithelium   d) elastic connective tissue

6. The part of the pharynx that is a passageway for air only is the:
   a) nasopharynx   b) oropharynx   c) laryngopharynx   d) tracheopharynx

7. Inhaled air passes from the trachea to the:
   a) primary bronchi   b) larynx   c) pharynx   d) secondary bronchi

8. Cartilage supports and keeps open all these structures except the:
   a) secondary bronchi   b) bronchioles   c) primary bronchi   d) larynx

9. The serous fluid between the pleural membranes keeps the membranes together and:
   a) exchanges gases   c) destroys pathogens
   b) creates friction   d) prevents friction

10. The primary bronchi and the pulmonary blood vessels enter the lung at the:
    a) apex   c) hilus on the medial side
    b) hilus on the lateral side   d) base

11. The tissue fluid that lines the alveoli is important to:
    a) prevent diffusion of gases   c) trap pathogens
    b) prevent friction   d) permit diffusion of gases

12. Within the alveoli, surface tension is decreased and inflation is possible because of the presence of:
    a) tissue fluid   c) pulmonary surfactant
    b) pulmonary blood   d) mucus

13. The respiratory centers in the brain are located in the:
    a) pons and cerebral cortex
    b) medulla and cerebral cortex
    c) hypothalamus and pons
    d) medulla and pons

14. During inhalation, the thoracic cavity is enlarged from top to bottom by contraction of the:
    a) external intercostal muscles, which move down
    b) diaphragm, which moves up
    c) diaphragm, which moves down
    d) internal intercostal muscles, which move up

15. In the alveoli, the partial pressures of oxygen and carbon dioxide are:
    a) low P_{O_2} and high P_{CO_2}
    b) high P_{O_2} and low P_{CO_2}
    c) high P_{O_2} and high P_{CO_2}
    d) low P_{O_2} and low P_{CO_2}

16. Intrapulmonic pressure is the air pressure within the:
    a) bronchial tree and alveoli
    b) intrapleural space
    c) mouth and nose
    d) rib cage and diaphragm

17. Irritants on the mucosa of the larynx are removed by:
    a) a deep breath   b) yawning   c) the sneeze reflex   d) the cough reflex

18. Most oxygen is transported in the blood:
    a) on RBC membranes
    b) in blood plasma as free oxygen
    c) bonded to hemoglobin in RBCs
    d) bonded to hemoglobin in blood plasma

19. Most carbon dioxide is transported in the blood:
    a) as hydrogen ions in the RBCs
    b) as bicarbonate ions in the plasma
    c) as CO_2 in the plasma
    d) as part of hemoglobin in RBCs

20. Internal respiration is the exchange of gases between the:
    a) systemic capillaries and body tissues
    b) pulmonary capillaries and alveoli
    c) alveoli and systemic capillaries
    d) pulmonary capillaries and body tissues

21. The factors that increase the release of oxygen from hemoglobin in systemic capillaries include all of these except:
    a) high temperature   b) low P_{O_2} c) high P_{CO_2} d) low temperature

22. The air that remains in the lungs after the most forceful exhalation is called:
    a) vital capacity
    b) tidal volume
    c) residual air
    d) leftover expiration

23. The gas that is the most important chemical regulator of respiration is:
    a) O_2, because if present in excess it lowers the pH of body fluids
    b) CO_2, because if present in excess it lowers the pH of body fluids
    c) O_2, because if present in excess it raises the pH of body fluids
    d) CO_2, because if present in excess it raises the pH of body fluids

24. The receptors that detect a decrease in the oxygen level of the blood are located in the:
    a) carotid and aortic bodies
    b) medulla
    c) pulmonary artery
    d) hypothalamus

25. If pneumonia decreases the exchange of gases in the lungs, the resulting pH imbalance is called:
    a) metabolic acidosis
    b) metabolic alkalosis
    c) respiratory acidosis
    d) respiratory alkalosis

26. The nasal mucosa has all these functions except:
    a) warming incoming air
    b) moistening incoming air
    c) increasing the oxygen content of the air
    d) sweeping mucus and pathogens to the pharynx

MULTIPLE CHOICE TEST #2

Read each question and the four answer choices carefully. When you have made a choice, follow the instructions to complete your answer.

1. Which statement is NOT true of the bronchial tree?
   a) the trachea branches into the right and left primary bronchi
   b) air is brought to the alveoli by the secondary bronchi
   c) the bronchioles have no cartilage in their walls
   d) ciliated epithelium in the trachea sweeps mucus and pathogens upward

   Reword your choice to make it a correct statement.

   _____

2. Which statement is NOT true of the larynx?
   a) it is an air passageway between the pharynx and the trachea
   b) the vocal cords are pulled together across the glottis when speaking
   c) the vagus and accessory nerves are the motor nerves for speech
   d) the epiglottis covers the top of the larynx during breathing

   Reword your choice to make it a correct statement.

   _____

3. Which statement is NOT true of gas exchange?
   a) in external respiration, oxygen diffuses from the alveoli to the pulmonary capillaries
   b) in internal respiration, carbon dioxide diffuses from the tissues to the systemic capillaries
   c) the blood that enters pulmonary capillaries has a low P_{CO_2}
   d) the blood that enters systemic capillaries has a high P_{O_2}

   Reword your choice to make it a correct statement.

   _____

4. Which statement is NOT true of the respiratory muscles?
   a) the external intercostal muscles pull the ribs up and out during inhalation
   b) the motor nerves to the diaphragm are called the diaphragm nerves
   c) the diaphragm contracts and moves down during inhalation
   d) the internal intercostal muscles pull the ribs down and in during a forced exhalation

   Reword your choice to make it a correct statement.

   _____

5. Which statement is NOT true of the nervous regulation of respiration?
   a) the apneustic center in the pons helps bring about exhalation
   b) the medulla contains an inspiration center and an expiration center
   c) the inspiration center in the medulla generates motor impulses that cause contraction of the diaphragm and external intercostal muscles
   d) sensory impulses from the baroreceptors in the lungs to the medulla help prevent overinflation of the lungs

   Reword your choice to make it a correct statement.

   _____

6. Which statement is NOT true of the chemical regulation of respiration?
   a) an increased blood level of CO_2 is detected by chemoreceptors in the medulla
   b) an increased blood level of CO_2 lowers the pH of the blood
   c) hypoxia is detected by the pulmonary and aortic chemoreceptors
   d) changes in the blood oxygen level do not affect pH

   Reword your choice to make it a correct statement.

   _____

7. Which statement is NOT true of the transport of gases in the blood?
   a) most CO_2 is carried as bicarbonate ions in the plasma
   b) hemoglobin in RBCs is able to transport oxygen because it contains copper
   c) oxygen is released from hemoglobin in tissues that have a low Po_2 and a high Pco_2
   d) the oxygen-hemoglobin bond is formed as blood passes through the pulmonary capillaries

   Reword your choice to make it a correct statement.

   _____

8. Which statement is NOT true of pulmonary volumes?
   a) tidal volume is the amount of air in one normal inhalation and exhalation
   b) residual air is important to provide for continuous gas exchange in the alveoli
   c) vital capacity is the deepest inhalation followed by a normal exhalation
   d) two factors that determine expected vital capacity are age and height

   Reword your choice to make it a correct statement.

   _____

9. Which statement is NOT true of inhalation and exhalation?
   a) the normal range of respirations per minute is 20–30
   b) normal exhalation is a passive process
   c) normal inhalation is an active process
   d) the elasticity of the lungs contributes to normal exhalation

   Reword your choice to make it a correct statement.

   _____

10. Which statement is NOT true of the respiratory system and acid-base balance?
    a) hyperventilating may bring about a mild respiratory alkalosis
    b) the respiratory system helps compensate for metabolic acidosis by decreasing the respiratory rate
    c) the respiratory system affects the pH because it regulates the amount of CO_2 in body fluids
    d) a pulmonary disease that interferes with gas exchange results in respiratory acidosis

Reword your choice to make it a correct statement.

_____

Chapter 16

The Digestive System

The digestive system consists of the organs that contribute to the physical and chemical breakdown of complex food molecules into simpler molecules. These simpler molecules are then absorbed into the blood and lymph to be transported to cells throughout the body. This chapter describes the digestive organs and the specific functions of each that contribute to digestion and absorption.

DIVISIONS OF THE DIGESTIVE SYSTEM

1. Match each division of the digestive system with the statements that apply to each.

   Use each letter once. One answer line will have four correct letters, and the other will have three correct letters.

   1) Alimentary tube _____

   2) Accessory organs _____

   A. Begins at the mouth
   B. Include the teeth, tongue, and salivary glands
   C. Includes the stomach, small intestine, and large intestine
   D. Include the liver, gallbladder, and pancreas
   E. No digestion takes place here
   F. Digestion does take place in some organs
   G. Ends at the anus

2. Name the parts of the alimentary tube in which digestion takes place. _____ , _____ , and _____

3. Name the part of the alimentary tube in which most absorption of nutrients takes place.

   _____

4. Below is a diagram of the digestive system.

   Label the parts indicated.

TYPES OF DIGESTION AND END PRODUCTS OF DIGESTION

1. Match each type of digestion with the proper descriptive statements.

   Use each letter once. Each answer line will have two correct letters.

   1) Chemical digestion _____
   2) Mechanical digestion _____

   A. Food is broken down to smaller pieces
   B. Food is changed to simpler molecules
   C. Accomplished by specific enzymes
   D. Creates more surface area for the action of digestive enzymes

2. Name the end products of digestion of:

   1) Fats: _____ and _____

   2) Proteins: _____

   3) Carbohydrates: _____

3. Other nutrients released during the digestive process are _____ ,

   _____ , and _____ .

ORAL CAVITY AND PHARYNX

1. a) The opening for food into the oral cavity is the _____ .

   b) The superior boundary of the oral cavity is the _____ .

2. Both the teeth and the tongue contribute to _____ digestion in the oral cavity by what

   we call _____ .

3. a) An individual develops two sets of teeth. The first set is called the _____ teeth

   and, if complete, consists of _____ (number) teeth.

   b) The second set is called the _____ teeth and, if complete, consists of

   _____ (number) teeth.

4. Match the following parts of a tooth with the proper descriptions.

   Use each letter once. Two answer lines will have two correct letters.

   1) Enamel _____
   2) Dentin _____
   3) Pulp cavity _____
   4) Periodontal membrane _____

   A. Forms the roots of a tooth and the interior of the crown
   B. Produces a bone-like cement to anchor the roots of a tooth
   C. Covers the crown of a tooth
   D. Lines the tooth sockets in the mandible and maxillae
   E. Forms a hard chewing surface
   F. Contains blood vessels and nerves

5. a) The tongue is also important for the sense of _____ .

   b) As the first step in swallowing, the tongue is elevated to push food toward the

   _____ .

6. Name the pairs of salivary glands with these locations:

   1) Below the floor of the mouth _____

   2) In front of the ears _____

   3) At the posterior corners of the mandible _____

7. The salivary glands are exocrine glands because they have _____ to take saliva to the

   _____ .

8. a) The digestive enzyme in saliva is _____ , which digests starch to

   _____ .

   b) The water of saliva is important to dissolve food so that it may be _____ and to

   moisten a mass of food so that it may be _____ .

9. The only eating-related function of the pharynx is _____ , which is a reflex regulated

   by a center in the _____ of the brain.

ESOPHAGUS

1. The esophagus takes food from the _____ to the _____ .

2. a) At the junction of the esophagus and the stomach is a circular smooth muscle called the

   _____ .

   b) Contraction of this sphincter prevents the backup of _____ into the

   _____ .

TYPICAL STRUCTURE OF THE ALIMENTARY TUBE

1. Match each layer of the alimentary tube with the proper descriptive statements.

   Use each letter once. Two answer lines will have three correct letters, and two will have two correct letters.

   1) Mucosa _____

   2) Submucosa _____

   3) External muscle layer _____

   4) Serosa _____

   A. Includes the epithelial tissue that lines the organ

   B. Above the diaphragm; made of fibrous connective tissue

   C. Made of areolar connective tissue

   D. Secretes mucus and digestive enzymes

   E. Made of two layers of smooth muscle

   F. Contains lymph nodules to destroy pathogens

G. Contains Meissner's plexus that regulates secretions of the mucosa

H. Contains Auerbach's plexus that regulates peristalsis

I. Below the diaphragm; is the mesentery

J. Provides mechanical digestion and peristalsis

STOMACH

1. The stomach is the sac-like portion of the alimentary tube that extends from the

_____ to the _____ .

2. Some digestion does take place in the stomach, which also serves as a _____ for food so that digestion takes place gradually.

3. a) The folds of the gastric mucosa that are present when the stomach is empty are called

_____ .

b) The glands of the stomach are called _____ , and their secretion is called

_____ .

4. Match each cell of the gastric pits with its proper secretion.

   Use each letter once.

   1) Mucus cells _____

   2) Chief cells _____

   3) Parietal cells _____

   A. Secrete pepsinogen, an inactive form of the enzyme pepsin

   B. Secrete hydrochloric acid, which activates pepsin

   C. Secrete mucus, which helps protect the gastric mucosa

5. a) The part of gastric juice that kills most microorganisms that enter the stomach is

_____ .

b) The part of gastric juice that digests proteins to polypeptides is the enzyme _____ .

6. a) Secretion of gastric juice may begin with the sight or smell of food. This is a

_____ (sympathetic or parasympathetic) response.

b) When food actually reaches the stomach, the gastric mucosa secretes the hormone

_____ , which stimulates the secretion of more gastric juice.

7. a) Mechanical digestion in the stomach is a function of the _____ layer of the wall of the stomach.

b) The pyloric sphincter is located at the junction of the pylorus of the _____ and the

_____ of the small intestine.

c) When the pyloric sphincter contracts, it prevents the backup of food from the

_____ to the _____ .

8. Below is a diagram of the stomach.

Label the parts indicated.

LIVER AND GALLBLADDER

1. The liver is located just below the _____ in the upper right and center of the

   _____ cavity.

2. a) The digestive function of the liver is the production of _____ , which contains bile

   salts that emulsify _____ .

   b) This is an aspect of _____ (mechanical or chemical) digestion.

3. Bile leaves the liver through the _____ duct, which joins the _____

   duct of the gallbladder to form the _____ duct, which carries bile to the

   _____ of the small intestine.

4. Bile also has an excretory function, because _____ and _____ are

   transported to the intestines to be eliminated in _____ .

5. a) The gallbladder is located on the undersurface of the _____ .

   b) State the two functions of the gallbladder. _____ and _____

6. a) The production of bile and the contraction of the gallbladder are regulated by hormones produced

   by the _____ .

   b) The hormone _____ stimulates production of bile by the liver.

   c) The hormone _____ stimulates contraction of the gallbladder.

7. Below is a diagram of the liver, gallbladder, and pancreas.

   Label the parts indicated.

PANCREAS

1. The pancreas is located in the upper abdominal cavity between the _____ and the

   _____ .

2. Pancreatic juices are carried by the main pancreatic duct to the _____ duct to the duodenum, which is their site of action.

3. a) Enzyme pancreatic juice contains several enzymes. The enzyme _____ digests polypeptides to shorter chains of amino acids.

   b) The enzyme _____ digests emulsified fats to _____ and

   _____ .

   c) The enzyme _____ digests starch to _____ .

4. Bicarbonate pancreatic juice contains sodium bicarbonate that neutralizes the hydrochloric acid from

   the _____ in the _____ (site of action).

SMALL INTESTINE

1. a) The small intestine is coiled within the abdominal cavity and is encircled by the

   _____ .

   b) The small intestine carries food from the _____ to the _____ .

2. a) The three parts of the small intestine, in order, are the _____ ,

   _____ , and _____ .

   b) The common bile duct enters which of these parts? _____

3. Which layer of the wall of the small intestine is responsible for mixing chyme with digestive

   secretions and for peristalsis? _____

4. Digestion of food is completed in the small intestine and requires _____ from the

   liver, _____ from the pancreas, and the enzymes produced by the small intestine itself.

5. a) The crypts of Lieberkuhn are the _____ of the small intestine.

   b) The secretion of these glands is stimulated by the presence of _____ in the duodenum.

6. a) The digestive enzymes produced by the small intestine are sucrase, maltase, and lactase, which

   digest _____ to _____ .

   b) Peptidases complete the digestion of peptide chains to _____ .

7. Efficient absorption in the small intestine requires a very large surface area, which is provided by several structural modifications of the small intestine. Match each structure with its proper description.

Use each letter once.

1) Plica circulares _____
2) Villi _____
3) Microvilli _____

A. Large folds of the mucosa and submucosa
B. Small projections of the mucosa
C. Microscopic folds of the cell membrane on the free surface of each columnar cell

8. The villi of the small intestine contain the vessels into which the end products (nutrients) of digestion are absorbed. Each villus contains a _____ , which absorbs the water-soluble nutrients and a _____ , which absorbs the fat-soluble nutrients.

9. Match each of the following nutrients with the vessel in the villi into which it is absorbed (a letter statement) and the mechanism of absorption (a number statement).

Each answer line will have one letter and one number.

1) Amino acids _____
2) Fat-soluble vitamins _____
3) Water-soluble vitamins _____
4) Fatty acids and glycerol _____
5) Monosaccharides _____
6) Positive ions _____
7) Negative ions _____
8) Water _____

Vessel
A. Capillary network
B. Lacteal

Mechanism
1. Active transport
2. Passive transport
3. Osmosis
4. Requires bile salts

10. a) The absorption of vitamin _____ requires the _____ factor produced by the stomach lining.

b) The absorption of calcium ions requires vitamin _____ and _____ hormone.

11. a) Blood from the capillary networks in the small intestine travels through the portal vein to the _____ before returning to the heart.

b) Lymph from the lacteals in the small intestine enters the blood in the _____ vein.

12. Below is a diagram of the villi of the small intestine.

    Label the parts indicated.

Arteriole
Lymph vessel
Venule

○ Capillary network
○ Lacteal
○ Goblet cell
○ Intestinal epithelium

REVIEW OF DIGESTION

1. Complete the following chart by naming the digestive secretion and its action for each organ listed in the column under the proper food type. If an organ does not contribute to the digestion of a food type, write "none." Several boxes have been completed to get you started.

Food Type

Organ	Carbohydrates	Fats	Proteins
Salivary glands	Amylase—digests starch to maltose		
Stomach		None	
Liver			None
Pancreas		Lipase—digests emulsified fats to fatty acids and glycerol	
Small intestine		None	

LARGE INTESTINE

1. The large intestine is also called the _____ and extends from the _____ of the small intestine to the _____ .

2. The first part of the colon is the _____ , to which the appendix is attached.

3. Number the parts of the colon in order, beginning with the cecum.

    ___1___ cecum   _____ descending colon

    _____ rectum   _____ anal canal

    _____ ascending colon   _____ transverse colon

    _____ sigmoid colon

4. The functions of the colon are:

   1) The absorption of _____ , _____ , and _____ .

   2) The elimination of _____ .

5. a) The normal flora of the colon are the _____ that live in the colon.

   b) One function of the colon flora is to inhibit the growth of _____ .

   c) The other function of the colon flora is to produce _____ , especially

   _____ .

6. a) The defecation reflex for the elimination of feces involves which part of the CNS?

   _____

   b) The stimulus for defecation is stretching of the _____ as peristalsis of the colon pushes feces into it.

7. Number the parts of the reflex arc for the defecation reflex in proper sequence.

   ____1____ stretch receptors in the rectum generate impulses

   _____ the rectum contracts, and the internal anal sphincter relaxes

   _____ sensory impulses travel to the spinal cord

   _____ motor impulses return to the smooth muscle of the rectum

8. Voluntary control of defecation is provided by the _____ , which contracts to close the anus.

9. Below is a diagram of the colon.

Label the parts indicated.

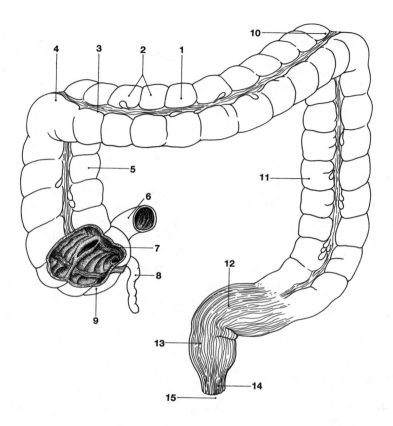

LIVER—OTHER FUNCTIONS

1. With respect to liver functions, match each of the following with the proper descriptive statement.

   Use each letter once.

   1) Transamination _____

   2) Glycogen _____

   3) Synthesis of clotting factors _____

   4) Beta-oxidation _____

   5) A, D, E, K, and B_{12} _____

   6) Fructose and galactose _____

   7) Synthesis of albumin _____

   8) Synthesis of enzymes _____

   9) Deamination _____

   10) Synthesis of lipoproteins _____

   11) Synthesis of bilirubin _____

   12) Cholesterol _____

   13) Iron and copper _____

   14) Kupffer cells _____

   A. To transport fats in the blood
   B. Monosaccharides that are changed to glucose
   C. To help maintain blood volume
   D. Formed from old RBCs and eliminated in feces
   E. The process in which the amino group is removed from an amino acid
   F. A steroid that is synthesized by the liver; excess is excreted in bile
   G. The process by which a fatty acid molecule is converted into two-carbon molecules
   H. Includes fibrinogen and prothrombin
   I. The form in which excess glucose is stored
   J. The process by which the non-essential amino acids are synthesized
   K. The macrophages of the liver that phagocytize pathogens
   L. To change harmful substances such as alcohol to less harmful ones
   M. The vitamins stored by the liver
   N. The minerals stored by the liver

CLINICAL APPLICATIONS

1. a) Mrs. L. is 50 years old and has been experiencing pain in the upper right abdominal quadrant after eating. Her doctor suspects that Mrs. L. has stones in which accessory organ of digestion?

   _____

   b) Such stones are usually made of what substance? _____

2. The pain of appendicitis would most likely be felt in which abdominal quadrant?

   _____

3. a) The term "peritonitis" means inflammation of the _____ .

   b) Describe the location of this membrane. _____

4. a) In the condition called heartburn, gastric juice damages the lining of the _____ .

   b) Name the sphincter that should prevent this. _____

MULTIPLE CHOICE TEST #1

Choose the correct answer for each question.

1. The vitamin produced by the normal flora of the colon in amounts sufficient to meet a person's daily need is:
   a) K   b) A   c) D   d) niacin

2. Backup of food from the small intestine to the stomach is prevented by the:
   a) lower esophageal sphincter   c) internal anal sphincter
   b) ileocecal valve   d) pyloric sphincter

3. All of the following are accessory organs of digestion except the:
   a) liver   b) salivary glands   c) stomach   d) pancreas

4. Mechanical digestion includes all of the following except:
   a) chewing   c) emulsification of fat by bile salts
   b) conversion of starch to maltose   d) contractions of the stomach

5. The hard chewing surface of a tooth is formed by:
   a) dentin   b) gingiva   c) bone   d) enamel

6. The only voluntary aspect of swallowing is:
   a) contraction of the pharynx   c) elevation of the soft palate
   b) peristalsis of the esophagus   d) elevation of the tongue

7. The functions of saliva include all of these except:
   a) taste   b) swallowing   c) starch digestion   d) protein digestion

8. A tooth is anchored in its socket in the jaw by the:
   a) root   b) pulp cavity   c) periodontal membrane   d) dentin

9. The layer of the alimentary tube that is responsible for peristalsis is the:
   a) serosa   b) external muscle layer   c) submucosa   d) mucosa

10. In the gastric mucosa, the parietal cells secrete:
    a) hydrochloric acid   b) pepsin   c) pepsinogen   d) complete gastric juice

11. The liver synthesizes all of these except:
    a) hemoglobin   b) fibrinogen   c) albumin   d) lipoproteins

12. When food reaches the stomach, secretion of gastric juice is stimulated by the hormone:
    a) epinephrine   b) secretin   c) gastrin   d) cholecystokinin

13. Bile is stored by the:
    a) common bile duct   b) gallbladder   c) liver cells   d) hepatic duct

14. Bile and pancreatic juices are carried to the duodenum by the:
    a) pancreatic duct   b) hepatic duct   c) cystic duct   d) common bile duct

15. Bicarbonate pancreatic juice is important to neutralize hydrochloric acid that enters the:
    a) pancreas   b) stomach   c) duodenum   d) esophagus

16. The digestion of protein involves all of these except:
    a) pepsin from the stomach   c) peptidases from the small intestine
    b) trypsin from the pancreas   d) amylase from the pancreas

17. The capillary networks and lacteals in the villi of the small intestine are important for:
   a) absorption of nutrients
   b) chemical digestion
   c) increasing surface area
   d) mechanical digestion

18. The absorption of amino acids and glucose into the capillary networks of the villi is accomplished by the process of:
   a) diffusion   b) active transport   c) passive transport   d) osmosis

19. The functions of the large intestine include all of these except:
   a) digestion of starch
   b) elimination of undigested material
   c) absorption of water
   d) absorption of vitamins and minerals

20. By the process of transamination, the liver synthesizes the:
   a) enzymes for detoxification
   b) non-essential amino acids
   c) essential amino acids
   d) clotting factors

21. The stimulus for the defecation reflex is:
   a) contraction of the rectum
   b) contraction of the internal anal sphincter
   c) stretching of the rectum
   d) relaxation of the internal anal sphincter

22. The liver stores all of these except:
   a) iron   b) glycogen   c) vitamins A and D   d) fat

23. The liver is stable to detoxify potentially harmful substances by means of the synthesis of specific:
   a) plasma proteins   b) lipoproteins   c) steroids   d) enzymes

24. Greater surface area in the small intestine is provided by all of these except:
   a) villi   b) microvilli   c) rugae   d) plica circulares

MULTIPLE CHOICE TEST #2

Read each question and the four answer choices carefully. When you have made a choice, follow the instructions to complete your answer.

1. Which statement is NOT true of the locations of digestive organs?
   a) the parotid glands are below the floor of the mouth
   b) the pancreas extends from the duodenum to the spleen
   c) the gallbladder is on the undersurface of the right lobe of the liver
   d) the part of the colon that follows the descending colon is the sigmoid colon

   Reword your choice to make it a correct statement.

   _____

2. Which statement is NOT true of the functions of the liver?
   a) fructose and galactose are changed to glucose
   b) bilirubin is synthesized and excreted into bile
   c) deamination is the first step in the use of excess amino acids for energy
   d) the process of beta-oxidation permits the use of starches for energy production

   Reword your choice to make it a correct statement.

   _____

3. Which statement is NOT true of digestive enzymes?
   a) amylase from the pancreas digests starch to maltose
   b) lipase from the pancreas digests fats to amino acids
   c) sucrase from the small intestine digests sucrose to monosaccharides
   d) pepsin from the stomach digests proteins to polypeptides

   Reword your choice to make it a correct statement.

   _____

4. Which statement is NOT true of the regulation of digestive secretions?
   a) gastrin stimulates the secretion of gastric juice
   b) increased secretion of saliva is a sympathetic response
   c) cholecystokinin stimulates contraction of the gallbladder
   d) secretin stimulates production of bile by the liver

   Reword your choice to make it a correct statement.

   _____

5. Which statement is NOT true of the digestive process?
   a) the end product of starch digestion is glucose
   b) mechanical digestion increases the surface area of food particles
   c) each digestive enzyme digests two types of foods
   d) emulsification of fats by bile salts is a form of mechanical digestion

   Reword your choice to make it a correct statement.

   _____

6. Which statement is NOT true of the teeth and tongue?
   a) both the teeth and the tongue are involved in chewing
   b) blood vessels and nerves are found in the enamel of a tooth
   c) chewing is an example of mechanical digestion
   d) the tongue is important for taste and for swallowing

   Reword your choice to make it a correct statement.

   _____

7. Which statement is NOT true of the passage of food through the alimentary tube?
   a) the pyloric sphincter prevents backup of small intestinal contents
   b) the ileocecal valve prevents the backup of feces from the colon
   c) swallowing propels food from the oral cavity through the pharynx and esophagus
      to the stomach
   d) the lower esophageal sphincter prevents backup of esophageal contents

   Reword your choice to make it a correct statement.

   _____

8. Which statement is NOT true of the stomach?
   a) hydrochloric acid destroys most microorganisms that enter the stomach because it has a pH of 7–8
   b) rugae are folds of the mucosa that permit expansion of the stomach
   c) pepsinogen is converted to pepsin by hydrochloric acid
   d) the smooth muscle layers of the stomach contract to mix food with gastric juice

   Reword your choice to make it a correct statement.

   _____

9. Which statement is NOT true of the villi of the small intestine?
   a) capillary networks absorb water-soluble nutrients
   b) blood from the capillaries of the villi flows through the portal vein to the liver
   c) villi are folds of the submucosa of the small intestine
   d) lacteals absorb the fat-soluble nutrients

   Reword your choice to make it a correct statement.

   _____

10. Which statement is NOT true of the liver and gallbladder?
    a) the common bile duct is formed by the hepatic duct and the accessory pancreatic duct
    b) the hepatic duct takes bile out of the liver
    c) the gallbladder stores bile and concentrates bile by absorbing water
    d) the cystic duct takes bile into and out of the gallbladder

    Reword your choice to make it a correct statement.

    _____

11. Which statement is NOT true of the small intestine?
    a) the small intestine is part of the alimentary tube
    b) the small intestine extends from the stomach to the colon
    c) enzymes are produced to complete the digestion of proteins and fats
    d) most absorption of nutrients takes place in the small intestine

    Reword your choice to make it a correct statement.

    _____

12. Which statement is NOT true of the colon?
    a) the internal and external anal sphincters surround the anus
    b) the ileum of the small intestine opens into the ascending colon
    c) the normal flora of the colon produce vitamins and inhibit the growth of pathogens
    d) the colon absorbs water, minerals, and vitamins

    Reword your choice to make it a correct statement.

    _____

Chapter 17

Body Temperature and Metabolism

This chapter describes the mechanisms of heat production and heat loss and the integration of these mechanisms to maintain a constant body temperature. Also in this chapter are simple descriptions of the metabolic pathways involved in the use of foods to produce ATP and a discussion of metabolic rate and the factors that affect energy and heat production.

BODY TEMPERATURE

1. a) State the normal range of human body temperature in °F: _____ to

   _____ , and in °C: _____ to _____ .

   b) The average body temperature is _____ °F or _____ °C.

2. For which two age groups is temperature regulation not as precise as it is at other times during life?

   _____ and _____

HEAT PRODUCTION

1. a) Heat is produced as one of the energy products of the process of _____ .

   b) The other energy product of this process is _____ .

2. a) The hormone that is the most important regulator of energy production is _____ ,

   produced by the _____ gland.

   b) This hormone increases heat production by increasing the rate of _____ within cells.

3. The hormone that increases the rate of cell respiration in stress situations is _____ ,

   produced by the _____ (gland).

4. a) Active organs produce significant amounts of heat because they are constantly producing

   _____ for their metabolic activities.

   b) The _____ produce about 25% of the total body heat at rest because they are

   usually in a state of slight contraction called _____ .

   c) Because it has so many important and continuous functions, the _____ produces
   about 20% of the total body heat at rest.

   d) Active organs do not "overheat" because the _____ that circulates through them
   carries heat to cooler parts of the body.

5. When food is consumed, more heat is produced as the digestive organs produce more ATP for

   _____ (name a process).

6. When a person has a fever, heat production _____ (increases or decreases) because
   metabolic rate is faster at higher temperatures.

HEAT LOSS

1. a) The major pathway of heat loss from the body is by way of the _____ because it
   covers the body surface.

   b) A secondary pathway of heat loss is by way of the _____ tract as heat is lost in
   water vapor in exhaled air.

   c) Minor pathways of heat loss are by way of the _____ and _____
   tracts, because urine and feces are at body temperature when excreted.

2. a) The temperature of the skin influences how much heat will be lost by the related processes of

   _____ , _____ , and _____ .

   b) Of these three processes, the one that involves air currents moving warmer air away from the skin

   is _____ .

   c) The processes of _____ and _____ both involve loss of heat to air
   or objects.

   d) In order for radiation and conduction to be effective heat loss mechanisms, the external

   environment must be _____ than the body temperature.

3. a) The temperature of the skin is determined by the flow of _____ through the skin.

   b) In the dermis, _____ will increase blood flow and heat loss, while

   _____ will decrease blood flow and help conserve heat.

4. a) In the process of sweating, excess body heat is lost as this heat _____ the sweat
   on the skin surface.

   b) Sweat is secreted by _____ sweat glands.

c) Sweating is not efficient when the atmospheric humidity is _____ but is efficient when the atmospheric humidity is _____ .

d) State the potential disadvantage of excessive sweating.

_____

REGULATION OF BODY TEMPERATURE

1. The part of the brain that may be likened to a thermostat and that regulates body temperature is the

_____ .

2. a) Specialized neurons in the hypothalamus detect changes in the temperature of the

_____ that circulates through the brain.

b) The hypothalamus receives sensory information about the environmental temperature from the

_____ in the skin.

3. Match each environmental situation with the proper responses brought about by the hypothalamus.

Use each letter once. Each answer line will have three correct letters.

1) Cold environment _____

2) Warm environment _____

A. Sweating increases
B. Vasodilation in the dermis
C. Muscle tone decreases to produce less heat
D. Vasoconstriction in the dermis
E. Shivering may occur to produce more heat
F. Sweating decreases

FEVER

1. A fever is an abnormally _____ body temperature and is caused by substances called

_____ that raise the setting of the hypothalamic thermostat.

2. a) Pyrogens that come from outside the body include _____ and

_____ .

b) Endogenous pyrogens are chemicals released during _____ .

3. a) When a pyrogen first affects the hypothalamus, the hypothalamic thermostat is reset

_____ (higher or lower), and the person feels _____ .

b) In order to raise the body temperature to the setting of the hypothalamic thermostat,

_____ will occur.

4. a) When the pyrogen has been destroyed, the hypothalamic thermostat is reset

_____ (higher or lower), and the person feels _____ .

b) At this time _____ will occur to lower the body temperature.

5. A fever may be beneficial because the metabolism of some _____ is inhibited by higher temperatures, and the activity of the person's own _____ is increased.

6. a) A very high fever may cause enzymes within cells to become denatured, which means they _____ , and as a result, cells may die.

   b) This is most serious in the _____ (organ) because _____ (cells) cannot reproduce to replace lost cells.

METABOLISM

1. The term for all the reactions that take place within the body is _____ .

2. a) The term for breakdown (or decomposition) reactions is _____ .

   b) The term for synthesis (or building) reactions is _____ .

   c) Which of these types of reactions requires energy (ATP)? _____

   d) Which of these types of reactions often releases energy that is used to synthesize ATP?

   _____

   e) The catalysts for many reactions in the body are specific proteins called _____ .

3. Complete the summary reaction of cell respiration:

   $C_6H_{12}O_6$ + _____ $\longrightarrow$ _____ + H_2O + _____ + _____
   (glucose)

4. The three stages of the cell respiration of a molecule of glucose are called _____ ,

   _____ , and _____ .

5. Match each statement about cell respiration with the proper stage.

   Use each letter as many times as it is correct (some lines will have two letters) for a total of 14 letters.

   A. Glycolysis   B. Krebs cycle   C. Cytochrome transport system

   1) _____ Takes place in the cytoplasm

   2) _____ Takes place in the mitochondria

   3) _____ Does not require oxygen

   4) _____ Requires oxygen

   5) _____ Glucose is broken down to pyruvic acid

   6) _____ A pyruvic acid molecule is broken down, and CO_2 is formed

   7) _____ Metabolic water is produced

   8) _____ A small amount of ATP is produced

9) _____ Most ATP is produced

10) _____ Energy is released by the reactions of the electrons of hydrogens with the cytochromes

11) _____ Lactic acid will be formed if no oxygen is present

6. a) The vitamins that are part of hydrogen carrier molecules are _____ and

_____ .

b) The vitamin necessary to remove CO_2 from pyruvic acid is _____ .

c) The minerals that are part of some of the cytochromes are _____ and

_____ .

PROTEINS AND FATS AS ENERGY SOURCES

1. a) When excess amino acids are used for energy production, the first step is deamination in which

the _____ group is removed.

b) The remaining carbon chain is converted to a molecule that can enter the _____ .

c) Such molecules may be a two-carbon _____ group or a three-carbon

_____ .

2. a) The end products of fat digestion are glycerol and fatty acids. To be used for energy production, a

three-carbon glycerol molecule is converted to _____ , which will enter the Krebs cycle.

b) To be used for energy production, a fatty acid is broken down in the process of

_____ into two-carbon _____ groups, which also enter the Krebs cycle.

3. a) Both amino acids and fatty acids may be converted by the liver into two- or four-carbon molecules

called _____ to be used for energy production.

b) The only non-carbohydrate molecules that can be converted to glucose to supply the brain are the

_____ .

ENERGY AVAILABLE FROM FOOD

1. The potential energy in food is measured in units called _____ or

_____ .

2. How many kilocalories are available in 1 gram of the following? carbohydrates _____ ,

fat _____ , and protein _____

SYNTHESIS USES OF FOODS

1. a) Excess glucose is stored as _____ in the liver and _____ , to be used for energy at a later time.

   b) Glucose is converted to _____ (monosaccharides), which are part of the nucleic acids _____ and _____ .

2. The primary uses for amino acids are the synthesis of the _____ amino acids and the synthesis of _____ .

3. Name three specific proteins and the cells (or organs) in which they are produced.

   a) _____ produced by _____

   b) _____ produced by _____

   c) _____ produced by _____

4. a) Fatty acids and glycerol may be used to synthesize _____ , which are then stored in adipose tissue.

   b) Fatty acids and glycerol may also be used to synthesize the _____ that are part of cell membranes.

   c) The acetyl groups obtained from fatty acids may be used by the liver to synthesize the steroid called _____ .

5. Name two other steroids that are synthesized from cholesterol, and name the organ that produces each.

   a) _____ produced by _____

   b) _____ produced by _____

METABOLIC RATE

1. a) Although metabolic rate means energy production, it is usually expressed as the production of which form of energy? _____

   b) The units to measure heat production are called _____ .

2. The energy production required simply to maintain life is called the _____ .

3. With respect to age, metabolic rate is highest in _____ and lowest in _____ .

4. Men usually have higher metabolic rates than do women because the hormone _____ increases the metabolic rate to a greater extent than does the hormone _____ .

5. The metabolic rate increases during stress situations because of the greater activity of the

_____ nervous system and the hormones _____ and

_____ .

6. Exercise increases the metabolic rate because of the greater activity of the _____ (organs).

CLINICAL APPLICATIONS

1. a) An abnormally high body temperature is called a _____ , and is caused by

   substances called _____ that affect the _____ .

   b) A low fever may be beneficial because some _____ are inhibited by a slightly higher temperature.

   c) A high fever may cause cells' enzymes to become denatured, which means _____ .

2. Name the vitamin whose deficiency would lead to:

   a) impaired blood clotting _____

   b) poor wound healing _____

   c) poor night vision _____

3. Name the mineral needed for each of these:

   a) part of hemoglobin _____

   b) part of vitamin B_{12} _____

   c) part of thyroxine _____

   d) part of cytochromes in cell respiration _____ and _____

MULTIPLE CHOICE TEST #1

Choose the correct answer for each question.

1. The hormone that is most important in the daily regulation of cell respiration is:
   a) insulin   b) thyroxine   c) epinephrine   d) growth hormone

2. Heat is distributed from active organs to cooler parts of the body by:
   a) the liver   b) blood   c) lymph   d) the kidneys

3. The average human body temperature in °F and °C is:
   a) 98.6°F/37°C   b) 97.6°F/35°C   c) 99.6°F/39°C   d) 97°F/36.6°C

4. In a cold environment, the arterioles in the dermis will:
   a) dilate to conserve heat   c) constrict to conserve heat
   b) dilate to lose heat   d) constrict to lose heat

5. When sweating takes place, excess body heat is lost in the:
   a) osmosis of sweat
   b) secretion of sweat
   c) evaporation of sweat
   d) filtration of sweat

6. When the body is at rest, the skeletal muscles produce a significant amount of heat because of:
   a) oxygen debt
   b) forceful contractions
   c) lactic acid production
   d) muscle tone

7. From the respiratory tract, a small amount of heat is lost in:
   a) exhaled water vapor
   b) inhaled water vapor
   c) inhaled oxygen
   d) exhaled carbon dioxide

8. The movement of air across the skin results in heat loss by the process of:
   a) conduction   b) convection   c) radiation   d) evaporation

9. The part of the brain that regulates body temperature is the:
   a) cerebrum   b) thalamus   c) hypothalamus   d) medulla

10. The body's response to a warm environment includes all of these except:
    a) increased sweating
    b) decreased muscle tone
    c) vasodilation in the dermis
    d) increased muscle tone

11. Chemicals produced during inflammation that cause fevers are called:
    a) endogenous pyrogens
    b) antibacterial pyrogens
    c) exogenous pyrogens
    d) pyrogenic pyrogens

12. A fever may be beneficial because:
    a) WBCs may be inhibited
    b) the growth of some pathogens may be inhibited
    c) RBCs are activated
    d) RBCs are inhibited

13. The term for synthesis reactions is:
    a) metabolism   b) catabolism   c) anabolism   d) metabolic rate

14. The Krebs cycle and the cytochrome transport system take place in which part of the cell?
    a) cytoplasm   b) ribosomes   c) nucleus   d) mitochondria

15. The most important synthesis uses for glucose are:
    a) pentose sugars and glycogen
    b) glycogen and polysaccharides
    c) fructose and pentose sugars
    d) fructose and glycogen

16. The most important synthesis uses for amino acids are:
    a) essential amino acids and enzymes
    b) proteins and non-essential amino acids
    c) proteins and essential amino acids
    d) enzymes and phospholipids

17. Most of the ATP produced during cell respiration is produced during which stage?
    a) glycolysis   b) Krebs cycle   c) cytochrome transport system   d) transamination

18. The carbon dioxide produced in cell respiration is produced in which stage?
    a) cytochrome transport system   b) deamination   c) glycolysis   d) Krebs cycle

19. All of these vitamins are necessary for cell respiration except:
    a) niacin   b) vitamin D   c) riboflavin   d) thiamine

20. The basal metabolic rate is the term for the body's heat production when the body is:
    a) in a stress situation
    c) exercising strenuously
    b) at rest
    d) performing light activity

21. In order to be used for energy production, amino acids may be changed to all of these except:
    a) acetyl groups   b) glucose   c) ketones   d) fatty acids

22. In order to be used for energy production, fatty acids and glycerol may be changed to all of these except:
    a) ketones   b) pyruvic acid   c) acetyl groups   d) glucose

MULTIPLE CHOICE TEST #2

Read each question and the four answer choices carefully. When you have made a choice, follow the instructions to complete your answer.

1. Which statement is NOT true of heat production?
    a) in stress situations, the hormone epinephrine increases heat production
    b) eating increases the activity of the digestive organs and increases heat production
    c) heat is an energy product of cell respiration, which is regulated primarily by thyroxine
    d) almost half the body's total heat at rest is produced by the liver and heart

    Reword your choice to make it a correct statement.

    _____

2. Which statement is NOT true of heat loss?
    a) radiation is an effective heat loss mechanism only when the environment is warmer than body temperature
    b) most heat is lost from the body by way of the skin
    c) excessive sweating may result in serious dehydration
    d) sweating is not an effective heat loss mechanism when the atmospheric humidity is high

    Reword your choice to make it a correct statement.

    _____

3. Which statement is NOT true of the body's responses in a warm environment?
    a) the hypothalamus initiates these responses as body temperature rises
    b) more heat will be lost as a result of vasoconstriction in the dermis
    c) sweating increases so that excess body heat will evaporate sweat on the skin surface
    d) muscle tone decreases so that less heat is produced

    Reword your choice to make it a correct statement.

    _____

4. Which statement is NOT true of the body's responses in a cold environment?
    a) putting on a coat is a behavioral response
    b) vasoconstriction in the dermis helps conserve heat

    c) sweating will decrease to help conserve heat
    d) shivering may occur as muscle tone decreases

Reword your choice to make it a correct statement.

_____

5. Which statement is NOT true of a fever?
    a) pyrogens activate the heat-conserving mechanisms of the hypothalamus
    b) high fevers may cause brain damage because carbohydrates become denatured
    c) pyrogens include bacteria, viruses, and chemicals released during inflammation
    d) a low fever may be beneficial because the activity of WBCs may be increased

Reword your choice to make it a correct statement.

_____

6. Which statement is NOT true of metabolic rate?
    a) heat production by the body at rest is called basal metabolic rate
    b) heat production is measured in kilocalories
    c) exercise and stress situations increase metabolic rate
    d) men and young children usually have lower metabolic rates than do women and elderly people

Reword your choice to make it a correct statement.

_____

7. Which statement is NOT true of carbohydrate metabolism?
    a) an important function of glucose is the synthesis of the pentose sugars
    b) the complete breakdown of glucose in cell respiration does not require oxygen
    c) the stages of the cell respiration of glucose are glycolysis, the Krebs cycle, and the cytochrome transport system
    d) 1 gram of carbohydrate yields 4 kilocalories of energy

Reword your choice to make it a correct statement.

_____

8. Which statement is NOT true of fat metabolism?
    a) 1 gram of fat yields 9 kilocalories of energy
    b) to be used for energy production, fatty acids are converted to acetyl groups
    c) fatty acids and glycerol are used to synthesize fats to be stored in the liver
    d) fatty acids and glycerol are used to synthesize phospholipids for cell membranes

Reword your choice to make it a correct statement.

_____

9. Which statement is NOT true of amino acid metabolism?
    a) 1 gram of protein yields 7 kilocalories of energy
    b) the liver synthesizes the non-essential amino acids
    c) most amino acids are used to synthesize the body's own proteins
    d) to be used for energy production, excess amino acids may be converted to pyruvic acid or to acetyl groups

Reword your choice to make it a correct statement.

_____

10. Which statement is NOT true of the stages of cell respiration?
    a) glycolysis takes place in the cytoplasm and does not require oxygen
    b) the Krebs cycle takes place in the mitochondria, and CO_2 is produced
    c) the cytochrome transport system takes place in the mitochondria, and metabolic water is produced
    d) most of the ATP produced in cell respiration is produced in the Krebs cycle

Reword your choice to make it a correct statement.

_____

Chapter 18

The Urinary System

The urinary system consists of the kidneys, ureters, urinary bladder, and urethra. This chapter describes the work of the kidneys in the formation of urine and the elimination of urine by the other organs of the urinary system. Of great importance is the formation of urine as it is related to many aspects of the homeostasis of body fluids.

FUNCTIONS OF THE KIDNEYS

1. The kidneys form urine from blood plasma and excrete _____ such as urea.

2. The kidneys regulate the electrolyte content of the blood by excreting or conserving

   _____ .

3. The kidneys regulate the pH of the blood by excreting or conserving ions such as

   _____ and _____ .

4. The kidneys regulate the volume of blood by excreting or conserving _____ .

5. By regulating all of these aspects of the blood, the kidneys also regulate these same aspects of

   _____ .

KIDNEYS—LOCATION AND EXTERNAL ANATOMY

1. The kidneys are located on either side of the _____ column in the upper abdominal

   cavity, _____ the peritoneum.

2. The upper part of the kidneys is protected by which bones? _____

3. a) Surrounding the kidneys is _____ tissue that acts as a cushion.

   b) The _____ is the fibrous connective tissue membrane that covers the adipose tissue and helps hold the kidneys in place.

4. a) On the medial side of each kidney is an indentation called the _____ .

   b) At this site, the _____ takes blood from the abdominal aorta into the kidney, and
   the _____ returns blood from the kidneys to the inferior vena cava.

5. Below is a diagram of the urinary system (left—male; right—female).

   Label the parts indicated.

KIDNEYS—INTERNAL STRUCTURE

1. Match each area of the kidney with the proper descriptive statements.

   Use each letter once. Two answer lines will have three correct letters, and the other will have two correct letters.

   1) Renal cortex _____

   2) Renal medulla _____

   3) Renal pelvis _____

   A. A cavity formed by the expansion of the ureter within the kidney at the hilus
   B. The outer layer of kidney tissue
   C. The inner layer of kidney tissue
   D. The calyces are funnel-shaped extensions of this part
   E. Urine enters from the papillae of the pyramids
   F. Consists of wedge-shaped pieces called renal pyramids
   G. Contains the loops of Henle and the collecting tubes of nephrons
   H. Contains the renal corpuscles and convoluted tubules of nephrons

2. Below are diagrams of a frontal section of the kidney and a microscopic section of the kidney.

   Label the parts indicated.

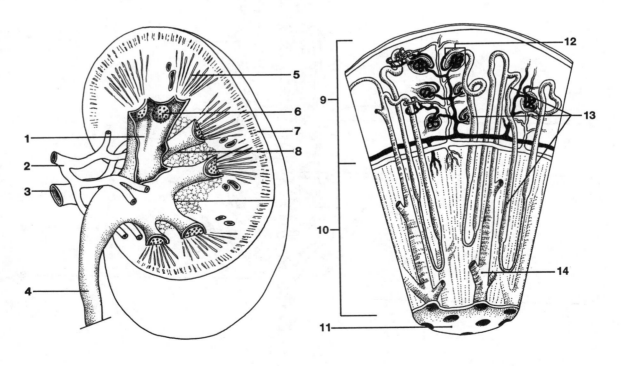

THE NEPHRON

1. a) Nephrons are the structural and _____ units of the kidneys.

   b) Each nephron consists of two major parts, called the _____ and the

   _____ .

2. A renal corpuscle consists of a capillary network called the _____ , which is

   surrounded by _____ , the expanded end of a renal tubule.

3. a) Blood enters the glomerulus from an _____ arteriole and leaves the glomerulus by

   way of an _____ arteriole.

   b) Which of these arterioles has the smaller diameter? _____

4. a) The inner layer of Bowman's capsule is very permeable because it has _____ .

   b) The outer layer of Bowman's capsule has no pores and is not _____ .

   c) The fluid that enters Bowman's capsule from the glomerulus is called _____ .

5. Number the parts of the renal tubule in the order that renal filtrate flows through them.

   _____ distal convoluted tubule

   _____ loop of Henle

   _____ collecting tubule

   _____ proximal convoluted tubule

6. Collecting tubules unite to form a papillary duct that empties urine into a calyx of the

   _____ .

7. The blood vessels that surround all the parts of a renal tubule are called the _____ ,

   and they carry blood that has come from an _____ arteriole.

8. Below is a diagram of a nephron.

   Label the parts indicated.

BLOOD VESSELS OF THE KIDNEY

1. a) The renal artery is a branch of the _____ .

   b) The renal vein takes blood to the _____ .

2. a) Number these blood vessels of the kidney in the order that blood flows through them. Begin at the renal artery and end at the renal vein.

   ___1___ renal artery   _____ small arteries in the kidney

   _____ small veins in the kidneys   _____ glomeruli

   _____ afferent arterioles   _____ peritubular capillaries

   _____ efferent arterioles   ___8___ renal vein

   b) In this pathway of blood flow, there are two sets of _____ in which exchanges take place between the blood and surrounding kidney tissue.

FORMATION OF URINE—GLOMERULAR FILTRATION

1. Glomerular filtration takes place in which major part of the nephron? _____

2. a) In glomerular filtration, blood pressure forces plasma, dissolved substances, and small proteins out of the _____ and into _____ .

   b) The fluid in Bowman's capsule is now called _____ .

   c) The components of blood that remain in the blood are _____ and _____ , because they are too _____ to be forced out of the glomerulus.

3. a) Are useful materials such as nutrients and minerals present in renal filtrate? _____

   b) Are waste products present in renal filtrate? _____

   c) Therefore, glomerular filtration is selective in terms of (choose one answer) _____ .

      1) usefulness—only waste materials enter the filtrate

      2) size—anything small or dissolved in blood plasma may enter the filtrate

      3) both of these

   d) Renal filtrate, therefore, is very similar to the _____ from which it is made, except that there is little protein and no _____ cells in filtrate.

4. a) The glomerular filtration rate (GFR) is the amount of renal filtrate formed by the kidneys in _____ (time) and is about 100 to 125 ml per minute.

   b) If blood flow through the kidneys decreases, the GFR will _____ .

   c) If blood flow through the kidneys increases, the GFR will _____ .

FORMATION OF URINE—TUBULAR REABSORPTION AND TUBULAR SECRETION

1. In the process of tubular reabsorption, useful materials are transported from the filtrate in the

   _____ to the blood in the _____ .

2. a) How much of the renal filtrate is reabsorbed back into the blood? _____ %.

   b) The filtrate that is not reabsorbed enters the renal pelvis and is then called _____ .

3. Name the mechanism by which each of these substances is reabsorbed from the filtrate back to the blood.

   a) Water _____   d) Negative ions _____

   b) Glucose _____   e) Small proteins _____

   c) Amino acids _____   f) Positive ions _____

4. a) There is a threshold level of reabsorption for glucose, amino acids, and vitamins. This means that

   there is a _____ to how much of each can be reabsorbed.

   b) For example, the threshold level for the reabsorption of glucose will be exceeded when the

   blood glucose level is too _____ (high or low) and results in a

   _____ (high or low) filtrate level of glucose.

   c) If the blood glucose level is normal, _____ (some, most, or all) of the glucose
   present in the filtrate will be reabsorbed.

5. a) The hormone that increases the reabsorption of sodium ions and the excretion of potassium ions

   is _____ .

   b) The hormone that increases the reabsorption of calcium ions is _____ .

6. a) In the process of tubular secretion, substances are transported from the blood to the

   _____ in the renal tubules.

   b) Waste products that may be secreted into the filtrate are _____ and

   _____ , as well as the metabolic products of _____ .

   c) In order to help maintain the normal pH of the blood, _____ ions may also be
   secreted into the renal filtrate.

7. a) The hormone aldosterone, by increasing the reabsorption of _____ ions, also

   increases the reabsorption of _____ by osmosis.

   b) This is very important to maintain blood _____ and blood _____ .

8. a) Antidiuretic hormone (ADH) directly increases the reabsorption of _____ by the
   distal convoluted tubules and collecting tubules.

   b) This reabsorption produces a urine that is more _____ (dilute or concentrated)
   than body fluids.

c) When ADH secretion decreases, _____ (more or less) water is reabsorbed, and the urine will be more _____ (dilute of concentrated).

9. a) The hormone ANH increases the excretion of _____ ions and _____ .

b) This will have what effect on blood volume? _____ On blood pressure? _____

10. Below is a diagram of the nephron.

   Name the substances reabsorbed or secreted by the mechanisms indicated.

Peritubular capillaries

Proximal convoluted tubule

Bowman's capsule

Filtration

Active transport
1. _____
2. _____
3. _____

Osmosis
1. _____

Pinocytosis
1. _____

Passive transport
1. _____

Glomerulus

Efferent arteriole

Secretion
1. _____
2. _____
3. _____
4. _____

Afferent arteriole

Distal convoluted tubule

Loop of Henle

Collecting tubule

THE KIDNEYS AND ACID-BASE BALANCE

1. a) If the body fluids are becoming too acidic, the kidneys will excrete more _____

    ions into the renal filtrate and will return more _____ and _____
    ions to the blood.

   b) This will _____ (raise or lower) the pH of the blood back toward normal.

2. a) If the body fluids are becoming too alkaline, the kidneys will excrete more

    _____ ions in the renal filtrate and return more _____ ions to the
    blood.

   b) This will _____ (raise or lower) the pH of the blood back toward normal.

OTHER FUNCTIONS OF THE KIDNEYS

1. a) The kidneys secrete the enzyme renin when blood pressure _____ .

   b) The cells that secrete renin are called _____ cells, which are located in the wall of

    the _____ arteriole.

   c) Renin starts the renin-angiotensin mechanism that results in the formation of

    _____ .

   d) State the two functions of angiotensin II. _____ and _____

   e) Both of these functions will _____ (raise or lower) blood pressure.

2. a) The kidneys secrete the hormone _____ when the body is in a state of hypoxia,

    which means _____ .

   b) This hormone then stimulates the _____ to increase the rate of production of

    _____ to increase the oxygen-carrying capacity of the blood.

3. The kidneys change the inactive forms of vitamin _____ to the most active form,

    which increases the absorption of _____ and _____ in the small
    intestine.

ELIMINATION OF URINE

1. a) The two ureters are located _____ the peritoneum of the dorsal abdominal cavity.

   b) Each ureter extends from the _____ of a kidney to the _____ side

    of the _____ .

   c) Peristalsis of the ureter propels urine into the bladder. Name the tissue in the wall of the ureter

    that is responsible for peristalsis. _____

2. a) The urinary bladder is located behind the _____ bones.

   b) In men, the bladder is superior to the _____ gland.

   c) In women, the bladder is inferior to the _____ .

3. The functions of the urinary bladder are to serve as a _____ for accumulating urine and to _____ to eliminate urine.

4. a) When the bladder is empty, the mucosa has folds called _____ .

   b) The epithelium of the bladder is _____ epithelium.

   c) Both of these permit _____ of the bladder without tearing the lining.

   d) The triangular area on the floor of the bladder that has no rugae is called the

   _____ .

   e) The boundaries of this area are formed by the openings of the two _____ and the

   _____ .

5. a) The smooth muscle layer of the wall of the bladder is called the _____ .

   b) Around the opening of the urethra, the detrusor muscle forms the _____ sphincter, which is _____ (voluntary or involuntary).

6. Below is a diagram of the urinary bladder.

   Label the parts indicated.

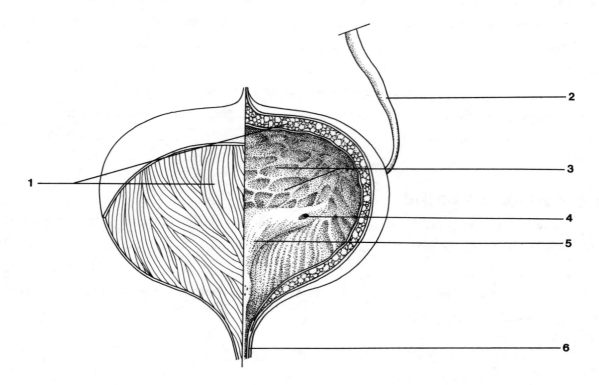

7. a) The urethra carries urine from the _____ to the _____ .

    b) In women, the urethra is _____ to the vagina.

    c) In men, the urethra extends through the _____ gland and the

       _____ and carries _____ as well as urine.

    d) Within the wall of the urethra is the _____ sphincter, which is

       _____ (voluntary or involuntary).

8. a) The term micturition reflex is another name for the _____ reflex.

    b) Which part of the CNS is directly involved in this reflex? _____

9. a) Number the following events of the urination reflex in the proper sequence.

      __1__ stretching of the detrusor muscle by accumulating urine

      _____ the detrusor muscle contracts, and the internal urethral sphincter relaxes

      _____ motor impulses along parasympathetic nerves return to the detrusor muscle

      _____ sensory impulses travel to the sacral spinal cord

      _____ stretch receptors in the detrusor muscle generate impulses

      __6__ the bladder is emptied

    b) Urination may be prevented by voluntary contraction of the _____ .

CHARACTERISTICS OF URINE

1. a) The normal range of urinary output in 24 hours is _____ .

    b) State one factor that may decrease urinary output. _____

    c) State one factor that may increase urinary output. _____

2. a) The yellow color of urine is often called _____ or _____ .

    b) Urine is usually _____ (clear or cloudy) in appearance.

3. a) The normal range of specific gravity of urine is _____ to _____ .

    b) Specific gravity is a measure of the _____ in urine and is an indicator of the

       _____ ability of the kidneys.

    c) Urine with a specific gravity of 1.023 is more _____ (dilute or concentrated) than
urine with a specific gravity of 1.015.

    d) State one factor that will result in the formation of a more concentrated urine.

    _____

4. The average pH of urine is _____ , but a pH range of _____ to

    _____ is considered normal.

5. Urine is approximately 95% _____ , which is the _____ for nitrogenous wastes and excess minerals.

6. Match each nitrogenous waste with its proper source.

   Use each letter once.

   1) Creatinine _____

   2) Uric acid _____

   3) Urea _____

   A. From the deamination of excess amino acids that are used for energy production
   B. From the use of creatine phosphate as an energy source in muscles
   C. From the decomposition of nucleic acids

7. If the blood levels of nitrogenous wastes are higher than normal, the kidneys are (choose one answer) _____.

   a) functioning properly   b) not functioning properly   c) working overtime

ABNORMAL CONSTITUENTS OF URINE

1. Match each abnormal constituent of urine with the proper reason for it.

   Use each letter once.

   1) Protein _____

   2) Blood _____

   3) Glucose _____

   4) Ketones _____

   5) Bacteria _____

   A. Infection somewhere in the urinary tract
   B. Increased use of fats and proteins for energy
   C. A higher than normal blood glucose level
   D. Bleeding somewhere in the urinary tract
   E. The glomeruli have become too permeable, allowing large molecules through

CLINICAL APPLICATIONS

1. A sharp blow to the back may dislodge a kidney, which is then called a "floating kidney." What tissues normally cushion the kidneys and keep them in place? _____ and

   _____

2. If a kidney stone (calculus) becomes lodged in a ureter, urine will not be able to reach the

   _____ , but will back up into the _____ of the kidney.

3. Choose your answers from: increase, decrease, remain the same.
   Following a severe hemorrhage:

   a) The FER would probably _____ .

   b) In turn, urinary output would then _____ .

   c) The blood level of waste products would then _____ .

MULTIPLE CHOICE TEST #1

Choose the correct answer for each question.

1. A renal corpuscle consists of:
   a) a glomerulus and peritubular capillaries
   b) a renal tubule and Bowman's capsule
   c) a glomerulus and Bowman's capsule
   d) a renal tubule and peritubular capillaries

2. The kidneys are located behind the:
   a) renal artery   b) peritoneum   c) spinal column   d) renal vein

3. All of these are found at the hilus of a kidney except the:
   a) renal artery   b) urethra   c) ureter   d) renal vein

4. The cavity within the kidney that collects urine is the:
   a) renal pelvis   b) urinary bladder   c) ureter   d) renal vein

5. The renal vein takes blood from the kidney to the:
   a) abdominal aorta   b) renal artery   c) superior vena cava   d) inferior vena cava

6. All of these are parts of the renal tubule except the:
   a) loop of Henle
   b) glomerulus
   c) proximal convoluted tubule
   d) distal convoluted tubule

7. If body fluids are becoming too acidic, the kidneys will excrete more of these ions in urine:
   a) sodium ions   b) bicarbonate ions   c) hydrogen ions   d) potassium ions

8. The hormone that directly increases the reabsorption of water by the kidneys is:
   a) ADH   b) aldosterone   c) PTH   d) ANH

9. The process of glomerular filtration takes place from the:
   a) glomerulus to Bowman's capsule
   b) renal tubule to peritubular capillaries
   c) Bowman's capsule to glomerulus
   d) peritubular capillaries to renal tubule

10. The process of tubular reabsorption takes place from the:
    a) glomerulus to afferent arteriole
    b) peritubular capillaries to renal tubule
    c) efferent arteriole to glomerulus
    d) renal tubule to peritubular capillaries

11. The renal pyramids make up the:
    a) renal cortex   b) renal pelvis   c) renal medulla   d) renal fascia

12. Renal filtrate differs from blood plasma in this way:
    a) only waste products are present in filtrate
    b) there are no nutrients in filtrate
    c) there is more protein in filtrate
    d) there are no blood cells in filtrate

13. When the blood level of oxygen decreases, the kidneys secrete:
    a) renin   b) aldosterone   c) angiotensin II   d) erythropoietin

14. When blood pressure decreases, the kidneys secrete:
    a) angiotensin II   b) renin   c) aldosterone   d) epinephrine

15. The part of the urinary bladder that actually eliminates the urine is the:
    a) detrusor muscle   b) trigone   c) rugae   d) transitional epithelium

16. Voluntary control of urination is provided by the:
    a) detrusor muscle
    b) external urethral sphincter
    c) spinal cord
    d) internal urethral sphincter

17. In tubular reabsorption, glucose and amino acids are reabsorbed by the process of:
    a) active transport   b) passive transport   c) pinocytosis   d) osmosis

18. The glomerular filtration rate will decrease if:
    a) the amount of waste products in the blood increases
    b) blood flow through the kidneys decreases
    c) blood flow through the kidneys increases
    d) the amount of waste products in the blood decreases

19. Urea is a nitrogenous waste product that comes from the metabolism of:
    a) nucleic acids   b) muscle tissue   c) amino acids   d) carbohydrates

20. Normal values for daily urinary output and pH of urine might be:
    a) 2.5 liters/3.0   b) 4.0 liters/6.5   c) 2.0 liters/9.0   d) 1.5 liters/6.0

21. Urine is propelled through a ureter by:
    a) striated muscle   b) ciliated epithelium   c) skeletal muscle   d) smooth muscle

22. The kidneys are protected from mechanical injury by the:
    a) pelvic bone and smooth muscle
    b) smooth muscle and rib cage
    c) adipose tissue and pelvic bone
    d) rib cage and adipose tissue

MULTIPLE CHOICE TEST #2

Read each question and the four answer choices carefully. When you have made a choice, follow the instructions to complete your answer.

1. Which statement is NOT true of tubular reabsorption and tubular secretion?
   a) water is reabsorbed by osmosis
   b) reabsorbed materials enter the glomerular capillaries
   c) creatinine and the metabolic products of medications may be secreted into the renal filtrate
   d) positive ions are reabsorbed by active transport, and negative ions and water follow

   Reword your choice to make it a correct statement.

   _____

2. Which statement is NOT true of hormone effects on the kidneys?
   a) ADH increases the reabsorption of water
   b) PTH increases the reabsorption of calcium ions
   c) aldosterone decreases the reabsorption of sodium ions
   d) ANH increases the excretion of sodium ions

   Reword your choice to make it a correct statement.

   _____

3. Which statement is NOT true of the urination reflex?
   a) the stimulus is stretching of the rugae of the urinary bladder by accumulating urine
   b) from the bladder, sensory impulses travel to the sacral spinal cord

    c) the detrusor muscle contracts to eliminate the urine
    d) the internal urethral sphincter relaxes to permit urination

Reword your choice to make it a correct statement.

_____

4. Which statement is NOT true of the location of the kidneys?
    a) the kidneys are posterior to the peritoneum
    b) the kidneys are medial to the spinal column
    c) adipose tissue surrounds the kidneys and cushions them
    d) the renal fascia is a fibrous connective tissue membrane that helps keep the kidneys in place

Reword your choice to make it a correct statement.

_____

5. Which statement is NOT true of a nephron?
    a) a glomerulus is surrounded by Bowman's capsule
    b) the proximal and distal convoluted tubules are found in the renal cortex
    c) the loops of Henle and collecting tubules are found in the renal pelvis
    d) all the parts of a renal tubule are surrounded by peritubular capillaries

Reword your choice to make it a correct statement.

_____

6. Which statement is NOT true of glomerular filtration?
    a) blood pressure in the glomeruli is high because the efferent arterioles are smaller in diameter than the afferent arterioles
    b) blood pressure in the glomeruli provides the force for filtration
    c) blood cells and large proteins remain in the blood in Bowman's capsule
    d) glomerular filtration increases if blood flow through the kidneys increases

Reword your choice to make it a correct statement.

_____

7. Which statement is NOT true of the characteristics of normal urine?
    a) specific gravity is a measure of the dissolved materials in urine
    b) cloudy urine may be an indicator of a urinary tract infection
    c) the volume of urinary output may be changed by factors such as excessive sweating or diarrhea
    d) glucose is present in urine only if the blood glucose level is too low

Reword your choice to make it a correct statement.

_____

8. Which statement is NOT true of the elimination of urine?
    a) a ureter carries urine from the renal pelvis to the urinary bladder
    b) the micturition reflex is a spinal cord reflex
    c) the urethra carries urine from the urinary bladder to the exterior
    d) the voluntary external urethral sphincter is in the wall of the ureter

Reword your choice to make it a correct statement.

_____

9. Which statement is NOT true of the kidneys?
   a) the kidneys change inactive forms of vitamin C to the active form
   b) when blood pressure decreases, the kidneys secrete renin to start the formation of angiotensin II
   c) in a state of hypoxia, the kidneys secrete erythropoietin to increase the rate of RBC production
   d) the kidneys help maintain normal blood volume and blood pressure

   Reword your choice to make it a correct statement.

   _____

10. Which statement is NOT true of the kidneys and regulation of the homeostasis of body fluids?
    a) the kidneys regulate blood volume by excreting or conserving water
    b) by regulating the composition of blood, the kidneys also regulate the composition of tissue fluid
    c) the kidneys excrete or conserve minerals to regulate the electrolyte balance of the blood
    d) the kidneys respond to a decreasing pH of the blood by excreting fewer hydrogen ions

    Reword your choice to make it a correct statement.

    _____

Chapter 19

Fluid-Electrolyte and Acid-Base Balance

The regulation of the water and mineral content of the body is the fluid-electrolyte balance, and the regulation of the pH of the body fluids is the acid-base balance. Some of this material has been part of previous chapters and is included in this chapter to provide a complete discussion of these important aspects of homeostasis.

WATER COMPARTMENTS

1. The water found within cells is called _____ fluid and is about

    _____ (fraction) of the total body water.

2. a) All the water found outside cells is called _____ fluid.

    b) This fluid may be given more specific names when found in specific locations. Name each of these fluids.

    1) _____ in tissue spaces between cells

    2) _____ in blood vessels

    3) _____ in lymph vessels

3. Match each of these specialized fluids with its proper location.

    Use each letter once.

    1) Cerebrospinal fluid _____

    2) Aqueous humor _____

    3) Synovial fluid _____

    4) Serous fluid _____

    A. Within the eyeball
    B. Between membranes such as the pleural membranes
    C. Around and within the CNS
    D. Within joint cavities

4. The two processes by which water moves from one compartment to another within the body are

    _____ and _____ .

WATER INTAKE AND OUTPUT

1. a) The body's major source of water is _____ .

   b) A secondary source of water is the water in _____ .

   c) A small amount of water is produced within the body as a product of the process of

   _____ .

2. a) The major pathway of water loss from the body is by way of the _____ system in

   the form of _____ .

   b) A secondary pathway of water loss is by way of the _____ in the form of

   _____ .

   c) Smaller amounts of water are also lost in _____ and _____ .

3. a) For healthy people, water intake should _____ water output.

   b) If sweating increases, what must be done to compensate? _____

   c) If fluid intake is excessive, however, _____ will increase to return the body's water
   content to normal.

REGULATION OF WATER INTAKE AND OUTPUT

1. The part of the brain that regulates the water content of the body is the _____ .

2. The term osmolarity means _____ .

3. The specialized cells in the hypothalamus that detect changes in the osmolarity of body fluids are

   called _____ .

4. a) When the body is dehydrated, the osmolarity of body fluids _____ (increases or
   decreases), because there is more dissolved material in proportion to water.

   b) In a state of dehydration, a person experiences the sensation of _____ and will

   _____ .

   c) As water is absorbed by the digestive tract, the osmolarity of the body fluids

   _____ (increases or decreases) toward normal.

5. a) The hormone _____ is produced by the hypothalamus and stored in the

   _____ pituitary gland.

   b) The function of ADH is to _____ by the kidneys.

   c) In what type of situation is ADH secreted? _____

   d) In this situation, ADH effects will cause urinary output to _____ .

6. a) The hormone _____ is produced by the adrenal cortex and increases the
   reabsorption of sodium ions by the kidney tubules.

b) How does this affect the reabsorption of water by the kidneys? _____ (increases or decreases)

c) State two types of situations that stimulate secretion of aldosterone.

1) _____

2) _____

7. If there is too much water in the body, the secretion of ADH will _____ (increase or decrease), and urinary output will _____ (increase or decrease).

8. If blood volume or BP increases, the heart will produce the hormone _____ , which will _____ (increase or decrease) the excretion of sodium ions and water.

ELECTROLYTES

1. When electrolytes are in water, they dissociate into their _____ .

2. Most electrolytes are _____ (organic or inorganic) molecules that include

_____ , _____ , and _____ .

3. a) Anions are _____ ions.

b) Give two examples. _____ and _____

c) Cations are _____ ions.

d) Give two examples. _____ and _____

4. a) By their presence in body fluids, electrolytes help create the _____ of these fluids and help regulate the _____ of water between water compartments.

b) Water will move by osmosis to a compartment with a _____ (greater or lesser) concentration of electrolytes.

5. Some electrolytes are structural components of tissues, such as _____ , or are part of proteins, such as _____ .

6. Match each body fluid with the statement that describes its electrolyte composition.

Use each letter once.

1) Intracellular fluid _____

2) Tissue fluid _____

3) Plasma _____

A. The most abundant cation is sodium, the most abundant anion is chloride, and there are few protein anions.

B. The most abundant cation is sodium, the most abundant anion is chloride, and there are many protein anions.

C. The most abundant cation is potassium, and the most abundant anions are phosphate and proteins.

REGULATION OF ELECTROLYTE INTAKE AND OUTPUT

1. We take in electrolytes as part of _____ and _____ .

2. a) Electrolytes are lost from the body in _____ , _____ , and

   _____ .

   b) The most abundant electrolytes in sweat are _____ and _____ .

   c) Electrolytes are present in urine when their blood levels are _____ (lower or higher) than the body's need for them.

3. Match each hormone with its proper effect(s) on electrolytes.

   Use each letter once. One answer line will have two correct letters.

   1) Aldosterone _____

   2) Calcitonin _____

   3) Parathyroid hormone _____

   4) ANH _____

   A. Increases the reabsorption of calcium and phosphorus from the bones to the blood
   B. Increases the removal of calcium and phosphorus from the blood and into bones
   C. Increases the reabsorption of sodium by the kidneys
   D. Increases the excretion of potassium by the kidneys
   E. Increases the excretion of sodium by the kidneys

ACID-BASE BALANCE

1. The pH of body fluids is regulated by three mechanisms: the _____ in body fluids,

   the _____ system, and the _____ .

2. a) The normal pH range of blood is _____ to _____ .

   b) The normal pH range of intracellular fluid is _____ to _____ .

   c) The normal pH range of tissue fluid is similar to that of _____ but is slightly more variable.

3. a) On the pH scale, a value of 7.0 is considered _____ .

   b) A pH below 7 is considered _____ , and a pH above 7 is considered

   _____ .

   c) Therefore, the pH of blood is slightly _____ , and the pH of intracellular fluid is

   slightly _____ or neutral.

BUFFER SYSTEMS

1. a) A buffer system consists of two chemicals: a weak _____ and a weak _____ .

   b) The chemicals of a buffer system react with _____ acids or bases to change them to substances that _____ (will or will not) have a great effect on pH.

2. The three buffer systems that help prevent drastic changes in the pH of the blood or other body fluids are the _____ , _____ , and _____ .

3. a) The bicarbonate buffer system consists of the weak acid _____ and the weak base _____ .

   b) If a potential pH change is caused by a strong acid, _____ will react with it to form a salt and the weak acid _____ , which has little effect on pH.

   c) If a potential pH change is caused by a strong base, _____ will react with it to form water and the weak base _____ , which has little effect on pH.

4. a) The phosphate buffer system consists of the weak acid _____ and the weak base _____ .

   b) This buffer system is important in the _____ (organs).

   c) To counteract increasing acidity, the kidneys will excrete which member of this buffer system in urine? _____

5. a) In the protein buffer system, an amino acid may act as either an _____ or a _____ .

   b) The _____ group of an amino acid acts as an acid because it can donate a _____ ion to the intracellular fluid.

   c) The _____ group of an amino acid acts as a base because it can pick up an excess _____ ion from the intracellular fluid.

6. How long does it take for a buffer system to react to prevent a great change in pH?

   _____

RESPIRATORY MECHANISMS TO REGULATE pH

1. The respiratory system has an effect on the pH of body fluids because it regulates the amount of _____ present in these fluids.

2. Carbon dioxide affects the pH of body fluids because it reacts with water and eventually forms _____ .

3. Match each respiratory pH imbalance with the statements that apply to each.

Use each letter once. Each answer line will have four correct letters.

1) Respiratory acidosis _____

2) Respiratory alkalosis _____

A. Caused by an increase in the rate of respiration
B. Caused by a decrease in the rate or efficiency of respiration
C. More CO_2 is retained within the body
D. More CO_2 is exhaled
E. Fewer H^+ ions are produced
F. More H^+ ions are produced
G. The pH of body fluids decreases
H. The pH of body fluids increases

4. To compensate for a metabolic acidosis, the respiratory rate will _____ (increase or decrease) to exhale _____ (more or less) CO_2 to _____ (increase or decrease) the formation of H^+ ions to _____ (raise or lower) the pH toward normal.

5. To compensate for a metabolic alkalosis, the respiratory rate will _____ (increase or decrease) to exhale _____ (more or less) CO_2 to _____ (increase or decrease) the formation of H^+ ions to _____ (raise or lower) the pH toward normal.

6. How long does it take for the respiratory system to respond to changes in pH?

_____

RENAL MECHANISMS TO REGULATE pH

1. To compensate for a state of acidosis, the kidneys will excrete _____ ions and will conserve _____ ions and _____ ions.

2. To compensate for a state of alkalosis, the kidneys will excrete _____ ions and _____ ions and will conserve _____ ions.

3. How long does it take the kidneys to respond to pH changes? _____

4. Number the pH-regulating mechanisms in the order of their greatest capacity (NOT speed) to correct an ongoing pH imbalance.

_____ Buffer systems

_____ Respiration

_____ Kidneys

CAUSES AND EFFECTS OF pH CHANGES

1. State a specific cause of respiratory acidosis. _____

2. State a specific cause of respiratory alkalosis. _____

3. State two specific causes of metabolic acidosis. _____

   and _____

4. State two specific causes of metabolic alkalosis. _____

   and _____

5. a) A state of acidosis has its greatest detrimental effects on the _____ .

   b) State two possible consequences of acidosis. _____

   and _____

6. a) A state of alkalosis affects both the _____ and _____ nervous
   systems.

   b) State two possible consequences of alkalosis. _____

   and _____

CLINICAL APPLICATIONS

1. Mrs. A. has congestive heart failure in which her right ventricle is not pumping efficiently. As a result,

   Mrs. A. has what is called _____ edema, which is an accumulation of tissue fluid that

   causes swelling that is most apparent in the _____ (part of the body).

2. As part of his physical fitness program, Mr. K. runs 5 miles a day. He did so on a hot August day and
   then felt very dizzy and weak. The probable cause of these symptoms was the loss of water and
   which electrolyte in sweat? _____

3. a) Variations in the blood level of potassium may have serious consequences. Both hypokalemia and

   hyperkalemia may affect the functioning of which vital organ? _____

   b) State a possible cause of hypokalemia. _____

4. Mr. S. is an elderly diabetic who sometimes forgets to administer his insulin. He is brought to the
   hospital in a state of ketoacidosis. You would expect which of these reports? (Choose the correct
   answer for each.)

1) Blood pH	a) 7.40	b) 7.35	c) 7.30
2) Respirations per minute	a) 40	b) 20	c) 10
3) Urine pH	a) 4.5	b) 6.5	c) 7.0

MULTIPLE CHOICE TEST #1

Choose the correct answer for each question.

1. Filtration forces water out of capillaries into tissue spaces, and the name for this water changes from:
   a) tissue fluid to lymph
   b) plasma to tissue fluid
   c) tissue fluid to plasma
   d) intracellular fluid to plasma

2. Most of the water output from the body is in the form of:
   a) sweat
   b) exhaled water vapor
   c) feces
   d) urine

3. Most of the water intake for the body is in the form of:
   a) fruits
   b) metabolic water
   c) beverages
   d) bread and cereal

4. All of these are cations except:
   a) bicarbonate ions
   b) sodium ions
   c) calcium ions
   d) potassium ions

5. The function of ADH is to:
   a) decrease the reabsorption of water by the kidneys
   b) increase the reabsorption of sodium ions by the kidneys
   c) decrease the water secreted in sweat
   d) increase the reabsorption of water by the kidneys

6. An electrolyte is a substance that, in solution, dissociates into its:
   a) positive atoms
   b) positive and negative ions
   c) negative molecules
   d) positive and negative bonds

7. Water will move by osmosis to an area where there are more:
   a) cells
   b) electrolytes
   c) water molecules
   d) membranes

8. Regulation of the water balance of the body is a function of the:
   a) thalamus
   b) cerebrum
   c) medulla
   d) hypothalamus

9. To compensate for a state of dehydration, urinary output will:
   a) decrease
   b) increase
   c) remain the same
   d) increase then decrease

10. The direct effect on the kidneys of the hormone aldosterone is to:
    a) decrease the reabsorption of sodium and the excretion of potassium
    b) increase the reabsorption of sodium and potassium
    c) increase the reabsorption of sodium and the excretion of potassium
    d) increase the excretion of sodium and potassium

11. Proteins are significant anions in which of these fluids?
    a) tissue fluid and lymph
    b) tissue fluid and intracellular fluid
    c) plasma and intracellular fluid
    d) lymph and cerebrospinal fluid

12. Extracellular fluid includes all of these except:
    a) water in capillaries
    b) water within cells
    c) cerebrospinal fluid
    d) tissue fluid

13. The absorption of calcium ions by the small intestine and kidneys is increased by:
    a) parathyroid hormone
    b) aldosterone
    c) calcitonin
    d) ADH

14. The normal pH range of blood is:
    a) 7.25–7.35
    b) 7.40–7.50
    c) 7.30–7.40
    d) 7.35–7.45

15. The mechanism with the greatest capacity to correct an ongoing pH imbalance is the:
   a) respiratory system   b) buffer systems   c) kidneys   d) digestive system

16. The mechanism that works most rapidly to correct a pH imbalance is the:
   a) kidneys   c) buffer systems
   b) respiratory system   d) none of these works rapidly

17. The part of the bicarbonate buffer system that reacts with a strong acid is:
   a) sodium bicarbonate   b) Na_2CO c) carbonic acid   d) H_2CO_3

18. An amino acid is able to buffer a strong acid when:
   a) the carboxyl group picks up an excess hydrogen ion
   b) the amine group picks up an excess hydrogen ion
   c) the carboxyl group gives off a hydrogen ion
   d) the amine group gives off a hydrogen ion

19. A state of acidosis affects the:
   a) digestive system, preventing the digestion of proteins
   b) CNS, causing muscle spasms and convulsions
   c) CNS, causing confusion and coma
   d) respiratory system, causing the respiratory rate to decrease

20. The respiratory system will help compensate for a metabolic acidosis by:
   a) decreasing the respiratory rate to exhale less CO_2
   b) increasing the respiratory rate to exhale more CO_2
   c) decreasing the respiratory rate to retain more CO_2
   d) increasing the respiratory rate to retain more CO_2

21. In order to compensate for acidosis, the kidneys will excrete:
   a) more hydrogen ions   c) fewer hydrogen ions
   b) more sodium ions   d) more bicarbonate ions

22. An untreated diabetic who is in a state of ketoacidosis will:
   a) be breathing slowly   c) be breathing rapidly
   b) excrete an alkaline urine   d) excrete a urine with a pH of 7

MULTIPLE CHOICE TEST #2

Read each question and the four answer choices carefully. When you have made a choice, follow the instructions to complete your answer.

1. Which statement is NOT true of hormone effects on fluid-electrolyte balance?
   a) PTH decreases the absorption of calcium ions by the small intestine
   b) ADH increases the reabsorption of water by the kidneys
   c) aldosterone increases the reabsorption of sodium ions by the kidneys
   d) ANH increases the excretion of sodium ions by the kidneys

   Reword your choice to make it a correct statement.

2. Which statement is NOT true of water compartments?
   a) water found in arteries and veins is called plasma
   b) the tissue fluid of the CNS is called cerebrospinal fluid
   c) the water found within cells is called intercellular fluid
   d) intracellular fluid is about two thirds of the total body water

   Reword your choice to make it a correct statement.

   _____

3. Which statement is NOT true of water intake and output?
   a) the metabolic water produced in cell respiration contributes to daily water intake
   b) most water lost from the body is in the form of feces
   c) most water intake is in the form of beverages
   d) the loss of water in sweat varies with the amount of daily exercise

   Reword your choice to make it a correct statement.

   _____

4. Which statement is NOT true of the regulation of the water content of the body?
   a) the osmoreceptors that detect changes in the water content of body fluids are in the hypothalamus
   b) a state of dehydration will bring about a decrease in urinary output
   c) the hormones that have the greatest effect on the water content of the body are aldosterone and PTH
   d) strenuous exercise that increases sweating will result in a sensation of thirst

   Reword your choice to make it a correct statement.

   _____

5. Which statement is NOT true of electrolytes?
   a) anions are negative ions such as chloride ions
   b) in water, electrolytes dissociate into their positive and negative ions
   c) some electrolytes are part of structural components of the body such as bones
   d) the electrolyte concentration in body fluids helps regulate the process of filtration

   Reword your choice to make it a correct statement.

   _____

6. Which statement is NOT true of buffer systems?
   a) the phosphate buffer system is one of the renal mechanisms for regulation of pH
   b) a buffer system consists of a weak acid and a weak base
   c) the buffer systems work very slowly to correct pH imbalances
   d) the bicarbonate buffer system is important in extracellular fluid

   Reword your choice to make it a correct statement.

   _____

7. Which statement is NOT true of the respiratory system and acid-base balance?
   a) if more CO_2 is retained in body fluids, more hydrogen ions will be formed
   b) respiratory compensation for metabolic acidosis involves decreasing respirations

c) respiratory acidosis may be the result of a severe pulmonary disease

d) the respiratory system begins to compensate for a pH imbalance within a few minutes

Reword your choice to make it a correct statement.

_____

8. Which statement is NOT true of the kidneys and acid-base balance?
   a) the kidneys begin to compensate for a pH imbalance within a few seconds to minutes
   b) to compensate for acidosis, the kidneys excrete more hydrogen ions
   c) to compensate for alkalosis, the kidneys retain more hydrogen ions within the body
   d) the kidneys have the greatest capacity to compensate for an ongoing pH imbalance

Reword your choice to make it a correct statement.

_____

9. Which statement is NOT true of the effects of pH imbalances?
   a) alkalosis affects peripheral neurons and causes muscle spasms
   b) untreated alkalosis may progress to convulsions
   c) acidosis affects the CNS and causes confusion
   d) untreated acidosis may progress to hyperactivity

Reword your choice to make it a correct statement.

_____

Chapter 20

The Reproductive Systems

This chapter describes the male and female reproductive systems, which produce the gametes that unite in fertilization to become a new individual. The female reproductive system has yet another function, that of providing a site for the developing embryo-fetus.

MEIOSIS

1. Meiosis is the cell division process that produces gametes, which are _____ and

   _____ .

2. a) The process of meiosis begins with one cell that has the _____ number of

   chromosomes, which is _____ for people.

   b) In meiosis, one cell divides _____ to form _____ new cells, each

   with the _____ number of chromosomes, which is _____ for

   humans.

3. a) When meiosis takes place in the ovaries, the process is called _____ .

   b) When meiosis takes place in the testes, the process is called _____ .

4. Match each process of meiosis with the proper descriptive statements.

   Use each letter once. Each answer line will have four correct letters.

   1) Spermatogenesis _____

   2) Oogenesis _____

   A. Begins at puberty and ends at menopause
   B. Begins at puberty and continues throughout life
   C. Requires the hormones FSH and testosterone
   D. Is a continuous process
   E. Requires the hormones FSH and estrogen
   F. Is a cyclical process
   G. Four functional cells are produced
   H. Only one functional cell is produced

5. a) If fertilization occurs, the _____ chromosomes of the sperm and the

_____ chromosomes of the egg will give the fertilized egg the diploid number of

chromosomes, which is _____ .

   b) State the term for a fertilized egg. _____

6. Below are diagrams showing spermatogenesis and oogenesis.

   Label the cells indicated.

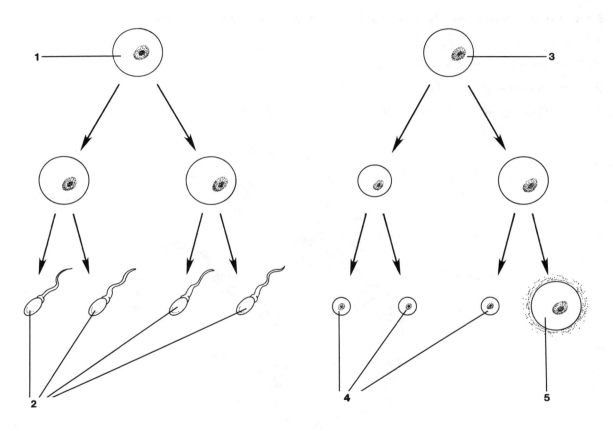

MALE REPRODUCTIVE SYSTEM

Testes and Sperm

1. a) The testes are suspended outside the abdominal cavity within the _____ .

   b) Viable sperm are produced only when the temperature of the testes is slightly

_____ than body temperature.

2. Within each testis, the interstitial cells produce the hormone _____ , and the process

of _____ takes place in the seminiferous tubules.

3. a) The stimulus for secretion of testosterone is the hormone _____ from the

   _____ gland.

   b) Testosterone is responsible for _____ of sperm.

   c) Testosterone also regulates the development of the male secondary sex characteristics. State two of

   these characteristics. _____ and _____

4. Below is a diagram of a sperm cell.

   Label the parts indicated and name the part with each of these functions.

   1) Provides motility _____

   2) Contains the 23 chromosomes _____

   3) Contains mitochondria that produce ATP _____

   4) Contains enzymes to digest the membrane of the egg cell _____

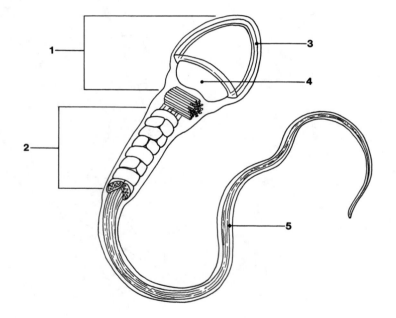

5. Below is a diagram of sections through a testis.

   Label the parts indicated.

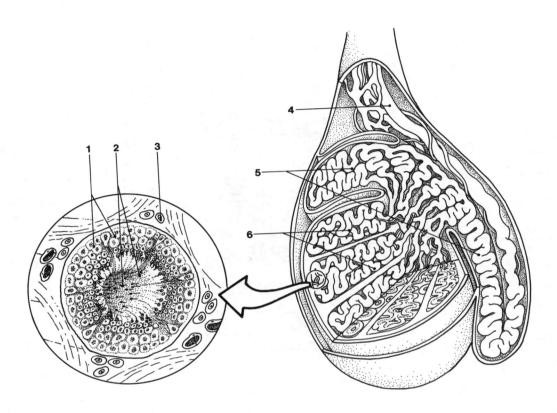

Epididymis, Ductus Deferens, and Ejaculatory Duct

1. a) The epididymis is a coiled tube on the _____ side of the testis.

   b) Within the epididymis, sperm complete their maturation, and their _____ become functional.

2. a) The ductus deferens is also called the _____ and carries sperm from the _____ to the _____ .

   b) The ductus deferens enters the abdominal cavity through the _____ canal, then curves over and down behind the _____ .

   c) The tissue in the wall of the ductus deferens that contracts to propel sperm to the ejaculatory duct is _____ .

3. The ejaculatory duct receives sperm from the _____ and the secretion of the _____ and empties these into the _____ .

4. Below is a diagram of the male reproductive system.

   Label the parts indicated.

Pubis _____   _____ Rectum

Urinary bladder _____   _____ 10

_____ 11

_____ 12

_____ 13

1 _____

2 _____   _____ Anus

3 _____   7

4 _____   8

5 _____   9

6

Seminal Vesicles, Prostate Gland, and Bulbourethral Glands

1. a) The two seminal vesicles are located posterior to the _____ , and their ducts join

   the _____ .

   b) The secretion of the seminal vesicles has an _____ pH to enhance sperm motility

   and contains _____ to nourish the sperm.

2. a) The prostate gland surrounds the first inch of the _____ , just below the

   _____ .

   b) The alkaline secretion of the prostate gland is important to maintain the _____ of

   sperm.

   c) The _____ muscle of the prostate gland contracts as part of

   _____ to expel semen from the urethra.

3. a) The bulbourethral glands are also called _____ .

b) The secretion of these glands has an _____ pH and is secreted into the _____ just before ejaculation.

4. All of these glands produce alkaline secretions. This is important to neutralize the _____ pH of the female _____ .

5. a) Semen consists of these secretions and _____ .

   b) The average pH of semen is _____ .

Urethra and Penis

1. a) The urethra carries semen from the _____ to the exterior.

   b) The first inch of the urethra is within the _____ , and the longest portion of the urethra is within the _____ .

2. The three masses of cavernous tissue within the penis consist of _____ muscle and connective tissue that contains large vascular channels called _____ .

3. During sexual stimulation, _____ impulses cause dilation of the penile arteries, and the _____ fill with blood, resulting in an erection.

4. The erect penis is capable of penetrating the female vagina to deposit semen. The expulsion of semen from the urethra is called _____ and is brought about by contraction of the _____ gland and peristalsis of the _____ .

Male Reproductive Hormones

1. a) Sperm production in the testes is initiated by the hormone _____ from the _____ gland.

   b) The maturation of sperm requires the hormone _____ from the testes.

2. The secretion of testosterone is stimulated by the hormone _____ from the _____ gland.

3. The hormone inhibin is secreted by the _____ , and its function is to decrease the secretion of _____ .

FEMALE REPRODUCTIVE SYSTEM

Ovaries

1. The ovaries are located in the _____ cavity on either side of the _____ .

2. The thousands of primary follicles in each ovary contain potential _____ .

3. a) The growth of ovarian follicles is stimulated by the hormone _____ from the _____ gland.

   b) This hormone also stimulates the follicle cells to secrete the hormone _____ .

4. A graafian follicle is a _____ follicle that ruptures and releases its ovum when stimulated by the hormone _____ from the _____ gland.

5. The hormone LH causes the ruptured follicle to become the _____ , which then begins to secrete the hormone _____ as well as estrogen.

6. Below is a diagram of the female reproductive system.

   Label the parts indicated.

Fallopian Tubes

1. The fallopian tubes may also be called _____ or _____ .

2. a) The lateral end of a fallopian tube encloses the _____ .

   b) The fringe-like projections of this end of the tube are called _____ and help pull the _____ into the tube.

3. To propel the ovum toward the uterus, the _____ layer of the fallopian tube contracts in peristaltic waves, and the _____ epithelium sweeps the ovum.

4. The union of sperm and egg is called _____ and usually takes place in the fallopian tube.

5. If a zygote does not reach the uterus but continues to develop within the fallopian tube, the pregnancy is called an _____ pregnancy.

Uterus

1. The uterus is located in the _____ cavity, medial to the _____ and superior to the _____ .

2. The body of the uterus is the large central portion. Above the body is the _____ of the uterus, and the lower portion that opens into the vagina is the _____ .

3. a) The epimetrium is a fold of the _____ that covers the uterus.

   b) The smooth muscle layer of the uterus is called the _____ .

   c) The lining of the uterus is called the _____ .

4. a) The endometrium consists of two layers. The _____ layer is the permanent, thin vascular layer next to the myometrium, and the _____ layer is regenerated and lost in each menstrual cycle.

   b) Name the two hormones that promote the growth of blood vessels in the functional layer.

   _____ and _____

5. a) What is the function of the endometrium? _____

   b) What is the function of the myometrium? _____

   c) Name the hormone that stimulates strong contractions of the myometrium at the end of pregnancy.

   _____

6. Below is a diagram of the female reproductive organs.

Label the parts indicated.

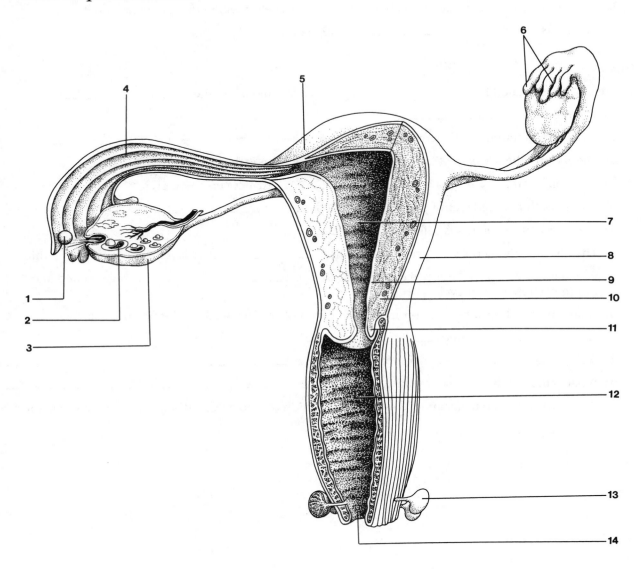

Vagina and Vulva

1. Match each structure with the proper descriptive statements.

   Use each letter once. One answer line will have three correct letters.

   1) Vagina _____

   2) Clitoris _____

   3) Labia majora and minora _____

   4) Bartholin's glands _____

   5) Vestibule _____

   A. The secretion keeps the mucosa of the vestibule moist
   B. Receives sperm from the penis during sexual intercourse
   C. Paired folds that cover the vestibule to prevent drying of the mucous membranes
   D. The birth canal and the exit for menstrual blood
   E. A small mass of erectile tissue that responds to sexual stimulation
   F. The area that contains the urethral and vaginal openings
   G. Contains bacteria (normal flora) that maintain an acidic pH that inhibits the growth of pathogens

Mammary Glands

1. a) The alveolar glands of the mammary glands produce _____ after pregnancy.

   b) Milk enters the _____ ducts, which converge and empty at the _____ of the breast.

2. During pregnancy, the alveolar glands are prepared for milk production by the hormones _____ and _____ , which are secreted by the _____ .

3. a) After pregnancy, the hormone _____ from the _____ gland stimulates production of milk.

   b) The hormone responsible for the release of milk from the mammary glands is _____ from the _____ gland.

4. a) The pigmented area around the nipple of the breast is called the _____ .

   b) Within the breast, the alveolar glands are surrounded by _____ tissue.

5. Below is a diagram of the mammary gland.

   Label the parts indicated.

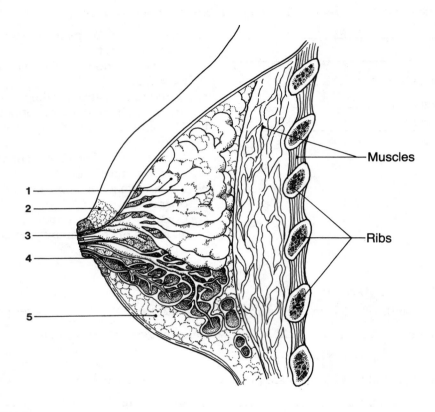

The Menstrual Cycle

1. The menstrual cycle requires hormones from the _____ and _____ and involves changes in the _____ and _____ (organs). The average menstrual cycle is approximately _____ days.

2. The hormones involved in the menstrual cycle are _____ and _____ from the anterior pituitary gland, _____ from the ovarian follicle, and _____ from the corpus luteum.

3. The three phases of the menstrual cycle are the _____ phase, the _____ phase, and the _____ phase.

4. a) The menstrual phase begins with the loss of the _____ layer of the endometrium; this is called _____ .

   b) During this phase, the hormone _____ stimulates the growth of several ovarian follicles.

5. a) During the follicular phase, the hormones _____ and _____ stimulate the growth and maturation of the ovum.

   b) The growth of blood vessels in the endometrium is stimulated by the hormone

   _____ .

   c) In ovulation, the hormone _____ causes a mature ovarian follicle to

   _____ and release its ovum.

6. a) During the luteal phase, the hormone _____ causes the ruptured follicle to

   become the _____ and secrete the hormone _____ .

   b) The hormone _____ stimulates further growth of blood vessels in the

   endometrium and promotes the storage of _____ .

7. If the ovum is not fertilized, a decrease in the hormone _____ causes the loss of the

   functional layer of the endometrium, and the cycle begins again with the _____
   phase.

CLINICAL APPLICATIONS

1. a) Mr. C. is 68 years old and tells his doctor that he is having increasing difficulty urinating. A

   possible cause of this is enlargement of the _____ gland.

   b) This enlargement is called _____ .

   c) This condition may make urination difficult because the prostate gland surrounds the first inch of

   the _____ .

2. a) Mr. and Mrs. D. ask their doctor for the most effective method of birth control. The doctor tells

   Mrs. D. that the surgical procedure called _____ would be very
   effective.

   b) In this procedure, the _____ are cut and tied.

   c) The doctor tells Mr. D. that the surgical procedure called a _____ is also a very
   effective method of contraception.

   d) In this procedure, the _____ are cut and tied off.

3. a) The usual site of fertilization is the _____ .

   b) A pregnancy in a site other than the uterus is called an _____ pregnancy.

4. In women after menopause, estrogen is no longer secreted. Consequences include loss of bone

   matrix, called _____ , and a higher blood level of _____ , which
   contributes to coronary artery disease.

MULTIPLE CHOICE TEST #1

Choose the correct answer for each question.

1. The process of meiosis produces _____ cells, each with the _____ number of chromosomes.
   a) 4/haploid   b) 2/haploid   c) 4/diploid   d) 2/diploid

2. The process of spermatogenesis produces:
   a) sperm cells, in cycles of 28 days
   b) sperm cells, from puberty to age 50
   c) only one functional sperm cell and three polar bodies
   d) sperm cells, from puberty throughout life

3. The process of oogenesis produces:
   a) an egg cell with the diploid number of chromosomes
   b) an egg cell approximately every 28 days
   c) egg cells and is stimulated by the hormones estrogen and progesterone
   d) egg cells from puberty throughout life

4. The hormones directly necessary for sperm production are:
   a) FSH and LH   c) testosterone and progesterone
   b) FSH and testosterone   d) LH and testosterone

5. The hormones directly necessary for egg cell production are:
   a) FSH and estrogen   c) LH and progesterone
   b) FSH and LH   d) estrogen and progesterone

6. The hormones directly necessary for the growth of blood vessels in the endometrium are:
   a) estrogen and progesterone   c) FSH and LH
   b) FSH and estrogen   d) LH and progesterone

7. The male reproductive duct that carries sperm from the epididymis into the abdominal cavity is the:
   a) ductus deferens   b) urethra   c) inguinal duct   d) ejaculatory duct

8. The part of a sperm cell that contains the 23 chromosomes is the:
   a) flagellum   b) acrosome   c) middle piece   d) head

9. The male reproductive gland that contributes to ejaculation is the:
   a) seminal vesicle   c) prostate gland
   b) Cowper's gland   d) bulbourethral gland

10. The male reproductive duct that carries semen through the penis to the exterior is the:
    a) ejaculatory duct   b) urethra   c) epididymis   d) ductus deferens

11. The parts of the testes that produce sperm are the:
    a) interstitial cells   c) seminiferous tubules
    b) rete testis   d) epididymides

12. The alkaline fluid of semen is important to neutralize the:
    a) acidic pH of the uterus   c) alkaline pH of the vagina
    b) acidic pH of the vagina   d) alkaline pH of the fallopian tube

13. The expulsion of semen from the urethra is called:
    a) secretion   b) ejaculation   c) erection   d) excretion

14. The layer of the uterus that will become the maternal portion of the placenta is the:
    a) epimetrium   b) myometrium   c) endometrium   d) serosa

15. The tissues of the fallopian tube that propel the ovum toward the uterus are:
    a) striated muscle and ciliated epithelium
    b) smooth muscle and simple squamous epithelium
    c) striated muscle and cuboidal epithelium
    d) smooth muscle and ciliated epithelium

16. The ovum matures and the endometrium develops during this phase of the menstrual cycle:
    a) the menstrual phase   c) the follicular phase
    b) the luteal phase   d) the ovarian phase

17. The vascular layer of the endometrium that is not lost in menstruation is the:
    a) basilar layer   c) functional layer
    b) myometrial layer   d) non-functional layer

18. One function of the hormone LH is to:
    a) cause rupture of the corpus luteum
    b) cause rupture of a graafian follicle
    c) cause a graafian follicle to secrete progesterone
    d) cause the corpus luteum to become a follicle

19. After pregnancy, the mammary glands are stimulated to produce milk by the hormone:
    a) estrogen   b) progesterone   c) oxytocin   d) prolactin

20. The parts of the vulva that cover the urethral and vaginal openings are the:
    a) clitoris and Bartholin's glands   c) labia minora and clitoris
    b) labia majora and minora   d) labia majora and Bartholin's glands

21. During the luteal phase of the menstrual cycle, the ruptured ovarian follicle becomes the:
    a) graafian follicle   c) corpus albicans
    b) primary follicle   d) corpus luteum

22. During the menstrual phase of the menstrual cycle, the functional layer of the endometrium is:
    a) regenerated by the basilar layer   c) stimulated to grow by estrogen
    b) lost in menstruation   d) stimulated to grow by progesterone

23. The site of fertilization is usually the:
    a) fallopian tube   b) vagina   c) uterus   d) ovary

24. A zygote is a:
    a) fertilized egg with 46 chromosomes   c) mature ovum with 46 chromosomes
    b) mature ovum with 23 chromosomes   d) fertilized egg with 23 chromosomes

MULTIPLE CHOICE TEST #2

Read each question and the four answer choices carefully. When you have made a choice, follow the instructions to complete your answer.

1. Which statement is NOT true of the locations of the female reproductive organs?
   a) the uterus is medial to the ovaries and inferior to the urinary bladder
   b) the ducts of Bartholin's glands open into the vaginal orifice
   c) the fallopian tubes extend from the ovaries to the uterus
   d) the vagina is anterior to the rectum and posterior to the urethra

   Reword your choice to make it a correct statement.

   _____

2. Which statement is NOT true of the locations of the male reproductive organs?
   a) the ductus deferens enters the abdominal cavity through the inguinal canal
   b) the testes are located in the scrotum medial to the upper thighs
   c) the urethra extends through the seminal vesicles and penis
   d) the epididymis is on the posterior side of a testis

   Reword your choice to make it a correct statement.

   _____

3. Which statement is NOT true of spermatogenesis and oogenesis?
   a) oogenesis is a cyclical process, and spermatogenesis is a continuous process
   b) both processes begin at puberty, but spermatogenesis ends at menopause
   c) spermatogenesis requires the hormones FSH and testosterone
   d) oogenesis requires the hormones FSH and estrogen

   Reword your choice to make it a correct statement.

   _____

4. Which statement is NOT true of the male reproductive ducts?
   a) the urethra carries semen to the exterior
   b) the epididymis carries sperm from the testis to the ductus deferens
   c) the ejaculatory duct carries sperm to the urethra
   d) the ductus deferens carries sperm from the urethra to the ejaculatory duct

   Reword your choice to make it a correct statement.

   _____

5. Which statement is NOT true of the male reproductive glands?
   a) the alkaline secretion of the prostate gland enters the urethra
   b) the secretion of the seminal vesicles is alkaline and contains glycogen
   c) the bulbourethral glands secrete an alkaline fluid into the urethra
   d) the prostate gland also contributes to ejaculation of semen

   Reword your choice to make it a correct statement.

   _____

6. Which statement is NOT true of the menstrual cycle?
   a) the follicular phase ends with ovulation
   b) the menstrual phase begins with the loss of the functional layer of the endometrium
   c) during the luteal phase, the corpus luteum begins to secrete progesterone
   d) the growth of blood vessels in the endometrium begins in the menstrual phase

   Reword your choice to make it a correct statement.

   _____

7. Which statement is NOT true of the uterus?
   a) the basilar layer regenerates the functional layer during each menstrual cycle
   b) the cervix is the narrow superior part that opens into the vagina
   c) the myometrium contracts for labor and delivery of the baby
   d) the fundus is the upper part between the openings of the fallopian tubes

   Reword your choice to make it a correct statement.

   _____

8. Which statement is NOT true of the mammary glands?
   a) the lactiferous ducts carry milk to the nipple
   b) milk production is stimulated by the hormone prolactin
   c) the alveolar glands produce milk after pregnancy
   d) the release of milk is stimulated by the hormone estrogen

   Reword your choice to make it a correct statement.

   _____

9. Which statement is NOT true of the ovaries and fallopian tubes?
   a) fimbriae are on the end of the fallopian tube that encloses the ovary
   b) fertilization of the ovum usually takes place in the fallopian tube
   c) an ectopic pregnancy occurs when the zygote becomes implanted in the uterus
   d) the ovum is swept toward the uterus by ciliated epithelium that lines the fallopian tube

   Reword your choice to make it a correct statement.

   _____

10. Which statement is NOT true of the testes?
    a) to produce viable sperm, the temperature of the scrotum must be slightly higher than body temperature
    b) spermatogenesis takes place in the seminiferous tubules
    c) the interstitial cells produce testosterone when stimulated by LH
    d) two of the target organs of testosterone are the testes themselves

    Reword your choice to make it a correct statement.

    _____

Chapter 21

Human Development and Genetics

This chapter describes the fundamentals of embryology and genetics. Embryology is the study of the development of a zygote into a functioning human being. This takes place during the 40 weeks of gestation. Genetics is the study of the inheritance of particular characteristics.

HUMAN DEVELOPMENT

Fertilization

1. The _____ of the sperm cell contains enzymes to digest the membrane of the egg cell to allow the entry of the sperm.

2. a) Fertilization is the union of the nuclei of the _____ and _____ .

   b) Each of these nuclei contains _____ chromosomes, and the zygote, therefore, has _____ chromosomes, the _____ number for people.

   c) Fertilization usually takes place within the female _____ .

3. The 23 pairs of chromosomes in the zygote consist of 22 pairs called _____ and one pair called the _____ .

4. Men have the sex chromosomes called _____ , and women have the sex chromosomes called _____ .

Implantation

1. a) The single-celled zygote divides by the process of _____ to form two cells.

   b) Further mitotic divisions are called _____ and produce four cells, then eight cells, and so on.

2. a) A solid sphere of embryonic cells is called a _____ .

   b) As mitosis continues, the solid sphere becomes hollow and is called the _____ .

3. a) The inner cell mass of the blastocyst contains the potential _____ .

   b) The outer layer of cells of the blastocyst is called the _____ , and it secretes

   enzymes to digest the surface of the _____ to permit _____ of the
   blastocyst in the uterus.

4. The trophoblast will eventually become the embryonic membrane called the _____ ,

   which in turn will develop into the fetal portion of the _____ .

5. Below is a diagram of the processes of fertilization through implantation.

   Label the parts indicated.

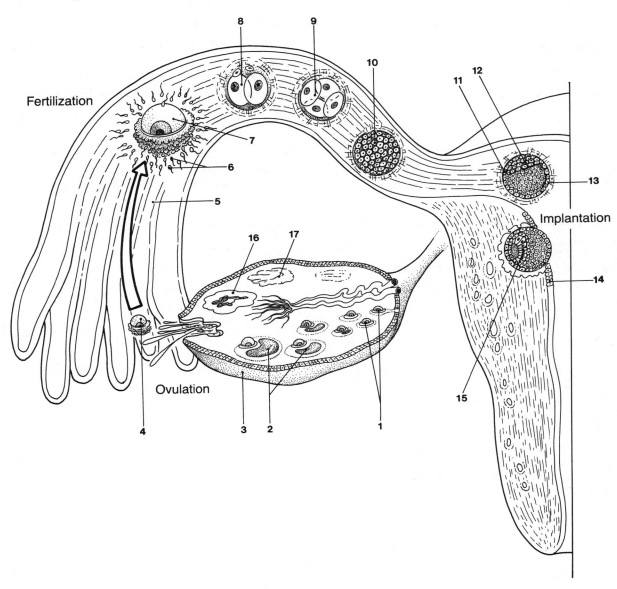

Embryo and Embryonic Membranes

1. About 2 weeks after fertilization, the embryonic disc develops three primary layers of cells. These layers are called the _____ , _____ , and _____ .

2. Name one tissue or part of the body that develops from each primary layer.

   1) Endoderm _____

   2) Mesoderm _____

   3) Ectoderm _____

3. Match each embryonic membrane with the proper descriptive statements.

   Use each letter once. Each answer line will have two correct letters.

   1) Amnion _____

   2) Chorion _____

   3) Yolk sac _____

   A. Contains fluid that absorbs shock around the embryo

   B. Forms the first blood cells for the embryo

   C. Develops small projections called chorionic villi

   D. Contains the fetal blood vessels that become part of the placenta

   E. Contains cells that will become oogonia or spermatogonia

   F. Contains fluid into which fetal urine is excreted

4. a) The period of embryonic growth ends at the _____ week of gestation.

   b) The period of fetal growth extends from week _____ to week _____ of gestation.

5. Below are diagrams of embryos at 2 weeks and 5 weeks of gestation.

   Label the parts indicated.

— 1

— 2

— 3

— 4

— 5

— 6

○ Embryo
○ Amnion
○ Chorion
○ Yolk sac

Two Weeks

— 7

— 8

— 9

— 10

— 11

— 12

— 13

Five Weeks

Placenta and Umbilical Cord

1. a) The maternal part of the placenta is formed by the _____ of the uterus.

    b) The fetal part of the placenta is formed by the _____ .

    c) The fetus is connected to the placenta by the _____ .

    d) It is in the placenta that _____ of materials take place between fetal blood and maternal blood.

2. In the placenta, fetal blood vessels are within maternal _____ , and there is no mixing of fetal and maternal blood.

3. The umbilical cord contains two umbilical _____ and one umbilical

    _____ .

4. a) The umbilical arteries carry blood from the _____ to the _____ .

    b) This blood contains _____ and _____ that diffuse into the maternal blood sinuses for elimination by the mother.

5. a) The umbilical vein carries blood from the _____ to the _____ .

    b) This blood contains _____ and _____ from the maternal blood to be brought to the fetus.

6. After the birth of a baby, the umbilical cord is cut, and the placenta is delivered as the

    _____ .

7. a) The placenta is the source of the hormones necessary to maintain pregnancy. The first hormone secreted is called hCG and is produced by the _____ of the embryo.

    b) Under the influence of hCG, the _____ in the maternal ovary continues to secrete

    the hormones _____ and _____ .

8. The hormones secreted by the placenta itself are _____ and _____ , and their secretion continues throughout gestation.

9. a) During pregnancy, estrogen and progesterone prevent the development of ovarian follicles by

    inhibiting the secretion of _____ and _____ from the anterior pituitary gland.

    b) Estrogen and progesterone also prepare the _____ for lactation after the birth of a baby.

    c) Progesterone is very important to prevent contractions of the _____ , which might otherwise result in a miscarriage.

Parturition and Labor

1. a) The term parturition means _____ .

    b) The term labor refers to the _____ that occurs during birth.

2. a) Toward the end of gestation, the myometrium begins to contract weakly because the secretion of _____ by the placenta begins to decrease.

   b) At this time, how is the fetus usually positioned in the uterus? _____

3. a) During the first stage of labor, contractions of the uterus force the _____ into the cervix.

   b) How does this change the diameter of the cervical opening? _____

   c) What happens to the amniotic sac? _____

   d) What happens to the amniotic fluid? _____

4. a) During the second stage of labor, the hormone _____ causes stronger contractions of the uterus.

   b) These strong contractions result in the delivery of the _____ .

5. a) During the third stage of labor, the uterus continues to contract and delivers the _____ .

   b) Further contractions of the uterus are very important to _____ the uterine blood vessels to prevent hemorrhage in the mother.

The Infant at Birth

1. a) The baby becomes independent of the mother when the _____ is cut.

   b) The baby begins to breathe as the blood level of _____ rises and stimulates the respiratory center in the _____ .

2. a) In the baby's heart, the _____ is closed as more blood returns to the left atrium.

   b) Just outside the heart, the _____ constricts.

   c) Both of these changes now permit more blood to flow to the baby's _____ .

3. A newborn baby may have mild jaundice because the _____ is not yet mature enough to excrete _____ efficiently.

GENETICS

Chromosomes and Genes

1. a) The human diploid number of chromosomes is _____ .

   b) The chromosomes are actually 23 pairs called _____ chromosomes.

   c) One member of each pair has come from the father and is called _____ .

   d) The other member of the pair has come from the mother and is called _____ .

   e) The chromosome pairs designated 1–22 are called _____ .

f) The remaining pair is called the _____ , which are XX for _____

and XY for _____ .

2. a) The hereditary material of chromosomes is _____ .

    b) The genetic code is the sequence of _____ in the DNA.

    c) A gene is the DNA code for _____ .

3. Match each genetic term with its proper definition.

   Use each letter once.

   1) Alleles _____

   2) Genotype _____

   3) Phenotype _____

   4) Homozygous _____

   5) Heterozygous _____

   6) Dominant allele _____

   7) Recessive allele _____

A. The expression of the alleles that are present; the appearance of the individual

B. Will appear in the phenotype only if two are present in the genotype

C. Will appear in the phenotype even if only one is present in the genotype

D. Having two similar alleles (genes) for one trait

E. The alleles that are present; the genetic make-up

F. The possibilities for the expression of a gene

G. Having two different alleles (genes) for one trait

Genetic Problems

1. Inheritance of dominant-recessive traits

   1) a) Mom has blond hair (recessive) and Dad has brown hair (dominant). If Dad is homozygous for this trait, what are the possibilities for their children? Use this Punnett square:

Mom _____

Dad _____

    b) Each child has a _____ % chance of having brown hair and a _____ % chance of having blond hair.

2) a) Mom has blond hair and Dad is heterozygous for brown hair. What are the possibilities for their children? Use this Punnett square:

Mom _____

Dad _____

b) Each child has a _____ % chance of having brown hair and a _____ % chance of having blond hair.

2. Inheritance of blood type—A and B alleles are co-dominant, and the O allele is recessive.

1) a) Mom has type O blood and Dad is heterozygous type A. What are the possible blood types for their children? Use this Punnett square:

Mom _____

Dad _____

b) Each child has a _____ % chance of having type O blood and a _____ % chance of having type A blood.

2) a) Both Mom and Dad have type AB blood. What are the possible blood types for their children? Use this Punnett square:

Mom _____

Dad _____

b) Each child has a _____ % chance of having type A blood, a _____ % chance of having type B, a _____ % chance of having type AB, and a _____ % chance of having type O.

3. Inheritance of sex-linked traits—The recessive gene is found only on the X chromosome, and there is no corresponding gene on the Y chromosome.

1) a) Mom is a carrier of red-green colorblindness and Dad is red-green colorblind. What are the possibilities for their children? Use this Punnett square:

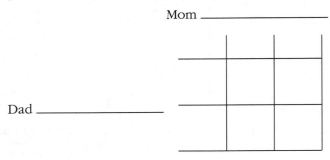

b) Each daugher has a _____ % chance of being colorblind and a _____ % chance of being a carrier of this trait. Each son has a _____ % chance of being colorblind and a _____ % chance of having normal color vision.

2) a) Mom is red-green colorblind and Dad has normal color vision. What are the possibilities for their children? Use this Punnett square:

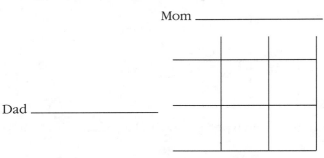

b) Each daughter has a _____ % chance of being colorblind and a _____ % chance of being a carrier of this trait. Each son has a _____ % chance of being colorblind and a _____ % chance of having normal color vision.

CLINICAL APPLICATIONS

1. a) Mrs. J. delivers her first baby at 36 weeks of gestation. The most serious problem for premature infants usually involves the _____ (organs), which may not yet be mature enough for normal inflation.

b) Mrs. J.'s baby has an Apgar score of 9, which means (choose one answer) _____ .

1) the baby requires immediate medical attention
2) the baby must be closely monitored because it is showing distress
3) the baby is responding well to its independent existence

2. a) Mrs. L. is 41 years old and pregnant with her third child. She has read that older women are more likely to have a child with Down syndrome. In this syndrome, the child has

_____ of chromosome #21 and as a result has some degree of

_____ retardation.

   b) Mrs. L.'s doctor tells her that the chromosome number of the fetus can be determined by a

   procedure called _____ that is performed at 16 to 18 weeks of gestation.

3. a) A cesarean section is the delivery of an infant by way of an incision through the

   _____ and _____ .

   b) State two reasons why a cesarean section may be preferable to a vaginal delivery.

   1) _____

   2) _____

MULTIPLE CHOICE TEST #1

Choose the correct answer for each question.

1. The embryonic stage that becomes implanted in the uterus is the:
   a) 4-cell stage   b) morula   c) blastocyst   d) 16-cell stage

2. The most superficial parts of the body develop from this primary layer:
   a) ectoderm   b) mesoderm   c) endoderm   d) outerderm

3. The chromosome number of a zygote is:
   a) 23, the haploid number   c) 23, the diploid number
   b) 46, the haploid number   d) 46, the diploid number

4. The average gestation period is approximately _____ weeks long, and the first _____ weeks are considered the period of embryonic growth.
   a) 46/12   b) 38/16   c) 42/4   d) 40/8

5. Both fetal and maternal tissues contribute to the formation of the:
   a) amnion   b) chorion   c) umbilical cord   d) placenta

6. The fetal vessel that carries oxygen and nutrients from the placenta to the fetus is the:
   a) aorta   b) umbilical vein   c) umbilical artery   d) chorionic vein

7. The fluid that surrounds the embryo-fetus and serves as a cushion is:
   a) plasma   b) amniotic fluid   c) intracellular fluid   d) chorionic fluid

8. The first blood cells for the fetus are formed by the:
   a) yolk sac   b) chorion   c) red bone marrow   d) spleen

9. The embryonic membrane that contributes to the formation of the placenta is the:
   a) amnion   b) umbilical cord   c) yolk sac   d) chorion

10. In the placenta, how are materials exchanged between mother and fetus?
    a) maternal blood enters fetal circulation   c) diffusion and active transport
    b) osmosis and filtration   d) fetal blood enters maternal circulation

11. During the third stage of labor:
    a) the infant is delivered
    b) the cervix dilates
    c) the placenta is delivered
    d) amniotic fluid exits through the birth canal

12. The second stage of labor includes all of these except:
    a) rupture of the amniotic sac
    b) delivery of the infant
    c) strong contractions of the myometrium
    d) secretion of oxytocin by the posterior pituitary gland

13. The first stage of labor includes all of these except:
    a) dilation of the cervix
    b) rupture of the amniotic sac
    c) weak contractions of the myometrium
    d) delivery of the infant

14. Pregnancy is maintained by these hormones produced by the chorion and placenta:
    a) estrogen, FSH, and LH
    b) hCG, estrogen, and progesterone
    c) oxytocin, hCG, and progesterone
    d) FSH, estrogen, and progesterone

15. A gene is the genetic code for one:
    a) cell   b) protein   c) DNA   d) RNA

16. With respect to a particular trait, the term genotype means:
    a) the sex chromosomes that are present
    b) the genetic makeup of the individual
    c) the appearance of the individual
    d) the haploid number of chromosomes

17. A pair of homologous chromosomes includes:
    a) two maternal chromosomes of the same number
    b) two paternal chromosomes of the same number
    c) a maternal and paternal chromosome of different numbers
    d) a maternal and paternal chromosome of the same number

18. A person who is heterozygous for a particular trait may have:
    a) two dominant genes
    b) two recessive genes
    c) a dominant gene and a recessive gene
    d) two sex-linked genes

19. With respect to a particular trait, the term phenotype refers to:
    a) the appearance of the individual
    b) the genetic makeup of the individual
    c) the diploid number of chromosomes
    d) the number of alleles present

20. The hereditary material of cells is contained in the:
    a) protein in the chromosomes
    b) DNA in the cell membrane
    c) protein in the nucleus
    d) DNA in the chromosomes

MULTIPLE CHOICE TEST #2

Read each question and the four answer choices carefully. When you have made a choice, follow the instructions to complete your answer.

1. Which statement is NOT true of the stages of labor?
    a) the amniotic sac ruptures during the second stage
    b) the placenta is delivered in the third stage

   c) the second stage ends with delivery of the infant
   d) the cervix dilates during the first stage

Reword your choice to make it a correct statement.

_____

2. Which statement is NOT true of embryonic membranes?
   a) the human yolk sac does not contain nutrients for the embryo
   b) the chorion will become part of the placenta
   c) the amnion contains amniotic fluid to cushion the fetus
   d) the first blood cells for the fetus are formed by the chorion

Reword your choice to make it a correct statement.

_____

3. Which statement is NOT true of the growth of the embryo-fetus?
   a) all the organ systems are established by the end of 8 weeks of gestation
   b) the heart begins to beat in the embryo stage
   c) the period of embryonic growth lasts from week 1 to week 18
   d) the last fetal organs to become functional are the lungs

Reword your choice to make it a correct statement.

_____

4. Which statement is NOT true of the placenta and umbilical cord?
   a) the umbilical vein carries oxygenated blood from the placenta to the fetus
   b) there is no mixing of fetal and maternal blood in the placenta
   c) the umbilical arteries carry blood with waste products from the fetus to the placenta
   d) within the placenta, fetal blood vessels are within the maternal arteries

Reword your choice to make it a correct statement.

_____

5. Which statement is NOT true of fertilization and implantation?
   a) the zygote undergoes a series of mitotic cell divisions called cleavage
   b) the embryonic stage that undergoes implantation is the morula
   c) the trophoblast of the blastocyst produces enzymes to digest the endometrium
   d) the zygote contains 23 chromosomes from the egg and 23 chromosomes from the sperm

Reword your choice to make it a correct statement.

_____

6. Which statement is NOT true of the hormones of pregnancy?
   a) The chorion produces hCG that stimulates the corpus luteum during early gestation
   b) no egg cells are produced during pregnancy because estrogen and progesterone inhibit the secretions of the anterior pituitary gland
   c) premature contractions of the myometrium are prevented by estrogen
   d) the mammary glands are prepared for lactation by estrogen and progesterone

Reword your choice to make it a correct statement.

_____

7. Which statement is NOT true of chromosomes and genes?
   a) a gene is the DNA code for one protein
   b) a homologous pair of chromosomes consists of one maternal and one paternal chromosome of the same number
   c) human cells have 22 pairs of autosomes and one pair of sex chromosomes
   d) the sex chromosomes are XX in men and XY in women

   Reword your choice to make it a correct statement.

   _____

8. Which statement is NOT true of the terminology of genetics?
   a) the expression of the alleles in the appearance of the individual is the genotype
   b) to be homozygous for a trait means to have two similar alleles
   c) to be heterozygous for a trait means to have two different alleles
   d) alleles are the possibilities for the ways a gene may be expressed in an individual

   Reword your choice to make it a correct statement.

   _____

9. Which statement is NOT true of inheritance?
   a) if a gene has more than two possible alleles, as in blood types, then there will be more than two possible phenotypes
   b) a dominant gene is one that appears in the phenotype of a heterozygous individual
   c) recessive genes may not appear in one generation but may reappear in individuals in the next generation
   d) a recessive gene is one that appears in the phenotype of a heterozygous individual

   Reword your choice to make it a correct statement.

   _____

10. Which statement is NOT true of inheritance of sex-linked traits?
   a) men cannot be carriers of sex-linked traits
   b) women who are carriers of sex-linked traits may pass the gene to a son or a daughter
   c) a son who inherits a sex-linked trait has inherited the gene from his father
   d) the genes for sex-linked traits are found only on the X chromosome

   Reword your choice to make it a correct statement.

   _____

Answer Key

Chapter 1

LEVELS OF ORGANIZATION

1. a) chemical
   b) any three of these: carbohydrates, lipids, proteins, nucleic acids
   c) any three of these: water, oxygen, carbon dioxide, calcium, iron (or any of the minerals)

2. a) organ system
   b) any three of the 11 organ systems: respiratory, skeletal, circulatory, nervous, digestive, muscular, reproductive, etc.

3. a) cellular   b) tissue   c) organ

4. 1) D, 1   2) A, 3   3) B, 2   4) C, 4

5. a) anatomy, physiology
   b) bones support (or protect) the body—they are very strong (or hard)

HOMEOSTASIS

1. health

2. stable (the same)

3. externally, internally

4. 1) food is digested into simple chemicals the body cells can use
   2) oxygen enters the blood to become available to cells
   3) take aspirin (take a nap)
   4) blood will clot to prevent extensive blood loss
   5) shivering will occur to produce heat (put on a coat)

TERMS OF LOCATION

1. below, or lower than
   superior

2. closer to the origin
   distal

3. toward the side
   medial

4. extending from the main part
   central

5. toward the surface
   deep

6. in front of, or toward the front
   posterior

7. behind, or toward the back
   ventral

8. within, or inside of
   external

BODY PARTS AND AREAS

1.
1) cranial	10) volar	19) plantar
2) orbital	11) deltoid	20) popliteal
3) nasal	12) pectoral	21) parietal
4) buccal	13) mammary	22) occipital
5) frontal	14) brachial	23) lumbar
6) temporal	15) iliac	24) sacral
7) cervical	16) inguinal	25) gluteal
8) axillary	17) femoral	26) perineal
9) umbilical	18) patellar	

2. 1) a) lateral   b) shoulder   c) neck
   2) a) proximal   b) thigh   c) knee
   3) a) posterior   b) back of the head
      c) small of the back
   4) a) ventral   b) chest
      c) navel
   5) a) superior   b) palm of hand
      c) sole of foot
   6) a) superficial   b) skin
   7) a) external   b) lungs
   8) peripheral, central

313

BODY CAVITIES

1. 1) C, G   2) A, D, H   3) B, C
   4) F   5) E, I, J

2. 1) thoracic cavity   5) cranial cavity
   2) abdominal cavity   6) spinal cavity
   3) pelvic cavity   7) dorsal cavity
   4) ventral cavity

BODY SECTIONS

1. 1) B   2) D   3) E   4) C   5) A

2. 1) midsagittal plane   4) frontal (coronal) plane
   2) sagittal plane   5) longitudinal section
   3) transverse plane   6) cross section

ORGAN SYSTEMS

1. 1) muscular   7) nervous
   2) circulatory   8) endocrine
   3) reproductive   9) lymphatic
   4) skeletal   10) digestive
   5) urinary   11) integumentary
   6) respiratory

2. 1) circulatory   11) endocrine
   2) urinary   12) reproductive
   3) nervous   or endocrine
   4) integumentary   13) respiratory
   5) respiratory   14) digestive
   6) muscular   15) muscular
   7) skeletal   16) nervous
   8) reproductie or   17) endocrine
      endocrine   18) circulatory
   9) digestive or   19) integumentary
      endocrine   20) digestive
   10) lymphatic or
      circulatory

CLINICAL APPLICATIONS

1. 1) the skin (and subcutaneous tissue)
   2) muscles of the abdominal wall
   3) peritoneum

2. meninges; brain and spinal cord
3. 1) the *kidneys* have stopped functioning
   2) the *heart* has stopped beating
   3) a blood vessel of the *lung*
   4) an unconscious state due to disease of the *liver*
   5) an erosion of the *stomach* lining
4. 1) stomach—upper left
   2) liver—upper right and left
   3) small intestine—all four
   4) large intestine—all four

MULTIPLE CHOICE TEST #1

1. a	5. b	9. a	12. b	15. a
2. d	6. b	10. c	13. b	16. d
3. d	7. c	11. d	14. b	17. b
4. a	8. d			

MULTIPLE CHOICE TEST #2

The letter of the correct choice is followed by the statement necessary to complete the answer. When an incorrect statement is to be corrected to make it true, the new (true) words are underlined.

1. d—the muscles are part of the organ level
2. c—the blood is a tissue
3. a
4. c—nerve tissue is specialized to generate and transmit impulses
5. c—internal changes do have effects on homeostasis
6. a—lines the abdominal cavity
7. b and e—the eyes and ears are lateral to the midline of the head
8. d—midtransverse section
9. d—a group of cells with similar structure and function is called a tissue
10. a—the diaphragm separates the thoracic and abdominal cavities

Chapter 2

ELEMENTS, ATOMS, AND BONDS

1. element

2. Fe—iron   Mg—magnesium
   Ca—calcium   N—nitrogen
   O—oxygen   S—sulfur
   C—carbon   Cl—chlorine
   H—hydrogen   Cu—copper
   K—potassium   Zn—Zinc
   Na—sodium   Co—cobalt
   I—iodine   Mn—Manganese
   P—phosphorus   F—fluorine

3. protons, neutrons, and electrons

4. a) electron, proton   b) neutron
   c) protons and neutrons
   d) protons and electrons   e) electrons

5. ion

6. molecule

7. ionic

8. covalent

9. a) any one of these: oxygen, carbon dioxide,
      nitrogen   b) water
   c) any one of these: sodium chloride, calcium
      chloride

10. ionic

11. covalent

12. 1) electron orbitals   4) electron orbitals
    2) protons   5) electron transfer
    3) protons

13. hydrogen

14. a) synthesis   b) decomposition

INORGANIC COMPOUNDS

1. water

2. a) dissolve
   b) any one of these: transport of nutrients in
      the blood, excretion of wastes in urine,
      senses of taste and smell

3. a) friction
   b) one of these: mucus in the digestive tract,
      synovial fluid in joints

4. excess body heat may be lost in the process of
   sweating

5. a) plasma   b) intracellular fluid
   c) lymph   d) tissue fluid
   e) 1. tissue fluid   2. intracellular fluid
      3. lymph   4. plasma

6. a) a gas   b) O_2
   c) cell respiration, ATP (energy)

7. a) cell respiration   b) CO_2 c) acidic

CELL RESPIRATION

1. CO_2 + H_2O + ATP + heat

2. CO_2 is exhaled; H_2O becomes part of
   intracellular water

3. ATP provides energy for cellular activities; heat
   contributes to a constant body temperature

TRACE ELEMENTS

1. 1) C   2) A   3) B, G, E
   4) D   5) B, F   6) H, E

ACIDS, BASES, AND pH

1. a) 0–14   b) 7   c) H^+, OH^-
   d) acidic   e) alkaline (basic)

2. a) pH 7.35–7.45   b) alkaline

3. buffers or buffer systems

4. have little or no effect on pH.

ORGANIC COMPOUNDS

1. 1) C   2) H   3) K   4) A
   5) F   6) J   7) B   8) I
   9) D   10) G   11) E

2. 1) D   2) G   3) I   4) B
   5) J   6) K, N   7) C   8) F
   9) A, L   10) E   11) H, M

CHEMICAL STRUCTURE—REVIEW

1. carbon, hydrogen, oxygen, nitrogen

2. a) amino acid   b) covalent

3. a) proteins
   b) any three of these:
      1) enzymes to catalyze reactions
      2) antibodies for defense against pathogens
      3) hemoglobin to carry oxygen
      4) muscle contraction
      5) some hormones
      6) structure of cells and tissues

4. carbon, hydrogen, oxygen

5. $C_6H_{12}O_6$

6. a) glucose   b) source of energy
   c) glycogen—storage form of excess glucose
      in the liver
      starch—an energy source in plant food
      cellulose—fiber to provide exercise for the
      colon; promotes peristalsis

ENZYMES

1. catalysts

2. 1) active site
   2) enzyme-substrate complex
   3) enzyme   4) product

3. shape

4. H^+, active site

DNA, RNA, AND ATP

1. pentose sugar, phosphate group, a nitrogenous
   base

2. 1) B, D   2) A, F   3) C, E

3. T is always paired with A; C is always paired
   with G

4. 1) C, E   2) A   3) B, D

CLINICAL APPLICATIONS

1. a) decrease, acidosis   b) a

2. d   3. b   4. a

MULTIPLE CHOICE TEST #1

1. b	5. a	9. d	13. e	17. d
2. b	6. b	10. b	14. d	18. d
3. a	7. c	11. a	15. d	19. b
4. d	8. c	12. b	16. c	20. a

MULTIPLE CHOICE TEST #2

*The letter of the correct choice is followed by the
statement necessary to complete the answer. When
an incorrect statement is to be corrected to make
it true, the new (true) words are underlined.*

1. b—water is a molecule made of two
   elements, hydrogen and oxygen

2. b—covalent bonds are <u>not</u> weakened when in
   a water solution

3. d—intracellular fluid is water found <u>within</u>
   cells

4. c—glucose is a <u>carbohydrate</u> (or <u>sugar</u>)
   molecule obtained from food

5. a—the heat energy produced <u>provides a
   constant body temperature</u>

6. b—iron is part of hemoglobin; calcium is part
   of bones and teeth; iodine is part of thyroxine

7. b—the normal pH range of blood is <u>7.35–7.45</u>

8. d—the excretion of waste products in urine
   depends on the <u>solvent</u> action of water

9. c—glycogen is a form of energy storage in the
   liver; true fats are a form of energy storage in
   adipose tissue; pentose sugars are part of
   DNA and RNA

10. a—hemoglobin transports <u>oxygen</u> in RBCs

11. a—all enzymes are <u>proteins</u>

12. c—<u>DNA</u> is the genetic code for our hereditary
    characteristics

13. d—it contains three <u>phosphate</u> groups

14. a—synthesis reactions involve the <u>formation</u>
    of bonds

Chapter 3

CELL STRUCTURE

1. 1) B, E, G, I   2) D, H   3) A, C, F, J
2. a) phospholipids, proteins, cholesterol
   b) 1) cholesterol   2) proteins
      3) proteins   4) phospholipids
      5) proteins
3. 1) cilia   7) nucleus
   2) microvilli   8) rough
   3) cell membrane   endoplasmic
   4) Golgi apparatus   reticulum
   5) smooth endoplasmic   9) ribosomes
      reticulum   10) mitochondrion
   6) centrioles   11) lysosome
4. 1) E, 6   2) A, 1   3) H, 8   4) B, 2
   5) G, 3   6) C, 7   7) F, 5   8) D, 4

CELLULAR TRANSPORT MECHANISMS

1. 1) C, 2   2) F, 1   3) A, 5   4) E, 7
   5) G, 3   6) D, 4   7) B, 6
2. 1) low O_2 2) high O_2 3) low CO_2
   4) high CO_2
3. 1) active transport   2) osmosis
   3) active transport
4. 1) the same   2) a higher
   3) a lower
5. 1) isotonic   2) hypotonic
   3) hypertonic

DNA AND THE GENETIC CODE

1. a) chromosomes   b) 46
2. two, double helix
3. thymine, guanine
4. protein
5. amino acids
6. a) three   b) triplet   c) codon

RNA AND PROTEIN SYNTHESIS

1. one
2. messenger, mRNA
3. uracil
4. nucleus, ribosomes
5. transfer, tRNA
6. codon
7. peptide, ribosomes
8. 1) mRNA   2) structural proteins
   3) enzymes
9. 1) nucleus   4) tRNA   7) ribosome
   2) DNA   5) amino acids
   3) mRNA   6) peptide bond

MITOSIS AND MEIOSIS

1. 1) A, B, G, H   2) C, D, E, F
2. each DNA molecule makes a copy of itself
3. 1) B, D, G   2) A, F   3) C, E
   4) H, I
4. 1) outer layer of skin—to replace cells that are
      worn off the skin surface
   2) red bone marrow—to replace RBCs that live
      only 120 days (or) stomach lining—to
      replace cells destroyed by the hydrochloric
      acid in gastric juice
5. a) nerve cells or muscle cells
   b) loss of these cells will have a permanent
      effect on the functioning of the organ of
      which they are a part
6. a) interphase   b) cytokinesis   c) anaphase
   d) metaphase   e) prophase   f) telophase
   sequence: a, e, d, c, f, b

CLINICAL APPLICATIONS

1. red bone marrow
2. a) the same   b) gain, osmosis, swell
3. a) mitosis   b) protein synthesis

MULTIPLE CHOICE TEST #1

1. b	5. d	9. c	13. a	17. b
2. b	6. b	10. c	14. c	18. a
3. a	7. a	11. d	15. d	19. b
4. d	8. b	12. c	16. d	20. b

MULTIPLE CHOICE TEST #2

The letter of the correct choice is followed by the statement necessary to complete the answer. When an incorrect statement is to be corrected to make it true, the new (true) words are underlined.

1. c—active transport—the movement of molecules from an area of lesser concentration to an area of greater concentration

2. d—ribosomes—the site of protein synthesis

3. b—DNA exists as a double strand of nucleotides called a double helix

4. c—amino acids are bonded to one another by peptide bonds

5. d—anaphase—the spindle fibers pull each set of chromosomes toward opposite poles of the cell

6. c—it is selectively permeable, meaning that only certain substances may pass through

7. a—nerve cells are unable to reproduce themselves

8. c—osmosis—the absorption of water by the small intestine

9. a—human cells in a hypertonic solution would shrivel (or) human cells in an isotonic solution would remain undamaged

Chapter 4

EPITHELIAL TISSUE

1. 1) columnar epithelium
   2) cuboidal epithelium
   3) simple squamous epithelium
   4) ciliated epithelium
   5) stratified squamous epithelium

2. 1) E, 1, 5, 8   2) A, 3, 9   3) F, 7
   4) D, 2, 6   5) C, 4, 11, 13   6) B, 10, 12

3. 1) A, 2   2) C, 3   3) B, D, 1

CONNECTIVE TISSUE

1. 1) B, 4, 8   2) E, 1   3) D, 7   4) G, 2, 9
   5) A, 3, 11   6) C, 5, 12   7) F, 6, 10

2. A) blood   B) adipose tissue
   C) areolar tissue
   D) fibrous connective tissue   E) bone
   F) cartilage

MUSCLE TISSUE

1. 1) SM   2) SK   3) SM   4) C
   5) SK   6) SK   7) C   8) SM
   9) SM   10) SK   11) C   12) SK
   13) SM

2. A) skeletal muscle   B) smooth muscle
   C) cardiac muscle

NERVE TISSUE

1. neurons, impulses

2. 1) cell body   2) nucleus   3) dendrites
   4) axon

3. a) away from   b) toward

4. a) Schwann cells   b) oligodendrocytes

5. a) synapse   b) neurotransmitters

6. brain and spinal cord (or peripheral nerves)

7. any two of these: sensation, movement, learning, memory

MEMBRANES

1. 1) B, C, D, F, H, J, L   2) A, E, G, I, K

2. a) 1. parietal pleura   2. visceral pleura
      3. peritoneum   4. mesentery
      5. visceral pericardium
      6. parietal pericardium

   b) parietal, visceral
   c) peritoneum, mesentery
   d) parietal, visceral

3. 1) F   2) G   3) A   4) B
   5) C   6) E   7) D

CLINICAL APPLICATIONS

1. blood supply

2. blood supply (or) capillaries

3. a) skeletal   b) heart

4. peritoneum, abdominal

5. synovial, cartilage

MULTIPLE CHOICE TEST #1

1. b	6. b	11. a	15. a	19. a
2. a	7. d	12. b	16. c	20. b
3. d	8. c	13. c	17. d	21. d
4. d	9. c	14. d	18. d	22. d
5. c	10. a			

MULTIPLE CHOICE TEST #2

The letter of the correct choice is followed by the statement necessary to complete the answer. When an incorrect statement is to be corrected to make it true, the new (true) words are underlined.

1. d—columnar epithelium that absorbs nutrients is found in the small intestine

2. b—cardiac muscle that pumps blood is found in the heart

3. a—peritoneum—lines the abdominal cavity

4. d—bones are moved by skeletal muscle

5. d—an example of an endocrine gland is the thyroid gland (or) an example of an exocrine gland is a salivary gland (sweat gland)

6. a—smooth muscle in the iris of the eye changes the size of the pupil

7. d—the axon of a neuron carries impulses away from the cell body

8. b—nutrients and waste products are transported by blood plasma

9. a—adipose tissue stores fat as a potential energy source

10. c—stratified squamous epithelium of the outer layer of the skin has dead cells on the surface

Chapter 5

GENERAL STRUCTURE AND FUNCTIONS

1. 1) B, 3   2) C, 1   3) A, 2

EPIDERMIS

1. a) stratum germinativum
   b) stratum corneum

2. a) keratin
   b) water, bacteria and chemicals (or water)

3. mitosis, stratum germinativum

4. tissue fluid, blister

5. a) melanin   b) ultraviolet rays
   c) protects living skin cells from further exposure to UV rays

DERMIS

1. 1) E   2) C   3) J   4) A   5) F
   6) I   7) D   8) H   9) G   10) K   11) B

2. a) pain
   b) touch, pressure, heat, and cold
   c) the skin of the palm has more receptors for touch

3. a) nails   b) keratin

4. a) cerumen   b) sebum   c) sweat

5. a) eyes or nose   b) head   c) keratin

6. arterioles

7. a) D, cholesterol, UV rays
   b) calcium and phosphorus

8. 1) epidermis
   2) dermis
   3) subcutaneous tissue
   4) sweat gland
   5) hair shaft
   6) stratum corneum
   7) stratum germinativum
   8) papillary layer
   9) sebaceous gland
   10) hair root
   11) hair follicle
   12) sensory receptor
   13) nerve
   14) vein
   15) artery

SUBCUTANEOUS TISSUE

1. superficial fascia

2. a) dermis and the muscles
   b) areolar connective tissue and adipose tissue

3. pathogens, breaks in the skin

4. a) fat, energy
   b) cushions bony prominences and provides insulation from cold

MAINTENANCE OF BODY TEMPERATURE

1. eccrine sweat, arterioles
2. a) warm   b) evaporation
3. a) constrict   b) decrease, retained
4. a) dilate   b) increase, lost
5. smooth muscle

CLINICAL APPLICATIONS

1. a) corneum
   b) infection, dehydration
2. eccrine sweat, rise (increase)

MULTIPLE CHOICE TEST #1

1. d	5. b	9. a	13. b	17. b
2. b	6. c	10. c	14. d	18. c
3. a	7. d	11. d	15. a	19. c
4. a	8. b	12. c	16. c	20. d

MULTIPLE CHOICE TEST #2

The letter of the correct choice is followed by the statement necessary to complete the answer. When an incorrect statement is to be corrected to make it true, the new (true) words are underlined.

1. b—adipose tissue stores <u>fat</u> as a form of potential energy
2. a—the epidermis is made of <u>stratified</u> squamous epithelium
3. d—secretion of sweat by eccrine sweat glands is important to <u>lose excess body heat</u>
4. c—melanocytes produce melanin that protects living skin layers from <u>ultraviolet rays</u>
5. d—in sweating, excess body heat is lost in the process of <u>evaporation</u> of sweat
6. c—the receptors in the <u>dermis</u> are for the cutaneous senses of touch, pressure, heat, cold, and pain
7. d—it is located between the stratum <u>germinativum</u> and the subcutaneous tissue
8. b—cholesterol in the skin is converted to vitamin <u>D</u>
9. b—the epidermis is the <u>outer</u> layer and the dermis is the <u>inner</u> layer
10. c—melanin

Chapter 6

FUNCTIONS OF THE SKELETON

1. red bone marrow
2. calcium
3. a) supports   b) muscles
4. a) mechanical injury   b) the skull protects the brain (or) the ribs protect the heart and lungs

BONE TISSUE

1. 1) C   2) D, F   3) A, E   4) B

CLASSIFICATION OF BONES

1. 1) D, 2, 4   2) C, 1, 3   3) A, 1, 3
   4) B, 1, 3
2. cartilage

3. periosteum, fibrous
4. blood vessels
5. a) tendons, ligaments
   b) fibrous connective tissue
6. 1) proximal epiphysis   7) spongy bone
   2) diaphysis   8) Haversian
   3) distal epiphysis   systems
   4) yellow bone marrow   9) Haversian canal
   5) marrow cavity   10) osteocytes
   6) compact bone   11) periosteum

EMBRYONIC GROWTH OF BONE

1. a) ossification   b) osteoblasts
2. a) fibrous connective tissue
   b) third, fibroblasts

3. a) fontanels
   b) 1. frontal bone
      2. anterior fontanel
      3. parietal bone
      4. posterior fontanel
      5. mandible
      6. sphenoid fontanel
      7. temporal bone
      8. occipital bone
4. fontanels permit compression of the infant's skull during birth
5. cartilage
6. diaphysis, epiphysis
7. epiphyseal discs
8. 1) cartilage production
   2) bone replaces cartilage
   3) bone replaces cartilage
   4) cartilage production
9. cartilage, bone
10. a) osteoclasts   b) yellow, adipose

FACTORS THAT AFFECT BONE GROWTH AND MAINTENANCE

1. 1) D   2) A   3) A   4) C
   5) C   6) B
2. 1) D, anterior pituitary gland
   2) F, pancreas
   3) A, thyroid gland
   4) B, thyroid gland
   5) E, parathyroid glands
   6) C, ovaries or testes
   7) calcitonin
   8) parathyroid hormone
   9) estrogen or testosterone
3. a) the mother, the father
   b) enzymes, cartilage and bone
4. a) bearing weight   b) calcium
   c) become brittle and fracture easily

THE SKELETON

1. a) axial, skull, rib cage
   b) appendicular, arms and legs
2. 1) rib cage   2) skull   3) hip bones
   4) scapula and clavicle

3. 1) clavicle
   2) scapula
   3) humerus
   4) radius
   5) ulna
   6) carpals
   7) metacarpals
   8) phalanges
   9) tarsals
   10) metatarsals
   11) phalanges
   12) frontal bone
   13) zygomatic bone
   14) maxilla
   15) mandible
   16) sternum
   17) rib
   18) vertebra
   19) hip bone
   20) sacrum
   21) coccyx
   22) femur
   23) patella
   24) tibia
   25) fibula

THE SKULL

1. 1) sphenoid bone
   2) lacrimal bone
   3) frontal bone
   4) coronal suture
   5) nasal bone
   6) zygomatic bone
   7) ethmoid bone
   8) conchae
   9) vomer
   10) maxilla
   11) mandible
   12) nasal bone
   13) lacrimal bone
   14) zygomatic bone
   15) maxilla
   16) frontal bone
   17) parietal bone
   18) coronal suture
   19) sphenoid bone
   20) squamosal suture
   21) temporal bone
   22) lambdoidal suture
   23) occipital bone
   24) external auditory meatus
   25) condyloid process
   26) mastoid process
   27) mandible
2. 1) mandible and maxillae
   2) temporal bone
   3) zygomatic bone
   4) maxillae and palatine bones
   5) ethmoid bone
   6) vomer and ethmoid bone
   7) lacrimal bone
   8) occipital bone, spinal cord
   9) sphenoid bone
   10) nasal bones
   11) a) maxillae, frontal, sphenoid, and ethmoid bones
       b) lighten the skull and provide resonance for the voice
3. parietal and temporal
4. parietal and occipital
5. parietal and frontal
6. parietal
7. a) malleus, incus, and stapes   b) hearing

THE VERTEBRAL COLUMN

1. support, spinal cord
2. a)
   1. atlas
   2. axis
   3. first thoracic
   4. intervertebral disc
   5. first lumbar
   6. sacrum
   7. coccyx
   8. cervical vertebrae
   9. thoracic vertebrae
   10. lumbar vertebrae
   11. sacrum
   12. coccyx

   b) 1) 7   2) 12   3) 5
   4) 5, sacrum   5) 4 or 5, coccyx
3. a) atlas, axis   b) pivot, side to side
4. posterior, thoracic
5. sacrum
6. a) body   b) cartilage
   c) absorb shock and permit movement
   d) symphysis

THE RIB CAGE

1. 1) first thoracic vertebra
   2) costal cartilage
   3) body of sternum
   4) xiphoid process
   5) floating ribs
   6) first rib
   7) manubrium
   8) true ribs
   9) seventh rib
   10) eighth rib
   11) false ribs
   12) 12th rib
   13) 12th thoracic vertebra
2. seven, three, two
3. heart and lungs
4. liver and spleen
5. up and out, expand (enlarge), lungs

THE SHOULDER AND ARM

1. scapula and clavicle
2. scapula
3. a) manubrium, scapula
   b) braces the scapula (keeps it back)
4. head, glenoid fossa, ball and socket
5. a) radius and ulna   b) ulna
6. a) humerus and ulna   b) hinge
7. a) pivot   b) palm up to palm down
8. a) carpals   b) eight   c) gliding
9. five, carpals, phalanges
10. a) saddle   b) rotation or gripping
11. a) two   b) three   c) 14   d) hinge

12. 1) acromial end
    2) acromion process
    3) coracoid process
    4) head of humerus
    5) humerus
    6) capitulum
    7) head of radius
    8) radius
    9) scaphoid
    10) trapezium
    11) trapezoid
    12) capitate
    13) lunate
    14) triquetrum
    15) pisiform
    16) hamate
    17) metacarpals
    18) phalanges
    19) clavicle
    20) sternal end
    21) glenoid fossa
    22) scapula
    23) trochlea
    24) semilunar notch
    25) ulna

THE HIP AND LEG

1. hip bone
2. acetabulum
3. a) ilium, ischium, and pubis   b) ilium
   c) sacroiliac   d) pubis
   e) pubic symphysis   f) ischium
4. a) femur   b) ball and socket
5. a) tibia and fibula   b) tibia
   c) muscle attachment
6. a) femur and tibia   b) hinge
7. a) tarsals   b) seven   c) calcaneus
8. five, tarsals, phalanges
9. a) 14   b) two   c) three
10. 1) ilium
    2) sacroiliac joint
    3) acetabulum
    4) ischium
    5) pubis
    6) sacrum
    7) coccyx
    8) pubic symphysis
11. 1) acetabulum
    2) head of femur
    3) greater trochanter
    4) neck of femur
    5) lesser trochanter
    6) femur
    7) medial condyles
    8) patella
    9) lateral condyles
    10) head of fibula
    11) tibial tuberosity
    12) tibia
    13) fibula
    14) medial malleolus
    15) lateral malleolus
    16) talus
    17) navicular
    18) cuneiforms
    19) cuboid
    20) metatarsals
    21) phalanges
    22) cuboid
    23) navicular
    24) talus
    25) calcaneus
    26) lateral malleolus

JOINTS (ARTICULATIONS)

1. **Name of Joint** **Movement Possible** **Examples (name two bones)**

   1) Suture   None—immovable   a. frontal and parietal bones
        b. parietal and temporal bones

   2) Symphysis   Slight movement   a. two vertebrae
        b. two pubic bones

   3) Hinge   Movement in one plane   a. humerus and ulna
        b. femur and tibia

   4) Gliding   Sliding movement   a. two carpals
   5) Saddle   Movement in all planes   a. carpometacarpal of the thumb
   6) Ball and socket   Movement in all planes   a. scapula and humerus
        b. hip bone and femur

   7) Pivot   Rotation   a. atlas and axis
        b. radius and ulna

   8) Condyloid   Movement in one plane with some lateral movement   a. mandible and temporal bone

SYNOVIAL JOINT STRUCTURE

1. 1) E   2) C   3) A   4) B   5) D
2. 1) joint capsule   4) articular cartilage
   2) bursa   5) synovial fluid
   3) synovial membrane   6) bursa

CLINICAL APPLICATIONS

1. a) epiphyseal disc   b) osteoblasts
2. osteoporosis
3. intervertebral
4. 1) cheek bone   5) collarbone and
   2) back of the head   top of the
   3) lower leg near the ankle   breastbone
   4) knee cap   6) lower jaw
        7) finger bones

MULTIPLE CHOICE TEST #1

1. d	5. d	9. a	13. c	17. b
2. b	6. c	10. b	14. d	18. b
3. b	7. b	11. c	15. a	19. b
4. d	8. a	12. b	16. c	20. b

MULTIPLE CHOICE TEST #2

The letter of the correct choice is followed by the statement necessary to complete the answer. When an incorrect statement is to be corrected to make it true, the new (true) words are underlined.

1. c—blood cells are produced by <u>red</u> bone marrow found in spongy bone
2. d—calcitonin <u>decreases</u> the reabsorption of calcium from <u>bones</u>
3. b—new bone matrix is produced by cells called <u>osteoblasts</u>
4. d—vitamin D is necessary for the absorption of calcium by the <u>small intestine</u>
5. b—the rib cage protects the <u>heart and lungs</u> (or <u>liver and spleen</u>)
6. b—synovial fluid <u>decreases</u> friction within the joint cavity
7. a—the hinge joint between the femur and <u>tibia</u> permits movement in one plane at the <u>knee</u>
8. b—the only movable joint is the condyloid joint between the temporal bone and the <u>mandible</u>
9. d—the hip bones articulate with the <u>sacrum</u>
10. b—the only weight-bearing bone in the lower leg is the <u>tibia</u>
11. b—during inhalation the ribs are pulled <u>up and out</u> to expand the lungs
12. d—there are <u>eight</u> carpals in each wrist and <u>14</u> phalanges in each hand

Chapter 7

MUSCLES AND MOVEMENT

1. bones, tendons
2. a) move the skeleton
   b) produce body heat
3. a) respiratory system   b) skeletal system
   c) nervous system   d) circulatory system

MUSCLE STRUCTURE

1. muscle cell
2. a) they become shorter   b) more
3. fascia, periosteum
4. a) joint   b) origin   c) insertion
   d) insertion

MUSCLE ARRANGEMENTS

1. a) opposite   b) the same (or stabilizing)
2. a) pull   b) push   c) pull
3. 1) to decrease the angle of a joint, extension
   2) to move a body part away from the midline, adduction
   3) to turn the palm down, suppination
   4) to lower the foot, dorsiflexion
4. a) frontal, cerebrum   b) cerebellum
5. 1) extension   7) flexion
   2) radius   8) radius
   3) biceps—relaxed   9) biceps—contracted
   4) scapula   10) scapula
   5) triceps—contracted   11) triceps—relaxed
   6) humerus   12) humerus

MUSCLE TONE AND EXERCISE

1. slight contraction
2. heat, body temperature
3. a) movement   b) no movement
   c) both   d) isotonic
   e) heart, respiratory
4. 1) improves coordination (or) helps maintain posture
   2) permits rapid muscle responses (or) produces body heat

MUSCLE SENSE

1. knowing where our muscles are without having to look at them
2. stretch receptors or proprioceptors
3. brain
4. a) parietal   b) cerebellum, coordination
5. permits us to accomplish everyday activities without having to constantly watch our movements

ENERGY SOURCES FOR MUSCLE CONTRACTION

1. a) ATP, creatine phosphate, glycogen
   b) ATP   c) glycogen
2. creatinine, kidneys
3. glucose
4. a) Glucose + $O_2 \rightarrow CO_2$ + H_2O + ATP + Heat   b) ATP
5. a) myoglobin   b) hemoglobin   c) iron
6. a) oxygen debt   b) lactic acid, fatigue
7. liver, glucose
8. a) water: becomes part of intracellular water
   b) heat: contributes to a constant body temperature
   c) carbon dioxide: is exhaled

MUSCLE FIBER—MICROSCOPIC STRUCTURE

1. neuron and a muscle cell
2. 1) B, C   2) D, E   3) A, F
3. 1) D   2) C   3) B   4) A
4. 1) sac of acetylcholine   5) synapse
   2) acetylcholine   6) sarcolemma
   3) acetylcholine receptors   7) myosin
   4) axon terminal   8) actin

SLIDING FILAMENT THEORY

1. 1) E   2) G   3) C   4) H   5) A
   6) F   7) B   8) D
2. tetanus

3. rapid nerve impulses sustain (or prolong) the state of contraction

EXERCISE—HOMEOSTASIS

1. 1) C, E   2) B   3) D, F   4) A
   5) G

MAJOR MUSCLES OF THE BODY

1. a) 1. masseter
      2. sternocleidomastoid
      3. deltoid
      4. pectoralis major
      5. biceps brachii
      6. brachioradialis
      7. rectus femoris
      8. sartorius
      9. vastus lateralis
      10. vastus medialis
      11. tibialis anterior
      12. external oblique
      13. rectus abdominus
      14. adductor longus
      15. gastrocnemius
      16. soleus

   b) 1. triceps brachii
      2. latissimus dorsi
      3. gluteus medius
      4. gluteus maximus
      5. biceps femoris
      6. soleus
      7. Achilles tendon
      8. trapezius
      9. deltoid
      10. teres major
      11. semimembranosus
      12. gastrocnemius

2. any three of these: biceps brachii and triceps brachii; quadriceps femoris and hamstring group; gastrocnemius and tibialis anterior; deltoid and pectoralis major; pectoralis major and latissimus dorsi; rectus abdominus and sacrospinalis group; adductor group and gluteus medius. There are others that are correct, if they have opposite functions.

3. 1) flexion of head
   2) extension of head
   3) flexion of arm
   4) abduction of arm
   5) extension of arm
   6) adduction of arm
   7) flexion of forearm
   8) extension of forearm
   9) flexion of leg
   10) extension of leg
   11) flexion of thigh
   12) extension of thigh
   13) abduction of thigh
   14) adduction of thigh

CLINICAL APPLICATIONS

1. a) nerves   b) paralyzed
   c) become smaller   d) atrophy
2. a) hamstring group   b) gastrocnemius
   c) trapezius

MULTIPLE CHOICE TEST #1

1. d   5. c   9. b   13. d   17. c
2. d   6. c   10. d   14. a   18. b
3. d   7. b   11. a   15. a   19. d
4. c   8. a   12. c   16. d   20. d

MULTIPLE CHOICE TEST #2

The letter of the correct choice is followed by the statement necessary to complete the answer. When an incorrect statement is to be corrected to make it true, the new (true) words are underlined.

1. d—unconscious muscle sense is integrated by the cerebellum
2. c—muscles are attached to bones by tendons, which are made of fibrous connective tissue
3. a—the deltoid is the shoulder muscle that abducts the arm
4. c—the pectoralis major is on the front of the chest and flexes the arm
5. d—muscle tone does depend on nerve impulses to muscle fibers
6. b—the direct energy source for contraction is ATP
7. c—the sarcolemma contains cholinesterase to inactivate acetylcholine
8. b—isotonic exercise is aerobic because it involves contraction with movement
9. b—some oxygen is stored in muscle by the protein myoglobin
10. d—within a muscle fiber, the sarcomeres all contract together

Chapter 8

NERVOUS SYSTEM DIVISIONS

1. brain and spinal cord
2. cranial nerves and spinal nerves
3. peripheral nervous system

NERVE TISSUE

1. neuron
2. 1) cell body   2) axon   3) dendrites
3. a) 1. synaptic knobs   9. cell body
      2. axon   10. nucleus
      3. myelin sheath   11. dendrites
      4. Schwann cell   12. neurolemma
      5. nucleus   13. axon
      6. cell body   14. myelin sheath
      7. dendrite   15. axon terminals
      8. synapse

   b) axon   c) cell body   d) dendrites
   e) synapse
   f) sensory neuron begins in receptors; motor
      neuron ends in muscle
4. a) Schwann cells   b) oligodendrocytes
   c) provides electrical insulation for neurons
5. a) nuclei and cytoplasm   b) regeneration
6. a) neurotransmitter, axon
   b) inactivator chemical   c) cholinesterase
7. 1) axon of presynaptic neuron 5) inactivator
   2) vesicles of neurotransmitter 6) receptor site
   3) neurotransmitter   7) sodium ion
   4) dendrite of postsynaptic
      neuron

NEURONS, NERVES, AND NERVE TRACTS

1. 1) B, D   2) C, F   3) A   4) G   5) E

THE NERVE IMPULSE

1. a) positive, negative   b) sodium
   c) potassium and negative   d) polarization
2. a) sodium, into   b) negative, positive
3. a) potassium, out of   b) repolarization
   c) positive, negative
   d) sodium and potassium pumps

THE SPINAL CORD AND SPINAL NERVES

1. 1) transmits impulses to and from the brain
   2) is the center for the spinal cord reflexes
2. a) vertebrae
   b) foramen magnum, first and second lumbar
      vertebrae
3. a) 1. dorsal root ganglion   4. central canal
      2. dorsal root   5. gray matter
      3. white matter   6. ventral root

   b) gray matter   c) dorsal root ganglion
   d) sensory, sensory   e) motor, motor
   f) white matter   g) sensory, toward
   h) motor, away from   i) central canal
4. 1) eight   2) 12   3) five   4) five   5) one
5. 1) thoracic   2) lumbar and sacral
   3) cervical (and first thoracic)   4) cervical

SPINAL CORD REFLEXES

1. an involuntary response to a stimulus
2. 1, 5, 4, 3, 2
3. 1) stretch receptor   7) synapse
   2) quadriceps femoris   8) gray matter
   3) sensory neuron   9) white matter
   4) femoral nerve   10) ventral root
   5) dorsal root ganglion   11) motor neuron
   6) dorsal root
4. stretching of a muscle, contraction of the same
   muscle
5. a) keep the body upright (maintain posture)
   b) protect the body from potential harm
   c) no conscious decision is required; that
      would take too much time

THE BRAIN

1. 1) H, N   2) B, L, O   3) K   4) A, P
   5) C, J   6) E, I, Q, S   7) M, R
   8) G   9) F   10) D
2. 1) C, F   2) A, B   3) E, G   4) D

3. 1) corpus callosum
   2) frontal lobe
   3) thalamus
   4) third ventricle
   5) hypothalamus
   6) pituitary gland
   7) brain stem
   8) midbrain
   9) pons
   10) medulla
   11) parietal lobe
   12) occipital lobe
   13) cerebellum
   14) fourth ventricle

4. 1) frontal lobe
   2) temporal lobe
   3) pons
   4) medulla
   5) parietal lobe
   6) occipital lobe
   7) cerebellum

5. cerebral cortex, cell bodies

6. a) lateral   b) fourth   c) third
   d) cerebral aqueduct

MENINGES AND CEREBROSPINAL FLUID

1. three

2. a) dura mater
   b) skull and vertebral canal   c) arachnoid
   d) pia mater; brain and spinal cord

3. arachnoid membrane, pia mater, cerebrospinal fluid

4. choroid plexuses, ventricles

5. 1) ventricles   2) subarachnoid space
   3) central canal   4) subarachnoid space

6. 1) exchanges nutrients and waste products between the CNS and blood
   2) absorbs shock (cushions) around the CNS

7. a) arachnoid villi, cranial venous sinuses
   b) the same as

8. 1) dura mater
   2) arachnoid membrane
   3) pia mater
   4) central canal
   5) subarachnoid space

9. 1) dura mater
   2) arachnoid membrane
   3) subarachnoid space
   4) pia mater
   5) lateral ventricle
   6) choroid plexus
   7) choroid plexus in third ventricle
   8) arachnoid villus
   9) cranial venous sinus
   10) cerebral aqueduct
   11) choroid plexus in fourth ventricle
   12) central canal

CRANIAL NERVES

1. 1) optic
   2) acoustic
   3) facial and glossopharyngeal
   4) olfactory
   5) acoustic
   6) facial and glossopharyngeal
   7) oculomotor, abducens, and trochlear
   8) vagus
   9) vagus
   10) vagus and accessory
   11) hypoglossal
   12) accessory
   13) oculomotor
   14) vagus and glossopharyngeal
   15) trigeminal
   16) facial
   17) trigeminal

2. 1) olfactory
   2) optic
   3) oculomotor
   4) trochlear
   5) trigeminal
   6) abducens
   7) facial
   8) acoustic
   9) glossopharyngeal
   10) vagus
   11) accessory
   12) hypoglossal

THE AUTONOMIC NERVOUS SYSTEM (ANS)

1. smooth, cardiac, glands

2. hypothalamus

3. a) sympathetic, stressful
   b) parasympathetic, non-stress

4. 1) P   2) S   3) S   4) P   5) P
   6) S   7) P   8) S

5. 1) thoracic spinal cord
   2) sympathetic preganglionic neuron
   3) sympathetic postganglionic neuron
   4) sympathetic ganglia
   5) lumbar spinal cord
   6) brain
   7) sacral spinal cord
   8) parasympathetic preganglionic neurons
   9) parasympathetic ganglion
   10) parasympathetic postganglionic neurons

6. **Visceral Effector**

	Parasympathetic Response	Sympathetic Response
1) stomach and intestines (glands)	increases secretions	decreases secretions
2) stomach and intestines (smooth muscle)	increases peristalsis	slows peristalsis
3) heart	decreases rate (to normal)	increases rate
4) iris	constricts pupil	dilates pupil
5) urinary bladder	contracts	relaxes
6) bronchioles	constrict (to normal)	dilate
7) salivary glands	increase secretion	decrease secretion
8) blood vessels in skeletal muscle	none	vasodilation
9) blood vessels in skin and viscera	none	vasoconstriction
10) sweat glands	none	increase secretion
11) liver	none	change glycogen to glucose

CLINICAL APPLICATIONS

1. a) meningitis   b) cerebrospinal fluid
2. a) frontal, left   b) motor speech area
3. a) sensation
   b) paralysis below the injury
   c) motor impulses from the brain cannot get to the muscles
4. a) medulla   b) occipital   c) cerebellum

MULTIPLE CHOICE TEST #1

1. c	6. a	11. c	16. a	21. c
2. a	7. b	12. c	17. b	22. a
3. a	8. d	13. c	18. b	23. c
4. d	9. d	14. b	19. b	24. a
5. b	10. d	15. d	20. c	

MULTIPLE CHOICE TEST #2

The letter of the correct choice is followed by the statement necessary to complete the answer. When an incorrect statement is to be corrected to make it true, the new (true) words are underlined.

1. c—CSF is reabsorbed into the blood in the cranial venous sinuses
2. d—regulates coordination (or) equilibrium (or) muscle tone
3. d—sensory neurons may also be called afferent neurons (or) motor neurons may also be called efferent neurons
4. c—visual area
5. b—the stimulus is detected by receptors
6. a—visual and auditory reflexes (or) equilibrium
7. c—the spinal cord extends from the foramen magnum to the disc between the first and second lumbar vertebrae
8. b—each spinal nerve has two roots; the dorsal root and the ventral, or motor, root
9. c—the nucleus is located within the cell body
10. b—the pia mater is the innermost layer and is on the surface of the brain and spinal cord
11. d—sense of smell
12. b—the parasympathetic division causes constriction of the bronchioles and increased peristalsis
13. b—during depolarization, sodium ions rush into the cell

Chapter 9

SENSORY PATHWAY

1. 1) receptors   3) sensory tracts
   2) sensory neurons   4) sensory area in
                       the brain

2. changes, impulses

3. receptors, central nervous system

4. central nervous system, brain

5. cerebrum (or) cerebral cortex

CHARACTERISTICS OF SENSATIONS

1. 1) D   2) A   3) B   4) C   5) E

CUTANEOUS SENSES

1. a) dermis of the skin
   b) changes in the external environment

2. a) pain   b) touch, pressure, heat, cold

3. parietal

4. organ, cutaneous

5. heart—left shoulder (or) gallbladder—right shoulder

MUSCLE SENSE

1. proprioceptors (stretch receptors), stretching

2. a) parietal   b) cerebellum

3. enables us to accomplish everyday activities without having to look at our muscles to see where a body part is

HUNGER AND THIRST

1. 1) B, C, E   2) A, D, F

TASTE AND SMELL

1. 1) B, D, E, G, H, J   2) A, C, F, I

2. 1) olfactory nerve   4) taste buds
   2) olfactory bulb   5) tongue
   3) olfactory receptors

THE EYE—STRUCTURES OUTSIDE THE EYEBALL

1. 1) D   2) G   3) F   4) C
   5) A   6) E   7) B

2. 1) eyelid   4) conjunctiva
   2) lacrimal gland 5) lacrimal sac
   3) lacrimal ducts   6) nasolacrimal duct

3. a) bones of the orbit   b) six
   c) move the eyeball

4. oculomotor, abducens, trochlear

THE EYE—EYEBALL

1. a) sclera, fibrous connective
   b) choroid layer   c) retina

2. 1) F   2) R   3) C   4) L
   5) A   6) Q   7) H   8) P
   9) E   10) B   11) D   12) K
   13) G 14) O 15) M 16) N
   17) I 18) J

3. 1) superior rectus 12) vitreous humor
       muscle   13) fovea
   2) ciliary body   14) optic nerve
   3) suspensory   15) retinal artery
       ligaments   and vein
   4) conjunctiva   16) optic disc
   5) cornea   17) retina
   6) iris   18) choroid layer
   7) lens   19) sclera
   8) pupil   20) Canal of
   9) aqueous humor   Schlemm
   10) anterior chamber 21) inferior rectus
   11) posterior chamber   muscle

4. 1) optic   2) oculomotor   3) sympathetic

5. a) occipital   b) binocular
   c) right side up

SUMMARY OF VISION

1. 1, 4, 6, 2, 7, 3, 5

THE EAR

1. hearing and equilibrium

2. outer ear, middle ear, inner ear

OUTER EAR

1. a) cartilage
   b) no, because it is not movable
2. a) temporal   b) ceruminous   c) cerumen

MIDDLE EAR

1. temporal, air
2. 1) B   2) E   3) A   4) C   5) D
3. 1) pinna (auricle)   8) vestibule
   2) ear canal   9) vestibular nerve
   3) ear drum   (eighth)
   4) malleus   10) cochlear nerve
   5) incus   (eighth)
   6) semicircular   11) cochlea
      canals   12) eustachian tube
   7) stapes

INNER EAR

1. temporal, membrane, fluid
2. 1) semicircular canals   2) cochlea
   3) utricle and saccule (or) vestibule
3. a) impulses
   b) acoustic (or) eighth cranial nerve
4. a) organ of Corti   b) fluid (endolymph)
   c) temporal
5. a) vestibule   b) gravity, head
6. a) three   b) movement
7. a) cerebellum, midbrain
   b) cerebrum (temporal lobe)
8. 1) semicircular canals   9) vestibular nerve
   2) ampulla   (eighth)
   3) utricle   10) cochlear nerve
   4) bony labyrinth   (eighth)
   5) perilymph   11) tympanic canal
   6) membranous   12) cochlear duct
      labyrinth   13) vestibular canal
   7) crista   14) cochlea
   8) saccule   15) round window
                         16) oval window

SUMMARY OF HEARING

1. 1, 5, 3, 8, 2, 4, 6, 7, 9

CLINICAL APPLICATIONS

1. a) aqueous humor   b) retina
2. malleus, incus, and stapes
3. conjunctiva, conjunctivitis
4. lens

MULTIPLE CHOICE TEST #1

1. d	5. b	9. d	13. c	17. b
2. d	6. b	10. b	14. d	18. b
3. c	7. a	11. a	15. c	19. c
4. c	8. a	12. b	16. d	20. d

MULTIPLE CHOICE TEST #2

The letter of the correct choice is followed by the statement necessary to complete the answer. When an incorrect statement is to be corrected, the new (true) words are underlined.

1. c—the ear drum is at the end of the ear canal
2. b—the auditory areas are in the temporal lobes
3. c—if too much light strikes the eye, the iris will constrict the pupil
4. c—the ear drum transmits vibrations to the malleus, incus, and stapes
5. d—the cranial nerves for the sense of smell are the olfactory nerves
6. a—the receptors for pain are free nerve endings in the dermis
7. c—the effect of a previous sensation on a current sensation is called contrast
8. d—the eyeball is moved from side to side by the extrinsic muscles
9. b—the cerebellum and the midbrain regulate the reflexes that keep us upright

Chapter 10

ENDOCRINE GLANDS

1. a) hormones, blood   b) target
   c) receptors
2. amines, proteins, and steroids
3. a) sphenoid   b) larynx   c) thyroid gland
   d) duodenum, spleen   e) kidneys
   f) uterus   g) scrotum
4. 1) anterior pituitary   7) parathyroid glands
   2) thyroid gland   8) thymus
   3) adrenal medulla   9) adrenal cortex
   4) testes   10) pancreas
   5) hypothalamus   11) ovaries
   6) posterior pituitary

THE PITUITARY GLAND

1. anterior pituitary, posterior pituitary
2. a) hypothalamus
   b) releasing, hypothalamus

Posterior Pituitary Gland

1. kidneys
2. a) increase, water
   b) decreases, increases
3. decreased
4. a) uterus and mammary glands
   b) smooth muscle (myometrium), baby,
      placenta   c) milk   d) hypothalamus

Anterior Pituitary Gland

1. a) 1) amino acids, proteins   2) mitosis
      3) fats
   b) GHRH   c) GHIH
2. a) thyroid gland   b) 1) thyroxine and T_3
   c) TRH
3. a) adrenal cortex   b) 1) cortisol   c) CRH
4. a) mammary glands   b) 1) milk
   c) hypothalamus
5. a) ovaries, testes   b) 1) egg cells, estrogen
   c) 1) sperm   d) GnRH
6. a) ovaries, testes
   b) 1) ovulation
      2) corpus luteum, progesterone

c) testosterone   d) GnRH
e) gonadotropic

THYROID GLAND

1. a) 1) proteins
      2) carbohydrates, fats, and amino acids
      3) physical, mental
   b) iodine   c) TSH, anterior pituitary
2. a) bones   b) 1) calcium and phosphate
   c) decreased   d) hypercalcemia

PARATHYROID GLANDS

1. a) bones, small intestine, kidney
   b) 1) calcium and phosphate
      2) small intestine   3) calcium
   c) increased, decreased
   d) hypocalcemia

PANCREAS

1. a) islets of Langerhans
   b) glucagon, insulin
2. a) liver
   b) 1) glycogen   2) fats and amino acids
   c) increased, food   d) hypoglycemia
3. a) 1) glucose   2) skeletal
      3) glucose, energy
      4) amino acids and fatty acids; proteins and
         fats
   b) decreased   c) hyperglycemia

ADRENAL GLANDS

1. adrenal cortex, adrenal medulla
2. epinephrine and norepinephrine, medulla
3. cortex, aldosterone
4. cortex, cortisol

ADRENAL MEDULLA

1. a) blood vessels
   b) 1) vasoconstriction
2. a) 1) increases rate   2) vasodilation

3) vasoconstriction
4) decreases peristalsis   5) dilation
6) conversion of glycogen to glucose
7) increases use
b) sympathetic   c) sympathetic, stressful

ADRENAL CORTEX

1. a) kidneys
   b) sodium, potassium
   c) 1) hydrogen (or K^+)
      2) sodium and bicarbonate   3) water
   d) blood pressure (or pH)
   e) sodium, potassium, blood pressure
2. a) 1) amino acids, fats   2) glucose
      3) anti-inflammatory
   b) ACTH, anterior pituitary

OVARIES

1. a) uterus, mammary glands (or) bones, adipose tissue
   b) 1) ovum   2) endometrium
      3) growth of duct system of mammary glands (or) fat deposition
      4) closure of the epiphyseal discs
   c) FSH, anterior pituitary
2. a) uterus, mammary glands
   b) 1) blood vessels, glycogen
      2) secretory cells
   c) LH, anterior pituitary

TESTES

1. a) testes, bones, muscles (or) reproductive organs
   b) 1) sperm   2) growth of reproductive organs (or) larynx, facial hair, muscles
      3) closure of the epiphyseal discs
   c) LH, anterior pituitary
2. a) anterior pituitary
   b) FSH, spermatogenesis
   c) increased testosterone

PROSTAGLANDINS

1. a) phospholipids   b) locally
2. three of these: blood clotting, pain mechanisms, digestive secretions, reproduction, inflammation, vasodilation or vasoconstriction

STIMULUS FOR SECRETION— SUMMARY

1. 1) E   2) A   3) J   4) D
    5) F   6) G   7) M   8) I
    9) B   10) H   11) M   12) C
   13) K   14) L   15) N   16) L

CLINICAL APPLICATIONS

1. parathyroid hormone
2. thyroxine
3. a) pancreas
   b) glucose
   c) diabetes mellitus
4. growth hormone

MULTIPLE CHOICE TEST #1

1. c	6. b	11. d	15. c	19. a
2. d	7. b	12. d	16. d	20. c
3. b	8. d	13. a	17. c	
4. a	9. c	14. b	18. b	
5. a	10. c			

MULTIPLE CHOICE TEST #2

The letter of the correct choice is followed by the statement necessary to complete the answer. When a statement is to be corrected to make it true, the new (true) words are underlined.

1. a—insulin causes the liver to change glucose to glycogen
2. a—GH increases the rate of mitosis in growing bones
3. d—FSH and LH are called gonadotropic hormones because their target organs are the ovaries or testes
4. b—insulin—hyperglycemia
5. d—epinephrine causes the liver to change glycogen to glucose
6. c—aldosterone increases the reabsorption of sodium ions
7. d—these hormones are actually produced by the hypothalamus
8. b—the thyroid gland is inferior to the larynx on the front of the trachea
9. d—secondary sex characteristics in men and women are regulated by testosterone and estrogen, respectively

Chapter 11

GENERAL FUNCTIONS OF BLOOD

1. 1) D, G   2) A, E, F   3) B, C

CHARACTERISTICS OF BLOOD

1. four to six
2. a) 38%–48%   b) 52%–62%
3. a) 7.35–7.45   b) alkaline
4. a) thickness (or resistance to flow)
   b) cells, plasma proteins (albumin)

BLOOD PLASMA

1. 91
2. a) dissolve   b) nutrients, waste products
3. a) bicarbonate   b) HCO_3^-
4. 1) A, D, F   2) A, C, G   3) B, E, H

HEMOPOIETIC TISSUES

1. blood cells
2. red bone marrow, lymphatic tissue
3. a) flat, irregular   b) spleen, lymph nodes
4. a) lymphocytes, monocytes
   b) red blood cells, white blood cells, platelets
5. 1) lymph nodes   4) spleen
   2) lymph nodes   5) red bone marrow
   3) red bone marrow

RED BLOOD CELLS

1. a) erythrocytes, red bone marrow
   b) a nucleus
   c) biconcave discs (or) thinner in the middle
      than at the edge

2. a) hemoglobin   b) iron
3. a) pulmonary (lungs), oxyhemoglobin
   b) systemic, reduced hemoglobin
4. a) stem cell   b) mitosis
5. 1) red blood cells   3) agranular WBC
   2) granular WBCs   4) platelets
6. a) oxygen   b) low blood oxygen level
   c) erythropoietin, RBC production
7. a) normoblast   b) reticulocyte
   c) mature RBCs, oxygen
8. a) protein, iron
   b) vitamin B_{12}, DNA
   c) stomach   d) vitamin B_{12}
9. a) 120
   b) liver, spleen, red bone marrow
   c) liver, hemoglobin
10. a) bilirubin   b) liver, bile   c) feces
11. a) whites of the eyes (or) light skin
    b) jaundice
12. 1) 4.5–6.0 million   2) 38–48
    3) 12–18

RED BLOOD CELL TYPES

1. ABO, Rh
2. A, B, AB, O

3.

	Type A	Type B	Type AB	Type O
Antigens present on RBCs	A	B	A and B	neither A nor B
Antibodies present in plasma	anti-B	anti-A	neither anti-A nor anti-B	both anti-A and anti-B

4. 1) A antigen   4) B antigen
   2) B antibody   5) A antibody
   3) A antigen   6) B antigen

5. a) positive; negative   b) no
   c) if an Rh negative person receives (or is exposed to) Rh positive blood

6. a) hemolysis
   b) kidneys, free hemoglobin

WHITE BLOOD CELLS

1. a) leukocytes   b) granular, agranular

2. a) red bone marrow
   b) neutrophils, eosinophils, basophils
   c) lymphatic
   d) lymphocytes, monocytes

3. nuclei

4. pathogens, immunity

5. 1) A   2) B   3) E   4) F
   5) C, G   6) D, H

6. 1) 5,000–10,000
   2) leukocytosis, infection
   3) leukopenia, radiation (or) exposure to certain chemicals or antibiotics

PLATELETS

1. thrombocytes, red bone marrow

2. megakaryocytes

3. a) prevention of blood loss
   b) vascular spasm, platelet plugs, chemical clotting

4. a) smooth muscle   b) serotonin, damage
   c) smaller, blood clot

5. a) capillaries   b) stick to the edges

6. 150,000–300,000

7. thrombocytopenia

CHEMICAL BLOOD CLOTTING

1. rough, rough

2. liver, blood plasma

3. a) K   b) bacteria, colon (large intestine)

4. calcium, bones

5. a) platelets, damaged tissues
   b) prothrombin activator
   c) prothrombin activator, thrombin
   d) thrombin, fibrin   e) fibrin

6. a) retraction, repair   b) fibrinolysis

7. a) simple squamous   b) heparin
   c) liver, thrombin

8. a) thrombus   b) embolism

CLINICAL APPLICATIONS

1. b—the WBC count is high

2. Factor 8, liver

3. a) erythroblastosis fetalis
   b) negative, positive, positive, positive
   c) RhoGam will destroy any Rh positive RBCs in maternal circulation to prevent maternal production of Rh antibodies

MULTIPLE CHOICE TEST #1

1. b	5. b	9. b	13. b	17. c
2. a	6. d	10. d	14. b	18. d
3. b	7. b	11. b	15. a	19. a
4. c	8. a	12. c	16. a	20. d

MULTIPLE CHOICE TEST #2

The letter of the correct choice is followed by the statement necessary to complete the answer. When an incorrect statement is to be corrected to make it true, the new (true) words are underlined.

1. d—oxygen is transported within RBCs

2. b—eosinophils help detoxify foreign proteins

3. c—the intrinsic factor is produced by the stomach lining to prevent digestion of vitamin B_{12}
4. b—prothrombin, fibrinogen, and other clotting factors are synthesized by the liver
5. c—type B has B antigens on the RBCs (or) type A has A antigens on the RBCs
6. b—Hb—12–18 grams/100 ml

7. a—the normal lifespan of RBCs is 120 days
8. b—gamma globulins are antibodies produced by lymphocytes
9. a—a normoblast is the last stage with a nucleus
10. d—heparin is produced by basophils
11. b—platelet plugs are useful only in capillaries
12. d—anemia—decreased RBC count

Chapter 12

FUNCTION AND LOCATION
1. pump blood
2. a) lungs, thoracic   b) diaphragm

PERICARDIAL MEMBRANES
1. three
2. fibrous, fibrous connective tissue
3. a) parietal   b) visceral, epicardium
4. prevent friction

CHAMBERS OF THE HEART
1. four, atria, ventricles
2. cardiac muscle, myocardium
3. a) endocardium, valves
   b) smooth, clotting
4. a) ventricles   b) interatrial septum
   c) interventricular septum

CHAMBERS—VESSELS AND VALVES
1. 1) D, 1   2) A, 4   3) B, 3
   4) C, 2
2. 1) superior vena cava
   2) right pulmonary artery
   3) right pulmonary veins
   4) coronary arteries
   5) right atrium
   6) inferior vena cava
   7) right ventricle
   8) aorta
   9) left pulmonary artery
   10) left pulmonary veins
   11) left atrium
   12) left ventricle

3. 1) C, 3   2) B, 2   3) A, 4
   4) D, 1
4. 1) superior vena cava
   2) right pulmonary artery
   3) pulmonary semilunar valve
   4) endocardium
   5) right atrium
   6) tricuspid valve
   7) inferior vena cava
   8) aorta
   9) pulmonary artery
   10) left pulmonary artery
   11) pulmonary veins
   12) left atrium
   13) bicuspid (mitral) valve
   14) aortic semilunar valve
   15) left ventricle
   16) papillary muscles
   17) interventricular septum
   18) epicardium
   19) right ventricle
   20) chordae tendineae
5. a) myocardium, ventricle
   b) fibrous connective, flaps of the AV valves
   c) contract
6. a) atrial natriuretic hormone, increases
   b) kidneys, decrease

CIRCULATION THROUGH THE HEART
1. a) lungs, body   b) body, lungs
2. 1, 2, 6, 7, 4, 9, 8, 10, 3, 5

CORONARY VESSELS
1. a) myocardium (heart)   b) oxygen
2. a) aorta   b) right atrium
3. a) heart muscle cells begin to die
   b) a blood clot (or atherosclerosis) in a coronary vessel

CARDIAC CYCLE AND HEART SOUNDS

1. heartbeat
2. a) contraction   b) relaxation
3. diastole, diastole
4. 1) 1   2) 3   3) 6   4) 2
   5) 4   6) 7   7) 5   8) 8
5. flows passively
6. is pumped
7. a) two   b) AV   c) semilunar
   d) heart murmur

CARDIAC CONDUCTION PATHWAY

1. a) impulses   b) no   c) rate
2. 1) SA node   2) AV node
   3) Bundle of His   4) bundle branches
   5) Purkinje fibers
3. 1) SA node   4) bundle branches
   2) AV node   5) Purkinje fibers
   3) bundle of His
4. rapid
5. SA node, AV node
6. Bundle of His, bundle branches, Purkinje fibers
7. a) ECG   b) arrhythmia
   c) fibrillation

HEART RATE

1. a) 60–80 beats per minute   b) pulse
2. higher, smaller
3. lower

CARDIAC OUTPUT

1. 1 minute
2. blood pressure, oxygen
3. a) 1 beat   b) 60–80 mL
4. stroke volume × pulse
5. 4.5 liters
   cardiac output = 75 × 60
6. 60 bpm
   6000 = 100 × pulse
   $\dfrac{6000}{100}$ = pulse

7. 12 liters
   c.o. = 100 × 120

REGULATION OF HEART RATE

1. a) medulla
   b) accelerator and inhibiting centers
2. a) increase   b) vagus, decrease
3. a) pressoreceptors, carotid, aortic
   b) chemoreceptors, carotid, aortic
4. a) glossopharyngeal   b) vagus
5. 1) glossopharyngeal nerves
   2) vagus nerve (sensory)
   3) vagus nerve (parasympathetic)
   4) sympathetic nerves
   5) carotid sinus and body
   6) aortic arch
   7) aortic sinus and body
6. 1) pressoreceptors, sinus
   2) glossopharyngeal
   3) accelerator, sympathetic
   4) increase, increase

CLINICAL APPLICATIONS

1. a) rapid, uncoordinated contractions
   b) pumping, decrease
2. a) SA node   b) slower   c) decrease
3. 1) heart murmur
   2) myocardial infarction
   3) coronary atherosclerosis

MULTIPLE CHOICE TEST #1

1. a	6. d	10. d	14. b	18. d
2. d	7. b	11. b	15. a	19. d
3. b	8. c	12. c	16. d	20. a
4. c	9. a	13. b	17. c	21. b
5. a				

MULTIPLE CHOICE TEST #2

The letter of the correct choice is followed by the statement necessary to complete the answer. When an incorrect statement is to be corrected to make it true, the new (true) words are underlined.

1. d—the visceral pericardium may also be called the epicardium
2. b—the left ventricle pumps blood into the aorta

3. a—the mitral valve prevents backflow of blood from the <u>left</u> ventricle to the <u>left</u> atrium

4. d—when the atria are in systole, the ventricles are in <u>diastole</u>

5. c—the <u>SA node</u> initiates each heartbeat

6. a—cardiac output is the amount of blood pumped by a ventricle in 1 <u>minute</u>

7. b—<u>sympathetic</u> impulses to the heart <u>increase</u> the heart rate (or) <u>parasympathetic</u> impulses to the heart decrease the <u>heart rate</u>

8. b—the heart rate will increase in response to <u>sympathetic</u> impulses

9. b—the coronary sinus empties blood from the myocardium into the <u>right</u> atrium

10. d—an athlete's heart rate is low because the heart's stroke volume is <u>higher</u>

Chapter 13

BLOOD VESSELS—STRUCTURE AND FUNCTIONS

1. a) capillaries   b) arteries   c) veins

2. a) lining, simple squamous epithelial
   b) prevents abnormal clotting

3. a) smooth muscle, elastic connective tissue
   b) help maintain diastolic blood pressure

4. a) outer, fibrous connective tissue
   b) prevents rupture of blood vessels

5. 1) A, E, F   2) B, C, D

6. a) anastomoses   b) alternate pathways

7. a) simple squamous epithelium
   b) exchanges

8. a) precapillary sphincters
   b) dilate, increase, oxygen

9. a) sinusoids
   b) liver, spleen, red bone marrow

10. 1) tunica externa   6) endothelial cells
    2) tunica media   7) capillary
    3) endothelial lining   8) precapillary sphincter
    4) valve   9) venule
    5) arteriole

EXCHANGES IN CAPILLARIES

1. 1) A, E, G   2) C, D   3) B, F

2. a) oxygen   b) plasma, nutrients
   c) CO_2 d) tissue fluid, waste products

PATHWAYS OF CIRCULATION

Pathway—Pulmonary Circulation

1. a) right, lungs   b) left

2. oxygen and carbon dioxide, capillaries, alveoli

Pathway—Systemic Circulation

1. a) left, body   b) right

2. capillaries, cells (or tissue fluid)

3. 1) abdominal   2) ascending
   3) thoracic   4) aortic arch

4. 1) heart   10) shoulder
   2) thigh   11) forearm
   3) arm   12) small intestine
   4) bronchioles   13) esophagus
   5) brain   14) brain
   6) kidneys   15) abdominal organs
   7) liver   16) knee
   8) chest wall   17) hip
   9) lower leg   18) foot

5. 1) occipital   18) posterior tibial
   2) internal carotid   19) maxillary
   3) vertebral   20) facial
   4) brachiocephalic   21) external carotid
   5) aortic arch   22) common carotid
   6) celiac   23) subclavian
   7) hepatic   24) pulmonary
   8) splenic   25) axillary
   9) left gastric   26) intercostal
   10) superior mesenteric   27) brachial
   11) abdominal aorta   28) renal
   12) common iliac   29) gonadal
   13) internal iliac   30) inferior mesenteric
   14) external iliac   31) radial
   15) femoral   32) ulnar
   16) popliteal   33) deep volar arch
   17) anterior tibial   34) superficial volar arch

6. 1) neck   5) hip   9) kidney
   2) armpit   6) forearm   10) shoulder
   3) leg and thigh   7) brain   11) arm
   4) lower body   8) upper body   12) thigh

7. 1) anterior facial
    2) superior vena cava
    3) axillary
    4) cephalic
    5) hemiazygos
    6) intercostal
    7) inferior vena cava
    8) brachial
    9) basilic
    10) gonadal
    11) superior mesenteric
    12) volar arch
    13) volar digital
    14) superior sagittal sinus
    15) inferior sagittal sinus
    16) straight sinus
    17) transverse sinus
    18) vertebral
    19) external jugular
    20) internal jugular
    21) subclavian
    22) brachiocephalic
    23) pulmonary
    24) hepatic
    25) hepatic portal
    26) left gastric
    27) renal
    28) splenic
    29) inferior mesenteric
    30) internal iliac
    31) external iliac
    32) femoral
    33) great saphenous
    34) popliteal
    35) small saphenous
    36) anterior tibial
    37) dorsal arch

Hepatic Portal Circulation

1. digestive organs and spleen
2. superior mesenteric, splenic
3. sinusoids, inferior vena cava
4. a) capillaries
   b) digestive organs and spleen, liver

5.

	Example 1	**Example 2**	**Example 3**
1)	glucose	alcohol	bilirubin
2)	small intestine	stomach	spleen
3)	excess stored as glycogen	detoxifies	excretes into bile

Fetal Circulation

1. placenta
2. a) oxygen—CO_2, nutrients, waste products
   b) diffusion, active transport
3. umbilical arteries, umbilical vein
4. a) fetus, placenta
   b) CO_2, waste products
5. a) placenta, fetus   b) oxygen, nutrients
6. ductus venosus, inferior vena cava
7. a) foramen ovale, right atrium, left atrium
   b) lungs
8. a) pulmonary artery, aorta
   b) permits most fetal blood to bypass the lungs

9. a) constricts   b) closed, constricts
    c) pulmonary
10. 1) aorta
    2) ductus arteriosus
    3) pulmonary artery
    4) foramen ovale
    5) inferior vena cava
    6) ductus venosus
    7) umbilical arteries
    8) umbilical vein
    9) placenta
    10) navel of fetus

BLOOD PRESSURE

1. blood vessels
2. mmHg (millimeters of mercury)
3. a) left ventricle   b) contracting
   c) relaxing
4. aorta (or arteries), veins
5. a) arterial, venous   b) filtration, rupture
   c) nutrients
6. a) right ventricle   b) prevent

Maintenance of Systemic Blood Pressure

1. a) heart   b) decrease, decrease
   c) 1) smooth muscle
      2) legs, compress (or squeeze)
      3) thoracic cavity, breathing, heart
2. increase
3. a) constriction   b) increase
   c) decrease
4. a) systole, diastole
   b) decreases, increases
5. a) blood cells, albumin (or plasma proteins)
   b) decrease   c) anemia, liver, albumin
6. a) decrease
   b) increased heart rate (or) vasoconstriction
7. 1) vasoconstriction
   2) increased heart rate and force of contraction
   3) kidneys, volume   4) kidneys, water
   5) sodium ions and water, decreases

Regulation of Blood Pressure

1. 1) forcefully
      a) increase, Starling's Law
   2) filtration
2. 1) medulla
      a) vasoconstrictor, vasodilator
      b) pressoreceptors

2) sympathetic
  a) more, raise
  b) fewer, lower

CLINICAL APPLICATIONS

1. a) 140 mmHg, 90 mmHg
2. a) arteriosclerosis   b) atherosclerosis

MULTIPLE CHOICE TEST #1

1. a	5. b	9. b	13. d	17. d
2. a	6. d	10. c	14. b	18. a
3. c	7. d	11. b	15. c	19. d
4. c	8. b	12. d	16. a	20. a

MULTIPLE CHOICE TEST #2

The letter of the correct choice is followed by the statement necessary to complete the answer. When an incorrect statement is to be corrected to make it true, the new (true) words are underlined.

1. c—the vein that takes blood into the liver is the <u>portal</u> vein
2. a—the foramen ovale permits blood to flow from the <u>right</u> atrium to the <u>left</u> atrium to bypass the fetal lungs
3. b—the lining of both arteries and veins is very smooth to <u>prevent abnormal clotting</u>
4. d—decreased venous return will result in <u>decreased</u> cardiac output
5. b—renal artery—<u>kidney</u>
6. c—carbon dioxide diffuses from <u>tissues to the blood</u>
7. d—the carotid pulse is felt at the <u>side of the neck</u>
8. d—the tissue in arteries and veins that constricts or dilates is <u>smooth muscle</u>
9. b—norepinephrine causes vasoconstriction, which <u>raises</u> BP
10. d—BP in the veins is <u>lower</u> than BP in the capillaries

Chapter 14

LYMPH AND LYMPH VESSELS

1. lymph
2. a) filtration, tissue fluid
   b) lymph capillaries
3. 1) D   2) F   3) A   4) E
   5) B   6) C

LYMPH NODES AND NODULES

1. lymphatic, lymphocytes and monocytes
2. a) plasma cells   b) macrophages
3. 1) B, C, 1, 2   2) A, D, 3, 4
4. 1) right lymphatic duct   6) axillary nodes
   2) right subclavian vein   7) spleen
   3) cervical nodes   8) cisterna chyli
   4) left subclavian vein   9) inguinal nodes
   5) thoracic duct

SPLEEN

1. a) abdominal, diaphragm, stomach
   b) ribs
2. lymphocytes and monocytes, blood
3. phagocytize, antibodies
4. red blood cells, bilirubin
5. a) lymph nodes and nodules
   b) liver and red bone marrow
6. red blood cells

THYMUS

1. fetus—child
2. below (inferior to)
3. lymphocytes
4. a) antigens, immunity   b) competence

IMMUNITY—ANTIGENS AND ANTIBODIES

1. pathogens, prevent
2. T cells and B cells
3. a) bone marrow
   b) bone marrow, thymus
   c) spleen, lymph nodes and nodules
4. self, foreign
5. a) protein   b) specific
   c) gamma globulins or immune globulins

MECHANISMS OF IMMUNITY

1. cell-mediated, humoral
2. a) foreign
   b) macrophages, helper T cells
3. destroy, immunity

CELL-MEDIATED IMMUNITY

1. 1) F   2) A   3) B   4) E
   5) D   6) C
2. 1) macrophage
   2) self-antigens
   3) foreign antigen
   4) helper T cell
   5) memory T cell
   6) cytotoxic T cell
   7) suppressor T cell
   8) cytotoxic T cell destroying foreign antigen
   9) macrophage phagocytizing foreign antigen

HUMORAL IMMUNITY

1. 1) C   2) G   3) A   4) E
   5) F   6) B   7) D
2. 1) macrophage   9) antigen-antibody
   2) self-antigens   complex
   3) foreign antigen   10) macrophage
   4) helper T cell   phagocytizing foreign
   5) activated B cell   antigen
   6) memory B cell   11) complement fixation
   7) plasma cell   12) suppressor T cell
   8) antibodies
3. a) antibodies   b) macrophages
4. a) macrophages   b) lysis (rupture)
5. a) yes   b) slow   c) small
   d) may develop the disease
6. a) memory   b) fast   c) large
   d) will not get the disease   e) vaccines

TYPES OF IMMUNITY

1. 1) C, 1   2) E, 2   3) A, 2
   4) D, 3   5) B, 3

CLINICAL APPLICATIONS

1. a) virus, HIV   b) helper
2. a) antibodies, memory
   b) The vaccine contains a harmless form of the measles virus, which allows the body to prepare its defenses against the real measles virus.
3. a) cervical lymph nodes
   b) macrophages

MULTIPLE CHOICE TEST #1

1. d	5. a	9. d	13. a	17. d
2. b	6. d	10. c	14. c	18. c
3. c	7. c	11. b	15. d	19. b
4. d	8. b	12. d	16. b	20. a

MULTIPLE CHOICE TEST #2

The letter of the correct choice is followed by the statement necessary to complete the answer. When an incorrect statement is to be corrected to make it true, the new (true) words are underlined.

1. b—antibodies are produced in the spleen by cells called fixed plasma cells
2. d—the three major paired groups are the cervical, axillary, and inguinal nodes
3. a—they are found below the epithelium of mucous membranes
4. c—lymph contains the lymphocytes (and monocytes) produced by the lymph nodes
5. a—the right lymphatic duct returns lymph to the right subclavian vein
6. d—a vaccine provides artificially acquired active immunity
7. c—T cells are the lymphocytes produced by the thymus
8. a—when an antibody is produced, it will bond to a specific foreign antigen
9. b—the foreign antigen is recognized by macrophages and helper T cells
10. b—opsonization is the labeling of foreign antigens by antibodies

Chapter 15

NOSE, NASAL CAVITIES, AND PHARYNX

1. hairs
2. a) nasal septum   b) ciliated
   c) 1) warms the air
      2) moistens the air
      3) cilia sweep mucus, dust, and pathogens to the pharynx
   d) smell
3. a) nasal cavities
   b) 1) frontal, sphenoid
      2) ethmoid, or maxillae
   c) lighten the skull (or) provide resonance for the voice
4. 1) B, C, F, G, I   2) D, E   3) A, H
5. larynx

LARYNX

1. a) pharynx, trachea   b) speaking
2. 1) E   2) A, F   3) B   4) D
   5) C
3. vagus and accessory
4. together, exhaled
5. 1) epiglottis   4) cricoid cartilage
   2) thyroid cartilage   5) tracheal cartilages
   3) vocal cords

TRACHEA AND BRONCHIAL TREE

1. larynx, primary bronchi
2. a) cartilage   b) keep the trachea open
   c) ciliated epithelium
3. a) trachea   b) two, three
4. a) bronchioles, cartilage   b) alveoli
5. 1) frontal sinus   11) primary bronchi
   2) nasal cavity   12) bronchioles
   3) nasopharynx   13) mediastinum
   4) adenoid   14) visceral pleura
   5) palatine tonsil   15) pleural space
   6) oropharynx   16) parietal pleura
   7) epiglottis   17) diaphragm
   8) larynx   18) pulmonary capillaries
   9) laryngopharynx   19) alveoli
   10) trachea

THE PATHWAY OF AIR

1. 1, 6, 8, 5, 2, 4, 10, 3, 7, 9, 11
2. 1) primary bronchi
   2) secondary bronchi
   3) bronchioles
   4) alveoli

PLEURAL MEMBRANES

1. a) visceral   b) parietal
2. a) prevents friction   b) together

LUNGS

1. a) rib cage
   b) mediastinum, heart   c) diaphragm
2. a) hilus   b) primary bronchus, pulmonary artery and veins
3. a) simple squamous epithelium
   b) simple squamous epithelium
   c) thin, diffusion (exchange) of gases
   d) elastic connective tissue
4. a) diffusion of gases
   b) pulmonary surfactant, inflation

MECHANISM OF BREATHING

1. a) ventilation   b) inhalation, exhalation
2. medulla and pons
3. 1) intercostal, intercostal
   2) diaphragm, phrenic
4. air pressure
5. 1) B, D   2) C, F   3) A, E

INHALATION (INSPIRATION)

1. 1, 4, 3, 6, 2, 5, 7
2. contraction, lungs

EXHALATION (EXPIRATION)

1. 1, 3, 5, 4, 2, 6
2. contraction
3. internal intercostal, down and in, abdominal, upward

EXCHANGE OF GASES

1. a) alveoli, blood   b) systemic capillaries
2. oxygen, carbon dioxide
3. a) 21%, 0.04%   b) 16%, 4.5%
4. partial pressure, P
5. a) 1. high P_{O_2} 2. low P_{O_2}; arrow from air to
       3. low   blood
         P_{CO_2} 4. high P_{CO_2}; arrow from
                  blood to air
   b) external   c) heart, left, body
6. a) 1. low P_{O_2} 2. high P_{O_2}; arrow from
       3. high P_{CO_2} blood to cells
                  4. low P_{CO_2}; arrow from
                    cells to blood
   b) internal   c) heart, right, lungs

TRANSPORT OF GASES IN THE BLOOD

1. a) red blood cells   b) iron, hemoglobin
   c) lungs
2. 1) low P_{O_2} 2) high P_{CO_2}
   3) high temperature
3. bicarbonate (HCO_3^-), plasma
4. hydrogen (H^+)

PULMONARY VOLUMES

1. 1) F   2) C   3) E   4) B
   5) A   6) D
2. gas exchange

NERVOUS REGULATION OF RESPIRATION

1. medulla and pons
2. a) inspiration   b) expiration
3. apneustic, pneumotaxic, exhalation
4. 12–20
5. baroreceptors, inspiration
6. a) emotional   b) voluntary
   c) holding one's breath (or) singing, breathing
   faster
7. a) medulla
   b) pharynx, larynx, or trachea
   c) explosive, mouth

8. a) medulla   b) nasal cavities
   c) explosive, nose

CHEMICAL REGULATION OF RESPIRATION

1. a) O_2 and CO_2 b) pH
2. 1) A, B   2) C, D
3. a) CO_2 b) pH
   c) residual, does not

RESPIRATION AND ACID-BASE BALANCE

1. CO_2
2. 1) B, D, E   2) A, C, F
3. any severe pulmonary disease: emphysema, pneumonia
4. prolonged hyperventilation
5. a) untreated diabetes mellitus, severe diarrhea or vomiting   b) increase, exhale
6. a) overingestion of antacid medication
   b) decrease, retain

CLINICAL APPLICATIONS

1. a) elastic connective, passive   b) exhale
2. cartilage
3. pulmonary edema, the heart
4. a) pneumonia   b) cilia

MULTIPLE CHOICE TEST #1

1. c	7. a	12. c	17. d	22. c
2. b	8. b	13. d	18. c	23. b
3. d	9. d	14. c	19. b	24. a
4. b	10. c	15. b	20. a	25. c
5. a	11. d	16. a	21. d	26. c
6. a				

MULTIPLE CHOICE TEST #2

The letter of the correct choice is followed by the statement necessary to complete the answer. When an incorrect statement is to be corrected to make it true, the new (true) words are underlined.

1. b—air is brought to the alveoli by the
   bronchioles

2. d—the epiglottis covers the top of the larynx during <u>swallowing</u>

3. c—the blood that enters pulmonary capillaries has a <u>high</u> P_{CO_2}

4. b—the motor nerves to the diaphragm are called the <u>phrenic</u> nerves

5. a—the apneustic center in the pons helps bring about <u>inhalation</u> (or) the <u>pneumotaxic</u> center in the pons helps bring about exhalation

6. c—hypoxia is detected by the <u>carotid</u> and aortic chemoreceptors

7. b—hemoglobin in RBCs is able to transport oxygen because it contains <u>iron</u>

8. c—vital capacity is the deepest inhalation followed by <u>the most forceful</u> exhalation

9. a—the normal range of respirations per minute is <u>12–20</u>

10. b—the respiratory system helps compensate for metabolic acidosis by <u>increasing</u> the respiratory rate (or) the respiratory system helps compensate for metabolic <u>alkalosis</u> by decreasing the respiratory rate

Chapter 16

DIVISIONS OF THE DIGESTIVE SYSTEM

1. 1) A, C, F, G   2) B, D, E

2. oral cavity, stomach, small intestine

3. small intestine

4. 1) teeth
   2) oral cavity
   3) tongue
   4) sublingual gland
   5) submaxillary gland
   6) parotid gland
   7) liver
   8) gallbladder
   9) common bile duct
   10) duodenum
   11) pyloric sphincter
   12) ascending colon
   13) jejunum
   14) ileum
   15) cecum
   16) appendix
   17) esophagus
   18) lower esophageal sphincter
   19) stomach
   20) transverse colon
   21) pancreas
   22) descending colon
   23) sigmoid colon
   24) rectum
   25) anal canal

TYPES OF DIGESTION AND END PRODUCTS OF DIGESTION

1. 1) B, C   2) A, D

2. 1) fatty acids and glycerol
   2) amino acids   3) monosaccharides

3. vitamins, minerals, water

ORAL CAVITY AND PHARYNX

1. a) mouth   b) hard palate

2. mechanical, chewing

3. a) deciduous, 20   b) permanent, 32

4. 1) C, E   2) A   3) F   4) B, D

5. a) taste   b) pharynx

6. 1) sublingual   2) parotid
   3) submandibular

7. ducts, oral cavity

8. a) amylase, maltose
   b) tasted, swallowed

9. swallowing, medulla

ESOPHAGUS

1. pharynx, stomach

2. a) lower esophageal sphincter
   b) stomach contents, esophagus

TYPICAL STRUCTURE OF THE ALIMENTARY TUBE

1. 1) A, D, F   2) C, G   3) E, H, J
   4) B, I

STOMACH

1. esophagus, small intestine

2. reservoir

3. a) rugae   b) gastric pits, gastric juice

4. 1) C   2) A   3) B

5. a) hydrochloric acid   b) pepsin

6. a) parasympathetic   b) gastrin
7. a) external muscle
   b) stomach, duodenum
   c) duodenum, stomach
8. 1) esophagus   8) circular muscle layer
   2) cardiac   9) oblique muscle layer
      orifice   10) body
   3) lesser   11) greater curvature
      curvature   12) rugae
   4) pyloric   13) pylorus
      sphincter
   5) duodenum
   6) fundus
   7) longitudinal
      muscle layer

LIVER AND GALLBLADDER

1. diaphgram, abdominal
2. a) bile, fats   b) mechanical
3. hepatic, cystic, common bile, duodenum
4. bilirubin, excess cholesterol, feces
5. a) liver   b) stores bile, concentrates bile
6. a) duodenum   b) secretin
   c) cholecystokinin
7. 1) gallbladder   7) hepatic duct
   2) cystic duct   8) stomach
   3) common bile duct   9) pyloric
   4) duodenum   sphincter
   5) opening of common   10) pancreas
      bile duct   11) main pancreatic
   6) liver   duct

PANCREAS

1. duodenum, spleen
2. common bile
3. a) trypsin
   b) lipase, fatty acids and glycerol
   c) amylase, maltose
4. stomach, duodenum

SMALL INTESTINE

1. a) large intestine
   b) stomach, large intestine
2. a) duodenum, jejunum, ileum
   b) duodenum
3. external muscle layer
4. bile, enzyme pancreatic juice
5. a) glands   b) food (chyme)
6. a) disaccharides, monosaccharides
   b) amino acids
7. 1) A   2) B   3) C
8. capillary network, lacteal
9. 1) A, 1   2) B, 4   3) A, 1
   4) B, 4   5) A, 1   6) A, 1
   7) A, 2   8) A, 3
10. a) B_{12}, intrinsic   b) D, parathyroid
11. a) liver   b) left subclavian
12. 1) villus   4) lacteal
    2) capillary network   5) goblet cell
    3) microvilli   6) intestinal gland

REVIEW OF DIGESTION

1.   Food Type

Organ	Carbohydrates	Fats	Proteins
Salivary glands	Amylase—digests starch to maltose	None	None
Stomach	None	None	Pepsin—digests protein to polypeptides
Liver	None	Bile salts—emulsify fats	None
Pancreas	Amylase—digests starch to maltose	Lipase—digests emulsified fats to fatty acids and glycerol	Trypsin—digests polypeptides to peptides
Small intestine	Sucrase, maltase, and lactase—digest disaccharides to monosaccharides	None	Peptidases—digest peptides to amino acids

LARGE INTESTINE

1. colon, ileum, anus
2. cecum
3. 1, 6, 2, 5, 4, 7, 3
4. 1) water, minerals, vitamins
   2) undigested food
5. a) bacteria   b) pathogens
   c) vitamins, vitamin K
6. a) spinal cord   b) rectum
7. 1, 4, 2, 3
8. external anal sphincter
9. 1) transverse colon   9) cecum
   2) haustra   10) splenic flexure
   3) taenia coli   11) descending colon
   4) hepatic flexure   12) sigmoid colon
   5) ascending colon   13) rectum
   6) ileum   14) anal canal
   7) ileocecal valve   15) anus
   8) appendix

LIVER—OTHER FUNCTIONS

1. 1) J   2) I   3) H   4) G
    5) M   6) B   7) C   8) L
    9) E   10) A   11) D   12) F
   13) N   14) K

CLINICAL APPLICATIONS

1. a) gallbladder   b) cholesterol
2. lower right quadrant
3. a) peritoneum
   b) lines the abdominal cavity
4. a) esophagus
   b) lower esophageal sphincter (LES)

MULTIPLE CHOICE TEST #1

1. a	6. d	11. a	16. d	21. c
2. d	7. d	12. c	17. a	22. d
3. c	8. c	13. b	18. b	23. d
4. b	9. b	14. d	19. a	24. c
5. d	10. a	15. c	20. b	

MULTIPLE CHOICE TEST #2

The letter of the correct choice is followed by the statement necessary to complete the answer. When an incorrect statement is to be corrected to make it true, the new (true) words are underlined.

1. a—the parotid glands are in front of the ears (or) the sublingual glands are below the floor of the mouth
2. d—the process of beta-oxidation permits the use of fatty acids for energy production
3. b—lipase from the pancreas digests fats to fatty acids and glycerol
4. b—increased secretion of saliva is a parasympathetic response (or) decreased secretion of saliva is a sympathetic response
5. c—each digestive enzyme digests only one type of food
6. b—blood vessels and nerves are found in the pulp cavity of a tooth
7. d—the lower esophageal sphincter prevents backup of stomach contents
8. a—hydrochloric acid destroys most microorganisms that enter the stomach because it has a pH of 1–2
9. c—villi are folds of the mucosa of the small intestine
10. a—the common bile duct is formed by the hepatic duct and the cystic duct
11. c—enzymes are produced to complete the digestion of proteins and carbohydrates (or) disaccharides
12. b—the ileum of the small intestine opens into the cecum

Chapter 17

BODY TEMPERATURE

1. a) 96.5–99.5°F, 36–38°C
   b) 98.6°F or 37°C
2. infants, elderly

HEAT PRODUCTION

1. a) cell respiration   b) ATP
2. a) thyroxine, thyroid   b) cell respiration
3. epinephrine, adrenal medulla
4. a) ATP   b) skeletal muscles, muscle tone
   c) liver   d) blood
5. peristalsis (or) production of enzymes
6. increases

HEAT LOSS

1. a) skin   b) respiratory
   c) urinary, digestive
2. a) radiation, conduction, convection
   b) convection   c) radiation, conduction
   d) cooler
3. a) blood
   b) vasodilation, vasoconstriction

4. a) evaporates   b) eccrine
   c) high, low   d) dehydration

REGULATION OF BODY TEMPERATURE

1. hypothalamus
2. a) blood   b) temperature receptors
3. 1) D, E, F   2) A, B, C

FEVER

1. high, pyrogens
2. a) bacteria, viruses   b) inflammation
3. a) higher, cold   b) shivering
4. a) lower, warm   b) sweating
5. pathogens (bacteria), white blood cells
6. a) lose their shape (become inactive)
   b) brain, neurons

METABOLISM

1. metabolism
2. a) catabolism   b) anabolism
   c) anabolism   d) catabolism
   e) enzymes
3. $C_6H_{12}O_6 + O_2 \rightarrow CO_2 + H_2O + ATP + Heat$
4. glycolysis, the Krebs (citric acid) cycle, the cytochrome transport system
5. 1) A   2) B, C   3) A   4) B, C
   5) A   6) B   7) C   8) A, B
   9) C   10) C   11) A

6. 1) niacin, riboflavin   2) thiamine
   3) iron, copper

PROTEINS AND FATS AS ENERGY SOURCES

1. a) amine (NH_2)   b) Krebs cycle
   c) acetyl, pyruvic acid
2. a) pyruvic acid   b) beta-oxidation, acetyl
3. a) ketones   b) amino acids

ENERGY AVAILABLE FROM FOOD

1. Calories, kilocalories
2. 4, 9, 4

SYNTHESIS USES OF FOODS

1. a) glycogen, skeletal muscles
   b) pentose sugars, DNA, RNA
2. non-essential, proteins
3. There are many possible answers:
   1) hemoglobin—RBCs
   2) antibodies—WBCs
   3) keratin—epidermal cells
   4) collagen—fibroblasts (tendons, ligaments)
   5) melanin—melanocytes
   6) albumin—liver
   7) and, others
4. a) true fats (triglycerides)
   b) phospholipids   c) cholesterol
5. 1) estrogen or testosterone—ovaries or testes
   2) cortisol or aldosterone—adrenal cortex

METABOLIC RATE

1. a) heat   b) kilocalories
2. basal metabolic rate (BMR)
3. children, the elderly
4. testosterone, estrogen
5. sympathetic, epinephrine, norepinephrine
6. skeletal muscles

CLINICAL APPLICATIONS

1. a) fever, pyrogens, hypothalamus
   b) pathogens
   c) they lose their shape and function
2. a) K   b) C or E   c) A
3. a) iron   b) cobalt   c) iodine
   d) iron and copper

MULTIPLE CHOICE TEST #1

1. b	6. d	11. a	15. a	19. b
2. b	7. a	12. b	16. b	20. b
3. a	8. b	13. c	17. c	21. d
4. c	9. c	14. d	18. d	22. d
5. c	10. d			

MULTIPLE CHOICE TEST #2

The letter of the correct choice is followed by the statement necessary to complete the answer. When an incorrect statement is to be corrected to make it true, the new (true) words are underlined.

1. d—almost half the body's total heart at rest is produced by the liver and skeletal muscles
2. a—radiation is an effective heat loss mechanism only when the environment is cooler than body temperature
3. b—more heat will be lost as a result of vasodilation in the dermis
4. d—shivering may occur as muscle tone increases
5. b—high fevers may cause brain damage because enzymes become denatured
6. d—men and young children usually have higher metabolic rates than do women and elderly people
7. b—the complete breakdown of glucose in cell respiration does require oxygen

8. c—fatty acids and glycerol are used to synthesize true fats to be stored in <u>adipose tissue</u>

9. a—a gram of protein yields <u>4</u> kilocalories of energy

10. d—most of the ATP produced in cell respiration is produced in the <u>cytochrome transport system</u>

Chapter 18

FUNCTIONS OF THE KIDNEYS

1. waste products
2. minerals
3. hydrogen ions, bicarbonate ions
4. water
5. tissue fluid

KIDNEYS—LOCATION AND EXTERNAL ANATOMY

1. spinal, behind
2. ribs
3. a) adipose   b) renal fascia
4. a) hilus   b) renal artery, renal vein
5. 1) vertebra: T-12   6) ureter
   2) vertebra: L-5   7) ilium
   3) sacrum   8) urinary bladder
   4) urethra in penis   9) urethra
   5) kidney

KIDNEYS—INTERNAL STRUCTURE

1. 1) B, H   2) C, F, G   3) A, D, E
2. 1) renal pelvis   8) calyx
   2) renal artery   9) renal cortex
   3) renal vein   10) renal medulla
   4) ureter   11) papilla
   5) renal pyramid   12) renal corpuscle
   6) papilla   13) renal tubule
   7) renal cortex   14) papillary duct

THE NEPHRON

1. a) functional
   b) renal corpuscle, renal tubule
2. glomerulus, Bowman's capsule

3. a) afferent, efferent   b) efferent arteriole
4. a) pores   b) permeable
   c) renal filtrate
5. 3, 2, 4, 1
6. renal pelvis
7. peritubular capillaries, efferent
8. 1) proximal convoluted tubule   6) efferent arteriole
   2) glomerulus   7) afferent arteriole
   3) Bowman's capsule (inner)   8) loop of Henle
   4) Bowman's capsule (outer)   9) collecting tubule
   5) distal convoluted tubule   10) peritubular capillaries

BLOOD VESSELS OF THE KIDNEY

1. a) abdominal aorta
   b) inferior vena cava
2. a) 1, 7, 3, 5, 2, 4, 6, 8
   b) capillaries

FORMATION OF URINE— GLOMERULAR FILTRATION

1. renal corpuscle
2. a) glomerulus, Bowman's capsule
   b) renal filtrate
   c) large proteins, blood cells, large
3. a) yes   b) yes   c) 2
   d) blood plasma, blood
4. a) 1 minute   b) decrease
   c) increase

FORMATION OF URINE—TUBULAR REABSORPTION AND TUBULAR SECRETION

1. renal tubule, peritubular capillaries
2. a) 99   b) urine
3. 1) osmosis   2) active transport
   3) active transport   4) passive transport
   5) pinocytosis   6) active transport
4. a) limit   b) high, high   c) all
5. a) aldosterone
   b) parathyroid hormone (PTH)
6. a) filtrate
   b) creatinine, ammonia, medications
   c) hydrogen
7. a) sodium, water   b) volume, pressure
8. a) water   b) concentrated
   c) less, dilute
9. a) sodium, water
   b) decrease volume, decrease BP
10. Active transport—1) glucose
    2) amino acids   3) positive ions
    Osmosis—1) water
    Pinocytosis—1) small proteins
    Passive transport—1) negative ions
    Secretion—1) creatinine   2) medications
    3) H^+ 4) ammonia

THE KIDNEYS AND ACID-BASE BALANCE

1. a) hydrogen (H^+), bicarbonate (HCO_3^-) and sodium (Na^+)   b) raise
2. a) bicarbonate (HCO_3^-), hydrogen (H^+)
   b) lower

OTHER FUNCTIONS OF THE KIDNEYS

1. a) decreases   b) juxtaglomerular, afferent
   c) angiotensin II
   d) increases vasoconstriction; increases secretion of aldosterone   e) raise
2. a) erythropoietin, low oxygen
   b) red bone marrow, RBCs
3. D, calcium, phosphate

ELIMINATION OF URINE

1. a) behind
   b) hilus (or pelvis), lower posterior, urinary bladder
   c) smooth muscle
2. a) pubic   b) prostate   c) uterus
3. reservoir, contract
4. a) rugae   b) transitional
   c) expansion   d) trigone
   e) ureters, urethra
5. a) detrusor
   b) internal urethral, involuntary
6. 1) detrusor muscle   4) opening of ureter
   2) ureter   5) trigone
   3) rugae   6) urethra
7. a) urinary bladder, exterior   b) anterior
   c) prostate, penis, semen
   d) external urethral, voluntary
8. a) urination   b) spinal cord
9. a) 1, 5, 4, 3, 2, 6
   b) external urethral sphincter

CHARACTERISTICS OF URINE

1. a) 1–2 liters
   b) excessive sweating or diarrhea
   c) excessive consumption of fluids
2. a) straw, amber   b) clear
3. a) 1.010–1.025
   b) dissolved materials, concentrating
   c) concentrated
   d) excessive sweating or diarrhea
4. 6, 4.8–8.0
5. water, solvent
6. 1) B   2) C   3) A
7. b

ABNORMAL CONSTITUENTS OF URINE

1. 1) E   2) D   3) C   4) B
   5) A

CLINICAL APPLICATIONS

1. adipose tissue, renal fascia
2. urinary bladder, renal pelvis

3. a) decrease   b) decrease
   c) increase

MULTIPLE CHOICE TEST #1

1. c	6. b	11. c	15. a	19. c
2. b	7. c	12. d	16. b	20. d
3. b	8. a	13. d	17. a	21. d
4. a	9. a	14. b	18. b	22. d
5. d	10. d			

MULTIPLE CHOICE TEST #2

The letter of the correct choice is followed by the statement necessary to complete the answer. When an incorrect statement is to be corrected to make it true, the new (true) words are underlined.

1. b—reabsorbed materials enter the peritubular capillaries

2. c—aldosterone increases the reabsorption of sodium ions

3. a—the stimulus is stretching of the detrusor muscle of the urinary bladder by accumulating urine

4. b—the kidneys are lateral to the spinal column

5. c—the loops of Henle and collecting tubules are found in the renal medulla

6. c—blood cells and large proteins remain in the blood in the glomerulus

7. d—glucose is present in urine only if the blood glucose level is too high

8. d—the voluntary external urethral sphincter is in the wall of the urethra

9. a—the kidneys change inactive forms of vitamin D to the active form

10. d—the kidneys respond to a decreasing pH of the blood by excreting more hydrogen ions

Chapter 19

WATER COMPARTMENTS

1. intracellular, two thirds

2. a) extracellular
   b) 1) tissue fluid   2) plasma
   3) lymph

3. 1) C   2) A   3) D   4) B

4. osmosis, filtration

WATER INTAKE AND OUTPUT

1. a) drinking liquids   b) food
   c) cell respiration

2. a) urinary system, urine   b) skin, sweat
   c) exhaled water vapor, feces

3. a) equal   b) drink more liquids
   c) urinary output

REGULATION OF WATER INTAKE AND OUTPUT

1. hypothalamus

2. the concentration of dissolved materials in a fluid

3. osmoreceptors

4. a) increases   b) thirst, drink liquids
   c) decreases

5. a) ADH, posterior
   b) increase the reabsorption of water
   c) dehydration   d) decrease

6. a) aldosterone   b) increases
   c) 1) low blood pressure
      2) low blood sodium level

7. decrease, increase

8. ANH, increase

ELECTROLYTES

1. positive and negative ions

2. inorganic, salts, acids, bases

3. a) negative   b) Cl^-, HCO_3^-, HPO_4^{-2}
   c) positive   d) Na^+, K^+, Ca^{+2}

4. a) osmolarity, osmosis   b) greater

5. bones, enzymes

6. 1) C   2) A   3) B

REGULATION OF ELECTROLYTE INTAKE AND OUTPUT

1. food, beverages
2. a) urine, sweat, feces
   b) sodium, chloride   c) higher
3. 1) C, D   2) B   3) A   4) E

ACID-BASE BALANCE

1. buffer systems, respiratory, kidneys
2. a) 7.35–7.45   b) 6.8–7.0   c) blood
3. a) neutral   b) acidic, alkaline
   c) alkaline, acidic

BUFFER SYSTEMS

1. a) acid, base   b) strong, will not
2. bicarbonate, phosphate, protein
3. a) H_2CO_3, $NaHCO_3$
   b) sodium bicarbonate, H_2CO_3
   c) carbonic acid, $NaHCO_3$
4. a) NaH_2PO_4, Na_2HPO_4
   b) kidneys   c) NaH_2PO_4
5. a) acid, base
   b) carboxyl (COOH), hydrogen
   c) amine (NH_2), hydrogen
6. less than a second

RESPIRATORY MECHANISMS TO REGULATE pH

1. CO_2
2. hydrogen ions
3. 1) B, C, F, G   2) A, D, E, H
4. increase, more, decrease, raise
5. decrease, less, increase, lower
6. a few minutes

RENAL MECHANISMS TO REGULATE pH

1. hydrogen, sodium, bicarbonate
2. sodium, bicarbonate, hydrogen
3. a few hours to days
4. 3, 2, 1

CAUSES AND EFFECTS OF pH CHANGES

1. emphysema, pneumonia, asthma
2. prolonged hyperventilation
3. kidney disease, untreated diabetes mellitus, vomiting or diarrhea
4. overingestion of antacids, vomiting of stomach contents
5. a) central nervous system
   b) confusion and disorientation, coma and death
6. a) central nervous system and peripheral nervous system
   b) muscle twitches, convulsions

CLINICAL APPLICATIONS

1. systemic, lower legs and ankles
2. sodium
3. a) the heart
   b) kidney disease (or) excessive vomiting or diarrhea
4. 1) c
   2) a (this is respiratory compensation for acidosis)
   3) a (the kidneys are excreting more hydrogen ions)

MULTIPLE CHOICE TEST #1

1. b	6. b	11. c	15. c	19. c
2. d	7. b	12. b	16. c	20. b
3. c	8. d	13. a	17. a	21. a
4. a	9. a	14. d	18. b	22. c
5. d	10. c			

MULTIPLE CHOICE TEST #2

The letter of the correct choice is followed by the statement necessary to complete the answer. When an incorrect statement is to be corrected to make it true, the new (true) words are underlined.

1. a—parathyroid hormone increases the absorption of calcium ions by the small intestine
2. c—the water found within cells is called intracellular fluid
3. b—most water lost from the body is in the form of urine

4. c—the hormones that have the greatest effects on the water content of the body are aldosterone and <u>ADH</u>

5. d—the electrolyte concentration in body fluids helps regulate the process of <u>osmosis</u>

6. c—the buffer systems work very <u>rapidly</u> to correct pH imbalances

7. b—respiratory compensation for metabolic acidosis involves <u>increasing</u> respirations

8. a—the kidneys begin to compensate for a pH imbalance within a few <u>hours to days</u>

9. d—untreated acidosis may progress to <u>coma</u>

Chapter 20

MEIOSIS

1. egg and sperm
2. a) diploid, 46   b) twice, four, haploid, 23
3. a) oogenesis   b) spermatogenesis
4. 1) B, C, D, G   2) A, E, F, H
5. a) 23, 23, 46   b) zygote
6. 1) primary spermatocyte   4) polar bodies
   2) sperm cells   5) ovum
   3) primary oocyte

MALE REPRODUCTIVE SYSTEM

Testes and Sperm

1. a) scrotum   b) lower
2. testosterone, spermatogenesis (meiosis)
3. a) LH, anterior pituitary   b) maturation
   c) two of these: growth of reproductive organs, growth of the larynx, growth of muscles, growth of facial and body hair
4. 1) flagellum   2) head
   3) middle piece   4) acrosome
   1. head   4. nucleus
   2. middle piece   5. flagellum
   3. acrosome
5. 1) spermatogonia   4) vas deferens
   2) sperm cells   5) epididymis
   3) interstitial cells 6) seminiferous tubules

Epididymis, Ductus Deferens, and Ejaculatory Duct

1. a) posterior   b) flagella
2. a) vas deferens, epididymis, ejaculatory duct
   b) inguinal, urinary bladder
   c) smooth muscle

3. ductus deferens, seminal vesicles, urethra
4. 1) penis   8) testis
   2) urethra   9) scrotum
   3) glans penis   10) seminal vesicle
   4) prepuce   11) ejaculatory duct
   5) urethral orifice 12) prostate gland
   6) epididymis   13) bulbourethral gland
   7) vas deferens

Seminal Vesicles, Prostate Gland, and Bulbourethral Glands

1. a) urinary bladder, ejaculatory ducts
   b) alkaline, fructose
2. a) urethra, urinary bladder   b) motility
   c) smooth, ejaculation
3. a) Cowper's glands   b) alkaline, urethra
4. acidic, vagina
5. a) sperm cells   b) 7.4

Urethra and Penis

1. a) ejaculatory ducts
   b) prostate gland, penis
2. smooth, blood sinuses
3. parasympathetic, blood sinuses
4. ejaculation, prostate, reproductive ducts

Male Reproductive Hormones

1. a) FSH, anterior pituitary   b) testosterone
2. LH, anterior pituitary
3. testes, FSH

FEMALE REPRODUCTIVE SYSTEM
Ovaries

1. pelvic, uterus
2. egg cells (ova)
3. a) FSH, anterior pituitary   b) estrogen
4. mature, LH, anterior pituitary
5. corpus luteum, progesterone
6. 1) fallopian tube   7) urethra
    2) ovary   8) vagina
    3) uterus   9) fimbriae
    4) clitoris   10) cervix
    5) labium minora   11) Bartholin's gland
    6) labium majora

Fallopian Tubes

1. uterine tubes, oviducts
2. a) ovary   b) fimbriae, ovum
3. smooth muscle, ciliated
4. fertilization
5. ectopic

Uterus

1. pelvic, ovaries, urinary bladder
2. fundus, cervix
3. a) peritoneum   b) myometrium
    c) endometrium
4. a) basilar, functional
    b) estrogen and progesterone
5. a) becomes the maternal placenta
    b) contracts for delivery of the baby and
       placenta   c) oxytocin
6. 1) ovum   8) body of uterus
    2) mature follicle   9) endometrium
    3) ovary   10) myometrium
    4) fallopian tube   11) cervix
    5) fundus   12) vagina
    6) fimbriae   13) Bartholin's gland
    7) uterine cavity   14) vaginal orifice

Vagina and Vulva

1. 1) B, D, G   2) E   3) C
    4) A   5) F

Mammary Glands

1. a) milk   b) lactiferous, nipple
2. estrogen, progesterone, placenta
3. a) prolactin, anterior pituitary
    b) oxytocin, posterior pituitary
4. a) areola   b) adipose
5. 1) glandular tissue   4) lactiferous duct
    2) areola   5) adipose tissue
    3) nipple

The Menstrual Cycle

1. anterior pituitary gland, ovaries, uterus, ovaries, 28
2. FSH, LH, estrogen, progesterone
3. menstrual, follicular, luteal
4. a) functional, menstruation   b) FSH
5. a) FSH, estrogen   b) estrogen
    c) LH, rupture
6. a) LH, corpus luteum, progesterone
    b) progesterone, glycogen
7. progesterone, menstrual

CLINICAL APPLICATIONS

1. a) prostate   b) prostatic hypertrophy
    c) urethra
2. a) tubal ligation   b) fallopian tubes
    c) vasectomy   d) ductus deferens
3. a) fallopian tube   b) ectopic
4. osteoporosis, cholesterol

MULTIPLE CHOICE TEST #1

1. a	6. a	11. c	16. c	21. d
2. d	7. a	12. b	17. a	22. b
3. b	8. d	13. b	18. b	23. a
4. b	9. c	14. c	19. d	24. a
5. a	10. b	15. d	20. b	

MULTIPLE CHOICE TEST #2

The letter of the correct choice is followed by the statement necessary to complete the answer. When an incorrect statement is to be corrected to make it true, the new (true) words are underlined.

1. a—the uterus is medial to the ovaries and underline{superior} to the urinary bladder

2. c—the urethra extends through the <u>prostate gland</u> and penis

3. b—both processes begin at puberty, but <u>oogenesis</u> ends at menopause

4. d—the ductus deferens carries sperm from the <u>epididymis</u> to the ejaculatory duct

5. b—the secretion of the seminal vesicles is alkaline and contains <u>fructose</u>

6. d—the growth of blood vessels in the endometrium begins in the <u>follicular</u> phase

7. b—the cervix is the narrow <u>inferior</u> part that opens into the vagina

8. d—the release of milk is stimulated by the hormone <u>oxytocin</u>

9. c—an ectopic pregnancy occurs when the zygote becomes implanted in the <u>fallopian tube</u>

10. a—to produce viable sperm, the temperature of the scrotum must be slightly <u>lower</u> than body temperature

Chapter 21

HUMAN DEVELOPMENT
Fertilization

1. acrosome

2. a) egg and sperm   b) 23, 46, diploid
   c) fallopian tube

3. autosomes, sex chromosomes

4. XY, XX

Implantation

1. a) mitosis   b) cleavage

2. a) morula   b) blastocyst

3. a) embryo
   b) trophoblast, endometrium, implantation

4. chorion, placenta

5. 1) primary follicles   10) morula
   2) maturing follicles   11) blastocyst
   3) ovary   12) inner cell mass
   4) ovum   13) trophoblast
   5) fallopian tube   14) endometrium
   6) sperm   15) embryonic disc
   7) ovum (zygote)   16) corpus luteum
   8) two-cell stage   17) corpus albicans
   9) four-cell stage

Embryo and Embryonic Membranes

1. ectoderm, mesoderm, endoderm

2. 1) lining of digestive organs, lungs
   2) skeletal muscles, bones
   3) epidermis, nervous system

3. 1) A, F   2) C, D   3) B, E

4. a) eighth   b) 9, 40

5. 1) endometrium   8) head of embryo
   2) chorion   9) amniotic sac
   3) yolk sac   10) umbilical cord
   4) embryonic disc   11) arm bud
   5) amnion   12) leg bud
   6) chorionic villus 13) placenta
   7) yolk sac

Placenta and Umbilical Cord

1. a) endometrium   b) chorion
   c) umbilical cord   d) exchanges

2. blood sinuses

3. arteries, vein

4. a) fetus, placenta
   b) CO_2, waste products

5. a) placenta, fetus   b) O_2, nutrients

6. afterbirth

7. a) chorion
   b) corpus luteum, estrogen, progesterone

8. estrogen, progesterone

9. a) FSH and LH   b) mammary glands
   c) myometrium

Parturition and Labor

1. a) birth   b) sequence of events

2. a) progesterone   b) head downward

3. a) amniotic sac   b) dilates (widens) it
c) it ruptures
d) it flows out through birth canal

4. a) oxytocin   b) baby

5. a) afterbirth (placenta)   b) compress

The Infant at Birth

1. a) umbilical cord   b) CO_2, medulla

2. a) foramen ovale   b) ductus arteriosus
c) lungs

3. liver, bilirubin

GENETICS

Chromosomes and Genes

1. a) 46   b) homologous pairs of
c) paternal   d) maternal
e) autosomes
f) sex chromosomes, women, men

2. a) DNA   b) bases   c) one protein

3. 1) F   2) E   3) A   4) D
5) G   6) C   7) B

Genetic Problems

1. 1) a)

Mom—bb

Dad—BB	b	b
B	Bb	Bb
B	Bb	Bb

b) 100% chance—brown hair, 0% chance—blond hair

2) a)

Mom—bb

Dad—Bb	b	b
B	Bb	Bb
b	bb	bb

b) 50% chance—brown hair, 50% chance—blond hair

2. 1) a)

Mom—OO

Dad—AO	O	O
A	AO	AO
O	OO	OO

b) 50% chance—type O, 50% chance—type A

2) a)

Mom—AB

Dad—AB	A	B
A	AA	AB
B	AB	BB

b) 25% chance—type A, 25% chance—type B
50% chance—type AB, 0% chance—type O

3. 1) a)

Mom—XcX

Dad—XcY	Xc	X
Xc	XcXc	XcX
Y	XcY	XY

b) daughter: 50% chance—colorblindness, 50% chance—carrier
son: 50% chance—colorblindness, 50% chance—normal color vision

2) a)

Mom—XcXc

Dad—XY	Xc	Xc
X	XcX	XcX
Y	XcY	XcY

b) daughter: 0% chance—colorblindness, 100% chance—carrier
son: 100% chance—colorblindness, 0% chance—normal color vision

CLINICAL APPLICATIONS

1. a) lungs   b) 3

2. a) three, mental   b) amniocentesis

3. a) abdominal wall, uterus
b) 1) fetal distress (or) poor fetal position (breech birth)

2) maternal pelvic outlet is too small to permit a vaginal delivery

MULTIPLE CHOICE TEST #1

1. c	5. d	9. d	13. d	17. d
2. a	6. b	10. c	14. b	18. c
3. d	7. b	11. c	15. b	19. a
4. d	8. a	12. a	16. b	20. d

MULTIPLE CHOICE TEST #2

The letter of the correct choice is followed by the statement necessary to complete the answer. When an incorrect statement is to be corrected to make it true, the new (true) words are underlined.

1. a—the amniotic sac ruptures during the first stage

2. d—the first blood cells for the fetus are formed by the yolk sac

3. c—the period of embryonic growth lasts from week 1 to week 8

4. d—within the placenta, fetal blood vessels are within maternal blood sinuses

5. b—the embryonic stage that undergoes implantation is the blastocyst

6. c—premature contractions of the myometrium are prevented by progesterone

7. d—the sex chromosomes are XX in women and XY in men

8. a—the expression of the alleles in the appearance of the individual is the phenotype

9. d—a recessive gene is one that appears in the phenotype only if the individual is homozygous

10. c—a son who inherits a sex-linked trait has inherited the gene from his mother